Return to Nature

THE FIVE PILLARS OF HEALING

JON BURRAS

Illustrations by Randy Burras

Library of Congress Control Number: 2011901187
ISBN: Hardcover   978-1-4568-5866-7
                 Softcover   978-1-4568-5865-0
                 Ebook   978-1-4568-5867-4

This book was printed in the United States of America.

To order additional copies of this book, contact:
Xlibris Corporation
1-888-795-4274
www.Xlibris.com
Orders@Xlibris.com
91697

Contents

EPILOGUE

Foreword

I did not want to write this book. I also did not want my fantasy of Santa Claus, the Easter Bunny and the Tooth Fairy to turn out to be a cruel joke played on me either. I did not want to be the one who points out the giant white elephant in the middle of the living room to recovering alcoholics and codependents. I had no desire to ask them to please stand up and take notice before the elephant sits on them. I did not want to be like one of those unpopular politicians whose opinions are not based on poll results or majority views, but who are merely telling the cold hard truth to those who wish not to hear it. Come election time, these mavericks are usually doomed.

No, I did not want to be one of those honest guys, the ones whom nobody likes. They are the ones who always have an opinion and are always ready and willing to share it. They will never keep their big mouths shut. They are always stirring up controversy somewhere. No, that is not who I wanted to be.

I always thought that my funeral would be filled with hundreds of people who had nothing but good things to say about me. "Oh, he was such a nice guy!" would be the chorus at my eulogy. "He always cooperated and never made trouble. He never said a bad thing about anyone. Everyone really liked him." That is who I was raised to be, one of the darned nicest guys to ever grace this planet.

No, I did not want to write this book, but somebody needed to write this book, and it might as well be me. When you work with pain and suffering day in and day out, you begin to ask some deep questions. One minute your client is alive, and the next minute cancer has claimed another life. You witness the fragmentation that happens after years of sexual abuse and mistreatment. You begin to challenge the years of traditional treatment and begin to notice how institutionalized practices may be doing more harm than good.

I did not want to be the bad guy, the bearer of bad news who gets blamed for breaking up the tea party. No, I wanted to be liked by everyone. But I feel like I have become like the owl in a way. The owl is able to see into the night's darkness. The owl is able to see where others are blinded. That is who I have become. I still cannot believe that others cannot see what I see. "Am I crazy for seeing this?" I have often asked myself. But I know now that I am not crazy for seeing what I see. I finally have the courage to speak up and stop being one of the nice guys.

Very few people are willing to address the sacred taboos: money, sex, politics, medicine, spirituality and religion. We walk around them with our self-imposed blinders on. These topics become just another white elephant carousing around the house. They have become the untouchables. I now have the courage to begin to address the sacred taboos.

I feel as if I am watching the parade go by and the emperor is wearing what he believes to be his new clothes. But the emperor is naked. He has no clothes on. Everyone else is helping the emperor maintain his illusion. Why won't someone tell him? I guess that is my job.

I did not write this book to change the world. I wrote this book to change myself. The world will have to change when it is ready. I have my hands full trying to change myself. In a way, this book has been a journey of my own self-exploration.

This book is just a story—my story. If you were to write this book, then it would look a bit different. This book would then be your story. Everything that I have learned and written about is my story, experiences and interpretation of what I believe the truth to be. I feel as if I have been given the picture of a large puzzle and it is up to me to find the missing pieces to make it all fit together. Well, this is the result of those pieces all coming together. Many times we get stuck staring at the same piece of the puzzle, failing to see the big picture. We have been dissecting and splitting ourselves into many different parts for many years now.

This book is about finding the relationship between those parts. By examining the relationship between the parts you will have a roadmap and a direction in which to travel. You will begin to understand why the model that we have been using for health is entirely outdated and needs to be replaced. And finally, you will realize that you do not have to continue to suffer. There is hope for all of us. The plan is simple. The tools remain easily at your finger tips.

When I started studying massage some years ago, I came to realize that massage was not enough. Receiving hands-on treatments helped for a time, but I wondered why many people were not getting better in the long run. I then made a commitment to explore the physiology of the body, from the anatomy of stress to the physiology of fascia. I soon discovered that wasn't the full answer either. Next I thought that the magical solution might lie in the world of spiritual communities. I was only disappointed to find that authentic and complete healing did not happen there either. It was only when I let go of spirituality as the one and only solution that the answers began to be revealed. I went on to study the world of psychology and all that it entails. I did not stop there. I kept adding bits and pieces along the way, from an in-depth analysis of addiction mythology to a thorough study on yoga's ability to open up energy flow in the body. I juggled inner child work with the evolution of the human brain.

Having perused through the halls of Western Medicine I had hoped to find answers. There I spent time in emergency rooms and observed how the body is treated like a machine. I have worked for the Red Cross and been certified as an Emergency Medical Technician. I have studied anatomy and physiology until I dropped. But through all this experience, I was not getting the full answer.

What I have learned is that traditional practices and beliefs about healing can often be very ineffective in the long run. Some of these treatments make us feel better for short periods of time, but they do not make a dent into the real sources of our pain and human suffering. Something else is needed. I often notice that if we misdiagnose the problem, we often seek out a faulty solution. Even in the world of healing, misinterpretation of the problem is very common.

The answer to healing reveals itself in the holistic relationship between the many aspects of ourselves, not in the dissection of ourselves into individual components. Our movement, thoughts and emotions have become splintered and we are often told that one has nothing to do with the other. In my view of the healing experience, they are all very much connected. This book is a result of identifying and reconnecting those many relationships. It is our relationship among our many parts that will make us whole again, not the separation of these parts.

Black and white thinking has taught us that it is only those "other" people who have the problems. We are told that somebody else is in need of help. We are often labeled as being either "sick" or "well." There is no in-between. This book conveys the idea that we are all part of the same human experience and we will continue to be subjected to the same laws of nature as long as we are alive on the planet Earth. Nobody can escape from what is natural.

No, I did not want to write this book and spoil my image of being the nice guy. Instead of being eulogized at my funeral for being so nice by hundreds, now maybe a few true friends and family will gather and say, "He sure spoke his truth." It may not make everyone happy to hear what I have to say, but that is not what I am after. Nice guys might draw the crowds because they say what people want to hear. It is the honest ones who speak from the heart who earn respect. And that is why I wrote this book.

Introduction

Your mind wanders aimlessly in your drug-induced state as your body lies on the operating table, numb and immobile. Today is the day that you will receive your new liver. This is the moment of truth. Will you make it through this ordeal, or is this the end? Will your body reject this new organ? Are you just kidding yourself and buying time until the inevitable comes?

How did you get into this predicament? Would your fate be different if you hadn't drunk so much alcohol over the years? Will you ever see your family and friends again after the anesthesia begins to take over? Your palms are dripping with sweat. You have never been so scared in your life.

Why did you make the choices that you made? You are looking for someone to blame for your misfortune. Why is this fate? What could you have done differently to avoid this horrible feeling of dread? Your mind is exhausted, looking for answers about why this has happened to you. The answers do not come. You are left believing that an unloving God is punishing you. You sink into despair.

There is another answer. This answer may not be the one you want to hear. Nevertheless, it will help explain your serious predicament. What is happening to you today is the result of many years of behavior and choices that you have made along the way. Nobody did this to you. Nobody is trying to punish you. You are here as a result of your own thoughts and actions.

You chose the events leading up to your liver failure. This episode in your life actually began much earlier, perhaps even as far back as your birth. Having controlling and militaristic parents set you up to bottle all your feelings inside. You never learned to release your emotions from your body. You trapped those feelings inside. When you entered your adolescent years, you were looking for a way out of your emotional jail. You accepted alcohol into your life as a permissible way to ease the pain. Your liver failure is the end product of many years of repressed feeling which led to a lifetime of drinking alcohol. You created this and no one else is to blame but you.

This man is not alone in his pain. Our addictions, illnesses and pain within our bodies are often not just random acts handed out like a prize in a cereal box. Instead, they are well thought out processes that develop over time. You may function rather well in society and go along with all of the standard rules of repression. Your neck might stiffen in your twenties. You begin to wear eyeglasses at age thirty. Bad knees show up at age forty. Arthritis sets in at age fifty. You now admonish yourself by saying, "If only I would have listened to the warning signs along the way."

Your TMJ (Temporal Mandibular Joint) Syndrome at age thirty-six might have begun at age three when your father sexually abused you. You may have believed that you would die if you talked back to your father or resisted his advances, so you kept all of the anger inside. Your neck and jaw have been like a coiled spring ever since. Finally, the grinding of your teeth has caused enough severe pain that you have begun to do something about it. You have been trying to stay so busy in order to not feel the pain. You missed all of the warning signs along the way and now are paying the price.

You may have developed endometriosis as a teenager. You are scheduled to have a hysterectomy. You are only thirty years old. Why has this happened to you? You might believe that it is a cruel act of fate, but there is more to the story. The fact that a Catholic monk wrote about the evils of the body eight hundred years ago may be directly linked to your own life, your family and your religious mythology. Ultimately, that mythology has settled into your body. You believe that you are a bad person for feeling sexual; thus you have stopped your sexual energy from flowing and have created your own disease. This is not an isolated case. This is what happens to most of us, black or white, rich or poor.

Your chronic back pain might have been developing ever since you were a young child. You might have been taught that good girls do not get angry. Once this pattern became set into place, you tightened up along your spine whenever a situation occurred where anger was the appropriate natural response. As a forty-year-old mother of three children, your back becomes extremely painful every time you have to visit your mother-in-law, a woman whom you despise greatly. You could never admit this to her face but your body sure is telling that story.

The key point is this. When we follow the laws of nature, we maintain optimum health and vitality. When we choose to disregard the laws of nature, we help to create our own stress, addictions and disease. We develop most addictions and many degenerative diseases because we have stored energy in our bodies. When we cannot feel and express what our natural human nature wants us to feel and express, we then store the energy of those feelings in our body. This is called repression.

Repression is often the result of false beliefs or mythologies that we have created about ourselves. It is these false beliefs that trigger our stress response. Our stress response is most often an imaginary experience that we believe will kill us. Because of our abandonment of natural laws, we help to create our own stress.

Chronic pain is often the result of repression. This pain is the direct result of our inability to allow ourselves to feel and to have a relationship with our pain. We have been asking for thousands of years the immortal question, "Why is there suffering?" In most cases, we create our own suffering. Illness, disease and addictions usually do not just happen by themselves. We are responsible for most of our suffering because we have lost our ability or willingness to be guided by nature and have become detached from our true identity as human beings. It is only by returning to nature that we can hope to heal our suffering, mend our contracted bodies and evolve to the next level of consciousness. When we reclaim our relationship with nature, we reclaim our health and vitality.

We do this by utilizing tools and principles that are found in nature. Nature will heal us, not necessarily scientific jargon found in the laboratory. In this book, we will begin to explore the **Five Pillars of Healing**. These pillars are **process work, bodywork, expansive movement, breath work** and **addiction recovery.** With the help of these five pillars, we will begin to heal as we reclaim our lost relationship with nature.

Most often we are not being victimized by a cruel God or a random act. Our body tells the story of our life. Let's begin to unravel the story and reclaim our health. Now is the time to begin the journey back to nature.

PART ONE

LOSING YOUR MIND

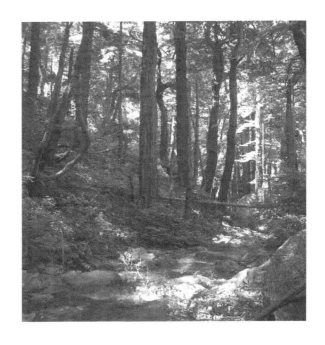

Nature's Way

When we honor the power of nature, we choose to work with the guidelines and laws of nature, rather than against them. These guidelines can be as simple as not building a house in a flood plain because the area is prone to floods. If you backpack in the mountains, you may wish to avoid setting up your tent near the river because the cool winds are drawn down as warm air rises. It is usually colder near the river than it is a short distance up the side of the mountain.

When the laws of nature guide us, we follow a built-in survival system. This survival system is commonly referred to as the *Stress and Relaxation Cycle*, which begins with our beliefs. We first acknowledge and respect the beliefs that nature teaches us; these natural beliefs will then help us react to life-threatening situations.

You might find yourself walking down a mountain trail and suddenly staring eye-to-eye with a giant grizzly bear. He is growling ferociously with his mouth foaming. Your nature-based beliefs alert you that there is danger present. You do not have to think twice about this. Your life may be in jeopardy. Your deep primal beliefs are activated. Your survival instincts take over. Your body immediately responds to this threat by activating the *Stress Response*, also called *Fight or Flight Response*. You are prepared for battle.

Suddenly the bear changes his mind and decides that he is not really interested in you or your peanut butter and jelly sandwich. He turns around and lumbers away. You are relieved. You catch your breath and let out a giant sigh of relief. Wiping the sweat from your brow, you enter a euphoric sense of relaxation. The danger is gone and you are safe now.

When we follow the laws of nature, we move through periods of stress that can last for moments or for extended periods of time. When the danger is gone, we enter into a state of relaxation. Relaxation means to feel safe. When guided by natural beliefs, honoring the laws of nature, the final end product is a state of relaxation.

We can observe this same response in animals. A dog will lie asleep on the floor. A strange noise is heard outside. Watch as the dog's ears perk up in quiet alertness. After a short time, there are no more sounds heard from outside. Soon the dog lowers his ears and resumes his afternoon nap. He goes back to relaxation when he feels safe and the danger is gone.

The Stress and Relaxation Cycle is a primal survival tool built into all species of animals, including human beings. The natural response to danger is self-preservation. Relaxation resumes when the danger passes and we can let down our guard. When we follow the laws of nature and the beliefs created within the natural world, the *Stress and Relaxation Cycle* becomes a natural and normal part of our daily lives.

Unnatural Stress Cycle

The cycle that most humans experience these days often looks quite different than the *Stress and Relaxation Cycle*. Most of the time, we engage in an *Unnatural Stress Cycle* based on false or magical beliefs. Our body still responds with the *Fight or Flight Response*. However, we seldom get to enjoy the final end product of relaxation. We seem to create a never ending circular stress cycle in ourselves.

Many of our beliefs are not based in nature but actually contradict the laws of nature. These unnatural beliefs contribute to the creation of imaginary life-threatening events that feel unsafe. For instance, being stuck in freeway traffic might feel like a bear is chasing you, based on the beliefs established in your mind. Feeling confined and imagining possibly arriving late to your destination becomes the same as being mauled by a wild animal.

The body goes into panic mode. The *Fight or Flight Response* is activated just as if we were in danger of losing our life. Our body's response is the same for an imaginary life-threatening event as for a real life-threatening event. Seldom do people die from being stuck in traffic. However, since the threat is perceived in the mind, it is more difficult to enter into the *Relaxation Response*.

Instead, we follow the path of pain and repression. We hold on to our fear. We tighten up to feel safe. We become frozen. In order to numb out the feelings that are overwhelming us, we choose addictions to eliminate the pain. We are still in our *Fight or Flight Response*, only now we choose something to obliterate the pain. We are still very much engaged in our battle, only this time the battle is raging in our own head.

As a final result of this unnatural cycle, as if the addiction response were not enough, we now have a greater likelihood of developing degenerative diseases. We have broken the natural cycle and now are frozen in terror. We do not feel safe. In fact, most of the time we strive to not feel anything at all. We have numbed out.

Since we have chosen to hold on to our pain and numb it out, we become bitter and resentful when a disease begins to take form within us. We are left speechless and yearn for answers. Blame is normally one of the first calls to response. We feel betrayed by a medical system that we have placed so much trust and confidence in to protect us.

When we adhering to the laws of nature we will create more health and wellness. But how can we follow these natural laws when we do not even know what they are anymore? The challenge to achieve our wellness is to acknowledge our foundation in nature and to listen and learn from nature about our natural beliefs. This process involves dropping down into our primal roots. This is a far cry from the rational mind's attempt to ascend to wellness through our intellect. By opening up to nature and our natural beliefs, we will begin to reverse a trend that has kept us numb and feeling unsafe.

STRESS PATHOLOGY CHART

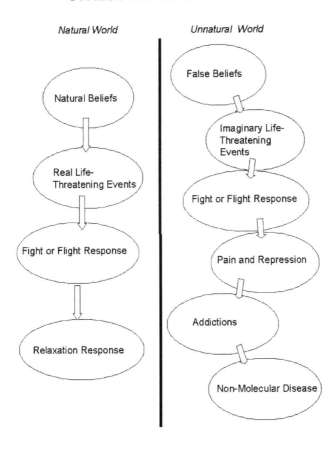

The Development of False Beliefs

In order to understand where our false beliefs originate, we must first grasp our historical perspective of the planet. The loss of our relationship with nature stems from the history of human civilization. Understanding our rise as a species and our changing relationship with the earth helps solve our present-day dilemmas.

Life began on our planet between 3.5 and 4.5 billion years ago. Primitive mammals evolved about 190 million years ago. It is estimated that the dinosaurs became extinct some 65 million years ago. Anthropoids, believed to be a semi-erect ape from which we evolved, began to appear about 60 million years ago. Present-day amphibians showed up around 20 million years ago, while the first recognizable human came into existence about 8 million years ago.

Humans began to walk upright 3.7 million years ago. About five hundred thousand years ago, present-day Homo sapiens emerged. Chellis Glendinning, author of *My Name is Chellis and I'm in Recovery from Western Civilization*, believes that we have been human in biological and psychological development for about one million years. Only in the last six or seven thousand years, civilizations as we know them today have emerged. In fact, until about five thousand years ago, history was passed down through verbal story telling. The last five thousand years have shown the rise of alphabets and the creation of written languages.

It was during these last five to ten thousand years that a basic belief began to emerge that human kind is not part of nature but is superior to nature. At the same time, patriarchy and male dominance over feminine values began to emerge. Women, children, animals and natural began to be dominated by the patriarchal way of thinking. Words, repression of emotions and rational thinking began to take a stronghold over intuition, sensation and expression of emotions.

We began to emerge from a species that was very much connected with nature to one that believed it was better than nature. Nature was now something that could be controlled. Human beings felt like they were the masters over nature. In *Animals and Women*, Marilyn French is quoted by the authors, Carol J. Adams and Josephine Donovan, as saying, "Patriarchy . . . , is an ideology founded on the assumption that man is distinct from the animals and superior to [them]."

For instance, domestication of animals began some ten thousand years ago, first with sheep and then with other animals. We began to emerge as an agricultural system and move out of the hunter-gatherer era. Animals were no longer regarded as a kindred species but something we could harvest and farm out. Pets evolved as our way to control other natural species. This separation from our natural roots has continued to gather momentum as we pursue unnatural practices, such as genetically altered food harvesting and cloning of animals. The farther that we moved away from our relationship with nature, the more boastful we became.

Our dominance over nature has created beliefs that mislead us into believing that we are not governed by the same laws that reside in the rest of nature. Many have come to believe that we are different and can make our own laws. Many of these new beliefs are actually false beliefs because they are contradictory to the laws of nature.

The *Unnatural Stress Cycle* begins with these false beliefs. Understanding our role in our process of stress, addictions and disease entails learning to unravel these false beliefs. In order to fully grasp the development of these false beliefs, it is imperative to see how our developing brain has contributed to this unnatural cycle. It is through the ascension of the human brain that we have been able to achieve much of our greatness as a species. It is also through this same brain that we have acquired our addictions, stress and false beliefs.

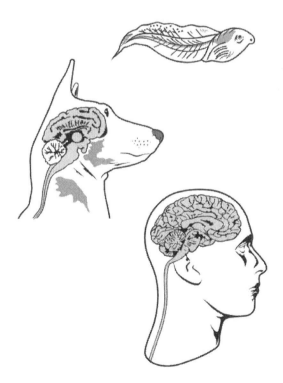

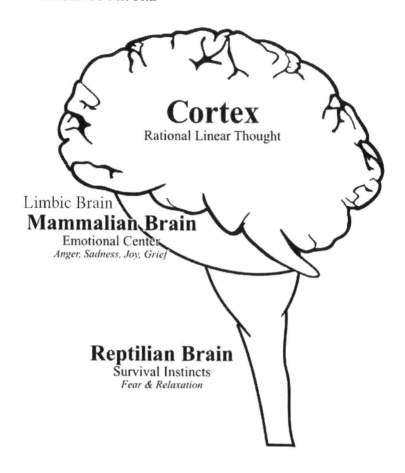

Cortex
Rational Linear Thought

Limbic Brain
Mammalian Brain
Emotional Center
Anger, Sadness, Joy, Grief

Reptilian Brain
Survival Instincts
Fear & Relaxation

BALANCED

BRAIN

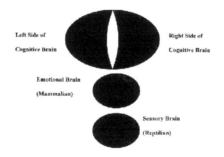

Left Side of
Cognitive Brain

Right Side of
Cognitive Brain

Emotional Brain
(Mammalian)

Sensory Brain
(Reptilian)

Evolution of the Brain

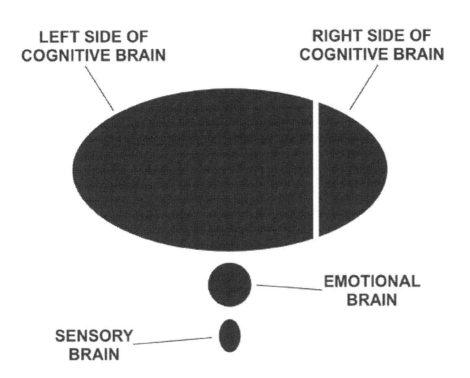

LEFT SIDE OF
COGNITIVE BRAIN

RIGHT SIDE OF
COGNITIVE BRAIN

EMOTIONAL
BRAIN

SENSORY
BRAIN

AVERAGE BRAIN USED

Our ascension as a dominant species can largely be attributed to the evolution of our brain. Our brain has changed much over the last couple of thousand years. Our brain is larger and more diverse than most other creatures in proportion to body weight and is separated into various sections. This structural brain separation is partly responsible for our belief that we are separate from nature.

From a biological and evolutionary perspective, human beings have three brains in distinct locations with different evolutionary functions. The fact that we have three separate brains helps to answer many questions about why humans are different from other species of animals.

These brains are called 1) the lower brain, 2) the middle brain, and 3) the Cognitive Brain. They are also known as the Reptilian Brain, the Limbic Brain (also known as the Emotional Brain or Mammalian Brain), and the Cortex, respectively. (The Cortex is also referred to as the Cognitive Brain.) Each of these brain centers has developed over millions of years in our human evolutionary pathway.

Our most primitive brain is called the Reptilian Brain, or the lower brain. This is located in an area at the base of the brain stem. All species with a spinal cord and a functioning brain have Reptilian Brains. A snake has a Reptilian Brain but so does a fish or spider.

In the evolution of species, the brain is the first growth to appear on the spinal cord. Essentially, a Reptilian Brain is just a bulge on the spinal column. The function of a Reptilian Brain is to keep one alive, whether that is a human or a tuna. This lower brain is responsible for our basic survival instincts. Basic sensory-motor functions like heart rate and respiration are located here. We also sense physical pain here. We are most connected to nature and our primal roots when we are experiencing life from this part of our brain.

The Mammalian Brain is located on top of the Reptilian Brain and is a later development in our species. Most mammals (like dogs) have a Mammalian Brain on top of their Reptilian Brain, whereas an insect only has a Reptilian Brain. When we experience emotions, we experience them here in our Mammalian Brain (also known as the Limbic Brain). Joy, sadness, anger and emotional pain are processed and experienced here.

As we evolved we did so from the center outward. Humans have another layer that resides on top of the emotional and the primitive brains. This is the thinking brain, or Cognitive Brain, where our organized brain activity occurs. Sometimes we refer to this area as the "Gray Matter," or Neo-cortex. It is our ability to reason and problem solve that makes our

Cognitive Brain such a powerful tool, and as a direct result, humans have been able to leap ahead of other species.

Candace Pert writes in *Molecules of Emotion,*

"It was NIMH researcher Paul MacLean who popularized the concept of the limbic system as the seat of the emotions. The limbic system was one constituent of his triune brain theory, which held that there are three layers to the human brain, representing different stages of humanity's evolution—the brainstem (hindbrain) or Reptilian Brain, which is responsible for breathing, excretion, blood flow, body temperature, and other autonomic functions; the limbic system, which encircles the top of the brainstem and is the seat of the emotions; and the cerebral cortex, in the fore brain, which is the seat of reason."

It is extremely important to understand the evolution of the human brain in order to comprehend the source of our false beliefs and the beginning of the Unnatural Stress Cycle. The fact that addictions are unique to the human species lies in the advancement of the Cognitive Brain, which is a dominant part of the human species. This rational part of our brain has learned to numb out emotions and sensations experienced by the lower two brains. Our Cognitive Brain has the ability to create false beliefs that are used to guide our lives.

The lower two brains have a purpose in our lives. They are present to keep us alive. Physical pain, which originates from the Reptilian Brain, is not an evil sensation. This pain is present as a messenger to tell us there is something wrong and that we need to stop and fix it or else we might die. The Reptilian Brain does not want you to die, so it gives you messages in the form of pain. "Hey, listen to me!" is what your Reptilian Brain is trying to say. As Peter Levine states in his book, *Waking the Tiger,* "The primitive world is still very much alive in us."

Our Cognitive Brain tends to take over and dominate the show. More specifically, the left side of our Cortex is primarily responsible for rational and logical thought, while the right side of the Cortex functions to stimulate our creativity and intuition. This gray matter seeks information to keep stimulating and growing.

This newer part of the brain can problem solve and can also find ways to numb out pain. This brain region can find a pill in the medicine cabinet or devise a mental technique that kills the painful message. It is here where the choice to be addictive is made to numb out any emotional pain.

The problem with this short cut to pain relief is that we have not learned what the messenger is trying to say. We have destroyed the messenger without resolving the conflict.

The Cognitive Brain is also responsible for destroying the painful messages coming from the middle brain. Some of the pleasant messages come through, like joy and excitement, but when our middle brain experiences sadness and grief, our Cognitive Brain does not want to have anything to do with it. The Cognitive Brain finds another creative manner in order to numb out the emotional pain being processed by the middle brain. Addictions are the result of our Cognitive Brain not allowing us to feel what the lower two brains are experiencing. This outer brain region might create busyness or a relationship with street drugs to prevent us from feeling our grief or sadness.

For instance, many times pain that originates from the Reptilian Brain is a warning sign of imminent danger. A chronic headache, inflammation, sharp back pain and hunger pains are clear warning signs. Most of the time we choose to ignore these signs and find addictions to numb out the pain.

Peter Levine writes in *Waking the Tiger,*

"Why don't humans just move into and out of these different responses as naturally as animals do? One reason is that our highly evolved neo-cortex (rational brain) is so complex and powerful that through fear and over-control it can interfere with the subtle restrictive instinctual impulses and responses generated by the reptilian core. In particular, the neo-cortex easily overrides some of our gentler instinctual responses-such as those guiding the healing of trauma through the discharge of energy. If the discharge is to serve its purpose, it must be initiated and driven by impulses from the reptilian brain. The neo-cortex must elaborate on instinctual information, not control it."

It seems that the lower two brains have been out-manned by the Cognitive Brain. Sensations like pain and emotions like hurt become numb through our larger Cognitive Brain. It is important to feel and experience these messages coming from our lower two brains for our own health and survival. When we can feel and experience these sensory and emotional impulses, we are honoring our relationship with nature.

Joseph Chilton Pearce, author of *Magical Child*, points out that up until the age of one year old we "are" our sensory experiences created by our lower brains. Our Cognitive Brain, which is responsible for our ego self, hasn't yet had a chance to develop. We "are" the experiences created by the lower brains, like hunger and pain. Once our Cognitive Brain develops, we have the ability to manufacture ways to numb out the feelings and sensations created by the lower two brains.

Descartes was mistaken when he so boldly proclaimed, "I think therefore I am." What he should have said is, "I think, I feel, I sense, I breathe and I move, therefore I am." We have come to identify who we are as our thoughts. Much of the time, these beliefs are false beliefs, drawing us away from nature.

The Cognitive Brain is a very powerful and creative device. It can create all sorts of painkilling effects for us. This part of our brain hungers for information. The more we continue to feed it with intellectual stimulation, the more it grows. As Peter Levine so eloquently states in *Waking the Tiger,* "Today, our survival depends increasingly on developing our ability to think rather than being able to physically respond."

The healing journey begins when we begin to balance our three brains. We must stop living solely in our thinking brain and attempt to integrate our feeling and sensing brains. Returning to nature means returning to beliefs rooted in nature. Our Cognitive Brain has so far managed to create beliefs that want to crush nature. Once again Peter Levine says it best:

"In our exploration of trauma we have learned about the primordial energies that reside within the reptilian core of our brains. We are not reptiles, but without clear access to our reptilian and mammalian heritage, we are not able to be fully human. The fullness of our humanity lies in the ability to integrate the functions of our triune brain.

We see that to resolve trauma we must learn to move fluidly between instinct, emotion, and rational thought. When these three sources are in harmony, communicating sensation, feeling, and cognition, our organisms operate as they were designed to."

It is our Cognitive Brain that has rationalized our world. This part of our brain has turned our culture into a warrior culture by rationalizing our existence. Our Cognitive Brain can easily justify the need to kill others by creating enemies and making them objects. For example, during the 1991 Gulf War, it is estimated that 100,000 Iraqi soldiers were killed on the battlefield. This was justified by the Cognitive Brain by labeling these soldiers as objects rather than as real human beings.

When the Cognitive Brain is constantly stimulated, it prevents us from relaxing, and our danger comes from within our own head. In response, we treat our bodies as warrior bodies and create an artificial enemy on the outside. As a result of our developed Cognitive Brain, we follow a thought pattern known as a "dominator." Under this way of thinking, we rationalize our need to plunder and subjugate nature and other human beings. We label external situations as "fearful" or needing to be "dominated" only because we are afraid at our own core of our existence.

Unfortunately, this way of thinking is not just limited to men. The feminist movement may have begun as an anti-war movement but eventually became something entirely different. The feminist movement ended up becoming a way for women to become dominators and warriors themselves. As women learned how to develop their Cognitive Brain and rational view of the world, things began to change. Women now can conquer and pillage as well—in sports, business, politics, and on the battlefield and other areas that were once reserved exclusively for the male gender.

The Cognitive Brain does not discriminate. Whether you are male or female, when you teach your Cortex to suppress what the Reptilian Brain and Emotional Brain are trying to convey you, many unnatural things begin to occur.

How Do We Acquire Our Beliefs?

Our beliefs are the cornerstone of our health and wellness. When we follow nature's guidance, we acquire beliefs that correspond to nature's rhythm. When we acquire beliefs that contradict nature, we set our natural flow off balance. In order to comprehend how this wayward cycle begins, we must first learn where our beliefs come from in the first place.

Our beliefs or mythologies are nothing more than an interpretation of the world around us. These beliefs are the stories that we tell ourselves in order to give meaning to our lives. When we interpret our world according to nature, we acquire natural beliefs. Our false beliefs arise when we interpret the world in a way that contrasts nature. Only by listening to nature and accepting our role as a part of nature will we begin to truly know what a natural belief is and what a false belief is.

We acquire our beliefs in one of four ways. The first way is through our own inner wisdom. This is the place where we listen to our inner parent tell us what we want and need. This is the voice that says, "I believe that I am hungry therefore I need to eat." This is our primal brain fully functioning.

When we are sad, our inner wisdom tells us to respond by crying. Watch a little girl who has a need. She is tired and needs to rest, but her mother continues to drag her around the mall. She cries and lies on the floor, responding naturally. She is respecting the beliefs originating from her brain. I am tired. I need to rest. I will cry to get my mother's attention. We are closest to nature when we follow our inner wisdom

The second way we acquire beliefs is through our own personal experience. When we are young and not yet fully developed, we do not understand much of the adult world. We encounter stresses and traumas throughout our young lives and we seek out meaning for what is happening to us. This search for meaning begins even as young as our womb experience. Many adults even report that they did not feel wanted when they were in the womb. Upon further investigation, they found out that their mother had tried to abort them. The belief that they were not wanted was validated. Even in the womb our beliefs begin to form as we seek answers to our world.

There is an interesting story about a client of mine named Rebecca. Rebecca told me about her and her son, James. She was baking cookies one day and her four year-old son James was asleep in the bedroom taking a nap. Rebecca noticed that she was short on ingredients for her recipe. She debated whether it would be safe to leave her son sleeping and sneak out to the store, which was just down the street. She justified to herself that she would only be gone for a few minutes.

This is what Rebecca did. She went out to the store and quickly returned. She was not gone long. To her horror she found that her son James had awoken and was distraught that his mother was not there. Nowhere in James' young mind could he comprehend that his mother just needed to buy some more ingredients. What James did was what most of us do when we attempt to interpret our world.

James created a belief. This belief was a false belief because it simply was not true. James believed that there was something wrong with him because he had been left alone. This is what is referred to as shame. In his mind, James made up a story in order to make sense of his world. In James's mind, being left was permanent. His mother was never coming back and it was his fault.

That was a horrible day in the life of young James and the story did not end there. As a young adult, James still suffered from abandonment issues. His false belief became a core identity issue and caused much stress and conflict as he struggled with shame and abandonment issues throughout his life.

Another client of mine tells a similar story. Angela grew up in a fairly rigid and conservative household. Emotional honesty was a rarity. One day as a thirteen year-old girl, Angela became really angry with her mother. She just let loose. This was not common. The next day Angela found her mother dead.

Angela went into psychogenic shock. She believed her anger had caused her mother's death. She did not really comprehend why her mother had died. The only way she could put meaning to this shocking event was to make up a story in her mind. Her false belief stated that expressing anger kills people. This was not the natural truth.

This false belief continued to torment Angela for years to come. When Angela first came to see me as a forty-five year old woman, she was suffering from severe migraine headaches, grinding of her teeth and significant jaw pain. She had also developed a significant addiction to street and designer drugs. Angela's repression of her anger was being stored within her body. Her false belief that anger kills was helping to create much of her own pain.

A hypothetical example may be that your parents are going through a divorce. With the limited information that you can comprehend as a young child, you falsely believe it is your fault that your parents are leaving each other and breaking up the family unit. You falsely believe that you did something wrong or there is something inherently wrong with you.

We can develop our beliefs at any age. Whenever we seek out an interpretation for something that is happening to us, we set out to discover answers. We experience many painful situations throughout life. We utilize a part of our higher thinking brain called the Magical Brain to help create a story that makes sense to us. It is these beliefs, many of them false beliefs, which become a large part of our identity.

Sarah was born into a family that was not very nurturing. Stoicism was the norm for this family. When Sarah was born, she was placed in a crib at night and most of the day. Nighttime was especially scary. She would cry all night long, and nobody came to pick her up. The family believed that they needed to train her to not be so needy. They wanted her to be emotionally strong.

Sarah cried every night for seven nights. She was terrified and felt alone in the world. She did not know that the big people were just down the hall. By the tenth night, Sarah gave up and stopped crying. She created a belief that she was not wanted and that the world was not a safe place. In order to survive her horror, she began to disassociate and leave her body. She could not feel pain or pleasure because she believed that the only way to survive was to take her presence someplace else.

As Sarah grew up, she seldom knew what she wanted or what she was feeling inside. She became so used to denying her needs and feelings that this denial became a normal reference point for her. Her false belief that the world was not a safe place continued to create her reality.

The third way we establish beliefs is through our peers. Our peers are people whom we respect and trust. They are our equals. From their experience we begin to establish our own beliefs.

For instance, there is a political election approaching. You are not very informed so you ask your peers for their opinions. You hope to create your own belief about a particular candidate. Using the information gathered from your peers, you begin to develop your own beliefs.

This belief may be true or false. If one of your peers does not like anyone who wears blue suits, he might make up a story that a particular candidate is a constant liar. You have to decide for yourself if this is the truth or if it is just someone else's Magical Mind creating a story based on his false beliefs.

Our peers are very instrumental in helping us establish our beliefs. The more we place our trust in our peers, the more we tend to respect their opinions. Often it is best to seek out a number of sources in order to establish our own beliefs. That way we can pick and choose what feels right and natural for us.

The fourth and often the most significant way we establish our beliefs is to acquire them from authority figures. An authority figure is any person, group, tradition or document that attempts to dictate our beliefs or opinions. Police officers, teachers, priests, gurus or political leaders can all be considered authority figures. Religious books such as the Talmud, Koran or the Bible could also be considered authority figures that help to shape one's beliefs.

Authoritarian systems work because of the trust placed in the authoritarian person, tradition or writing. The authoritarian figure is expected to have a final answer; the last word stops with the authoritarian. Over many eons, humans have discovered that this type of system brings order to their lives.

The problem arises when we begin to realize that many times our authoritarian figures are mistaken. The guidance we expect from them is often not nature-based. Rather, much of the time these beliefs being passed down are actually false beliefs or stories that have been made up. The authority figure may draw us farther away from our natural roots because this false belief is the reference point for the authority figure himself. We often gravitate toward authority figures to tell us what to think and how to feel. When we lose the ability to honor our own natural beliefs, we tend to place our trust in authority figures even more.

False beliefs do not just appear out of nowhere. These beliefs are either passed down to us through authority figures—chieftains, shamans, priests, rabbis, scholars, politicians, celebrities, etc., or we create a false belief for ourselves based on the knowledge that we have at the present time.

People in positions of power tend to establish mythologies for the rest of us. A news director will dictate how the rest of us become interested in top news stories. From car chases to political scandals, a news director will create belief systems for others to follow due to his position of power. A scholar can do the same thing just by writing a book.

For instance, E. M. Jellinek is credited with starting the mythology of alcoholism as a medical disease. Herbert Fingarette writes in *Heavy Drinking,*

> *"Jellinek, then a research professor in applied physiology at Yale University, was a distinguished biostatistician and one of the early leaders in the field of alcohol studies. In his first paper he presented some eighty pages of elaborately detailed description, statistics, and charts that depicted what he considered to be a typical or average alcoholic career. Jellinek cautioned his readers about the limited nature of his data, and he explicitly acknowledged differences among individual drinkers. But from the data's "suggestive" value, he proceeded to develop a vividly detailed hypothesis."*

It was Jellinek who set the stage, however shortsightedly, for the future of alcohol research and, subsequently, all theory about addiction. Fingarette states, "In 1960 Jellinek published *The Disease Concept of Alcoholism,* a book that eventually became the canonical scientific text for the classical disease concept."

There is a mystique that we attach to authority figures. We assume their knowledge comes from a "special" source. There is a backlash if we question where the authority gets his power. If we question the Catholic Church on its role as absolute authoritarian, we may be labeled as a "heretic." In the past, heretics were sentenced to death for questioning. Many authoritarian systems have a built in self-defense mechanism. They usually do not allow their beliefs to be questioned.

Don Johnson writes in *Body* about a man named Charles,

> *"Charles case also illustrates what I mean by authoritarianism: a belief system holding that we must depend on the judgments of publicly designated experts for reliable decisions about personal and social life. Those experts, moreover, are thought to derive their authority not from the community they serve but from sources outside that community. Presidents and party chairmen derive their authority from classified knowledge kept from ordinary people for the purposes of 'national security.' Scientists and physicians derive their claims from privileged access to experimental data and technical language. Popes, ayatollahs, and gurus are specially illuminated from above."*

Much of the time, a belief originates in the authority figure's magical mind. Illumination from above is nothing more than someone deciding that a belief system is true. If our view of nature is distorted, then our interpretation of our beliefs will also be fuzzy.

It was Sigmund Freud who developed much of the early work on the psychology of the brain. Freud theorized that most of our dysfunction or "defense mechanisms" could be traced back to our sexual issues. While this may sometimes be true, this Freudian belief has largely been discredited as being false by most current authorities. Yet Freud acted as an authority figure and many people went along with his guesses about why we do what we do. Most of Freud's theories have been disproved, including "Castration Anxiety" and "Penis Envy." Freud was given free rein to dictate our belief systems. In hindsight, we were misguided by a man, who, however well intentioned, was very wrong.

John Calvin, one of the leaders of the Protestant Reformation, was a workaholic. According to Leonard Shlain in *The Alphabet Versus the Goddess*, "Calvin was a workaholic who seldom took a day off or asked for a holiday. He praised hard work as a defense against the devil's schemes." Because of his authoritarian position, the concept of the Puritan Work Ethic was created. Many of us still follow this credo. We believe that if we are not busy, the devil will take over our mind. Benedict, a monk of the Middle Ages, had already laid fertile ground for this belief. According to Shlain, Benedict wrote, "Idleness is the enemy of the soul."

Our Unnatural Stress Cycle can be traced back to our relationship with our beliefs. Many times the beliefs that we carry correspond to what is actually happening in our natural world. Often they do not. It is these false beliefs that cause us so much pain in our lives.

It does not matter whether we created these beliefs ourselves in our attempt to give meaning to our world or if these beliefs were handed down by centuries-old tradition. A false belief will cause us to engage in a spiral of pain and repression. Learning to heal begins when we can identify the beliefs that are not rooted in nature and accept beliefs that bring us back to our natural roots.

Magical Thinking and False Beliefs

Human beings are unique because we have a brain capable of creating stories. In our search to explain our world, we often make up a story that corresponds with what is actually happening in nature.

The fact that an apple falls from a tree is one such example. The apple falls to the ground because a force called gravity is drawing the weight of the apple downward. In this case, the explanation for what is happening to the apple corresponds to the reality in nature. This is called congruence. Much of the time, the stories we create in order to explain our world are more fantasy oriented. These stories originate from our magical mind. Seldom do stories fabricated in the magical mind correspond to the actual events in nature. These stories are referred to as magical thinking.

Our belief systems are established from the information that is available to us at the time. We perceive our environment and attempt to resolve conflicts with the experiences and information that make sense to us. As children, when most of our belief systems were being formulated, we lived in a world of magical thinking. This world of magical thinking is the world of fantasy and illusion. Our beliefs spring from a mind that spends much of the time in fantasy.

We have a rich capacity to imagine and play. When we are engaged in our world of fantasy, we operate in another world. In this world we are not concerned with saving for our college tuition or retirement. Teddy bears and imaginary friends are real to us. There is no question regarding their authenticity. Our mind interprets their existence as a very real part of our lives.

Wonderful phenomena occur in the world of magical thinking. A child's mud pie becomes a pancake. A cardboard box is now a fort. A doll becomes a best friend who never leaves the child's side. A four-year-old believes that if he digs a hole in the backyard, he will reach China before lunchtime. Since a child's logical mind is still developing, the world of magical thinking becomes a big part of his reality. Children learn to interpret the world and the events around them to the best of their ability. A young child's reality, however, is often through a veil of illusion and magical thinking.

Our own ability to think magically has given rise to many great artists and storytellers. From *The Wizard of Oz* to *Mary Poppins*, many marvelous fantasies have been created out of someone's magical thinking. We can be forever entertained at a magic show with a real magician because we magically believe that the elephant is really disappearing right before our eyes. Magical thinking gives us answers to questions that we cannot logically rationalize at the time.

Magical thinking is a part of our brain's function and plays an important role in our lives. Magical thinking can spark a new idea for a bridge or building. It might also inspire a fabulous painting or spectacular circus act. Magical thinking might help us to solve a problem or seek a new solution.

While magical thinking is a wonderful place for children and artists to spend their time, there is a downside to this place. While many of us believe that we have grown up and left our childish belief systems behind, this is not always the case. Adults are just as capable of magical thinking as a young child might be. In fact, much of our adult beliefs about ourselves and the world around us originate from our ability to think magically. Even as adults we are still enshrouded in the world of magical thinking.

For instance, magical thinking is the belief that causes many of us to run out and buy a lottery ticket. We already have our winnings spent before the numbers are even drawn. Magical thinking occurs when we believe that an abusive relationship will change or go away by itself. In fact, magical thinking is the guiding factor in much of our lives because we are still thinking like children.

Magical thinking occurs very often in sports. How often do you see a team praying before a sporting event? (This was especially true when I played sports at a Catholic high school and competed against "public schools.") Magical thinking was used to drum up a sense of superiority. My team magically believed that we would win the contest because we had

God on our side. We were the "good guys" and the other team members were "pagans," or non-believers. This is what we magically believed in our minds.

Superstition is one aspect of magical thinking. When we begin to examine our superstitions, we also begin to unravel our world of magical thinking. How many people fervently "knock on wood" when they do not want to jinx themselves? This practice is really saying, "I believe that there are spirits in this wood that will bring me good luck." When someone sneezes, how many of us say, "God bless you?" Without stopping to question our actions, we are thinking magically that the devil enters the body when someone sneezes. By blessing the person who sneezes, we hope to erase any opportunity for the devil to harbor within. This was an old practice that began many years past and continues strongly, even to this day.

Spilling salt, black cats and Friday the 13th are other reminders of how magical thinking permeates our life. Have you ever seen a hotel or an elevator with a 13th floor? Many people place a special "corner-stone" in their new dwelling, signifying hope and safety for years to come. We magically believe that if we name our sports teams after an animal, then we will take on the characteristics of that animal.

Magical thinking is a way to interpret the world by telling ourselves a story. For instance, most people consider a dog's bark disturbing. But when an owl makes a noise, it becomes a "mystical" experience. When a wolf makes noises we think of vampires and werewolves. When birds make noise we magically think of this as "singing."

We magically believe what we hear from folktales (magical stories passed down through the generations), entertainment (a movie about singing birds) or through our own creation. It is magical thinking that encourages us to believe that when the sun sets every evening it goes inside a box, or goes "night-night." Our rational mind knows that the earth is just turning away from the sun and in twelve hours or so, the earth's rotation will allow the sun to shine again. Our magical beliefs, dating back thousands of years before we knew about the relationship between the sun and the earth, tell us that the sun goes to sleep for the evening. In the same manner, when we build a pier out over the ocean or a lake, we magically want to believe that we are walking on water.

Our ability to think magically can become a prime factor in our lives, from how we choose relationships to how we worship our god. Magical thinking becomes a prime initiator of false beliefs or beliefs that are not rooted in nature. False beliefs become the myths or lies that we continue to tell ourselves day in and day out.

Magical thinking allows us to live a life of fairy tales and fairy princesses. Our fantasy of Santa Claus and the Easter Bunny come from our world of magical thinking. We wish to believe there is a magical figure that leaves presents under our tree and is always there to protect us. We wish that this person is always good and has many surprises for us. This gives us hope and excitement when the rest of our lives might not be so fulfilling.

Since magical thinking helps to initiate beliefs that are not rooted in nature, they often cause detriment to our lives. Magical thinking becomes a reference point from which many of us see the world. Faced with a real crisis, we are often awakened from our magical world. We might leave our world of illusion and be greeted by strong emotions stemming from our primal roots.

Choosing a mate is often based on magical thinking. Here are a couple of examples of this. A classic magical belief when two people "fall in love" is that they were drawn together by Cupid's arrow. Joyce Block writes in *Family Myths,*

"The Greeks invented the god Eros, whom the Romans named Cupid, to explain the seemingly arbitrary and irrational nature of sexual love. By this poetic device, they solved the great mystery of why we love the ones we do by not solving it at all but, rather, by declaring that there is no logic, no predictable pattern, and that even gods and goddesses fall victim to the whims of an impulsive and mischievous little boy whose motives are rarely pure. Once we are struck by Cupid's golden arrow, there is no choice but to surrender to the mysterious force that propels us toward our fated lover. And, once afflicted, we surely cannot pause to consider questions of pain and pleasure, let alone evaluate whether the rewards of love are worth the risks."

Not only are we magically drawn to the fantasy belief of Cupid, we have also created other fantasies about why we choose our lovers. Many are drawn to the belief in "soul mates," a common New Age belief. We believe that we were together in a past life or our souls are meant to travel this world together. We so strongly desire meaning as to why we are drawn to someone that we unknowingly call upon our magical mind to determine that meaning for us.

A modern, scientific magical belief tells us that "chemistry" draws lovers together. The implication is that something in our cells exudes an odor or attraction for the other person. Realistically, compared to other mammals, we are very poor smellers. This is another magical belief, this time from the scientific way of thinking, which attempts to duplicate the Cupid belief.

Joyce Block in *Family Myths* says it this way:

"We refer to 'chemical reactions,' 'electrical sparks,' and other intangible happenings to explain why we 'fall' in and out of love, or why we find one person irresistibly attractive and another not at all."

As long as we have false beliefs about ourselves, we will continue to live magically in our fantasy world. We continue to choose partners who fulfill our chosen fantasies. If you are a "helpless maiden" you will seek a hero to rescue you. Many of us have a romantic fantasy about Mom or Dad. We continue to seek partners who play the mother or father role for us.

In spite of the fantasy world of celebrity gossip TV shows or bewitching matchmakers, we choose our partners for very real reasons. We find someone who has a quality that is familiar to us or a quality that we have repressed. For instance, if I live my life as a "good boy" and follow all the rules, I might choose a "bad girl" who is used to breaking rules. Since I have repressed my ability to rebel and break some rules, I now live my life with someone who is able to rebel. This brings balance back to my life. This is called "attraction of opposites."

We also choose partners by familiar qualities. If I am a religious person, I might find another religious person as a mate. We have something in common. If you are afraid to be alone, you might find another person who shares the same fear. The foundation for your partnership might then become, "As long as we are together then we are both safe."

Many times we form partnerships based on similar addictions. A person with an addiction to alcohol might choose another alcoholic, so they can hang out at the bars together. The method of forming partnerships is very much of this world and very real. Magical thinking has clouded a very real selection method.

Joyce Block says it very eloquently in *Family Myths,*

"To the extent that we are wedded to our personal mythologies, we must seek out companions who will confirm our fantasized images of

ourselves. Only fellow conspirators can aid us in our self-deceptions and fill up the vacuum that our self-betrayals have left us with. We develop special antennae that pick up signals that may be invisible to the untrained eye as we go in search of our 'other halves,' and find husbands, wives, and lovers who seem to embody what has been forbidden us."

Our love life is not the only place where we can get lost in magical thinking. Magical thinking is a cross-cultural phenomenon. The more rooted in fantasy, the stronger magical thinking might be for a particular culture. From kissing the Blarney stone in Ireland to getting to heaven by controlling the senses (a Hindu belief), we are alike in many ways. Many Latin American cultures believe in "sustos." These are tormenting spirits that are believed to invade when something bad happens. If your house burns down because you left a candle unattended, it is because the evil spirits came in and caught your house on fire.

Magical thinking can also be seen in the *folk science* of astrology. Through a well-designed mathematical system, astrologers teach that the position and movement of the stars affect our lives. The stars are believed to be in charge of everything from our business pursuits to our love life. Astrology gave solutions to those seeking answers when it was first introduced thousands of years ago. What we knew was that the stars changed positions. We also recognized that events happened here on earth. Magical thinking comes into play when we believe in the link between the stars and their shaping our daily lives. Just because the stars are moving in the night sky does not necessarily mean that the movement is affecting our love life here on earth—unless you choose to think magically.

Yes, we are affected somewhat by the movement of other bodies in space. The movement of the moon affects the flow of ocean tides. We are part of the energy that makes up the grand universe, but we are not affected that significantly. Let's imagine that someone on the opposite side of the earth dies. This affects you in some way. The planet weighs less and there is more oxygen in the air for the rest of us to breathe. But the changes would hardly be noticed. The same is true for astrology. It is a time honored magical belief that is very popular with those who choose to think magically.

Astrology was created when it was believed that the sun revolved around the earth. Today we know that is not so. It is the earth that revolves around the sun. The magical belief system is still alive and well and dictates many people's lives. The reading of the morning horoscope indicates how the day will proceed. Will you fall in love today? Should you be extremely careful crossing streets? Should you sell off some stocks today? Astrology becomes another authoritarian system used to guide our lives because we have lost our ability to trust our own natural beliefs and our own inner wisdom. "Blame it on the stars," becomes the motto.

Magical thinking is at the foundation of the Chinese belief system called Feng Shui. Incorporated into a scheme of home decorating, this philosophy relishes in magical thinking. Feng Shui wishes to blame the placement of the furniture in your home for how you feel inside.

For instance, if you place a set of concrete lions outside your front door, the lions are not supposed to be placed facing each other. Rather the lions need to be placed facing outward to ward off any possible intruders or enemies. One has to believe "magically" that 1) there are magical demons and goblins wanting to enter your home, and 2) that a concrete statue has the power to protect you and your home from any danger. This type of thinking sounds like something that originated in a children's movie.

Our religious beliefs are also deeply rooted in magical thinking. If you were an alien from another planet and came down to witness many of our religious practices, you would think we had all lost our minds on this planet.

Take for instance the Muslim holy shrine in Mecca. Hundreds of years ago a black meteor fell to earth. The people at the time believed that this black rock was a sign from the heavens. This idea was based on the limited scientific information about meteors at the time. The people of this age believed the meteor was a gift from God. They built a temple around the black rock for people to worship. In fact, written Muslim law decrees that each and every Muslim *must* make a pilgrimage to Mecca in order to worship this holy rock at least once in his lifetime. Today, even with the knowledge of what we know about meteors falling to earth, thousands of people *still* journey to Mecca each year to participate in this "holy" pilgrimage.

The Christian religion is no different when it comes to magical thinking. The ritual of baptism is a magical belief that states that we are all born with a black mark on our soul. The act of sprinkling "holy" water on the initiate will erase this black mark.

The ritual of a priest in fancy robes saying some words over a piece of bread and a glass of wine is another example of a Christian magical belief. A common belief among Christians is that the bread and wine are transformed into the body and blood of Christ through this ceremony. There is little distinction between this ritual and a child's mud pie being real.

It is magical thinking that causes a Hindu to bathe in the Ganges River to cleanse his soul or a Christian to cut down a pine tree and bring it into his home, hoping that Santa Claus will slide down the chimney and leave presents for all. A Jew magically believes that his prayers will be answered and his suffering diminished by placing a hand-written prayer in the Wailing Wall, a stone wall in Jerusalem.

Even the oldest and far reaching religions can be subject to magical thinking. Buddhism and Taoism are two such examples. Magical thinking occurs when a Tibetan Buddhist walks around all day repeating a mantra in hopes of enlightenment. It is these daily incantations that are needed to ward off the demons that lurk in the shadows.

Lewis M. Hopfe writes in *Religions of the World*, "Taoism is mainly associated with ignorance, superstition, and magical attempts to prolong life."

Religion is a wonderful place to foster magical thinking. We are all looking for hope and are all so vulnerable. We utilize our Cognitive Brain to create these wonderful stories for us in order to give our lives meaning. We feel safe when we have a magical story to protect us.

It is magical thinking that prevents a Christian from eating meat during Lent or a Muslim to abstain from eating, smoking, sex, or any pleasure during daylight hours for the entire month of Ramadan. The concepts of karma and sin are other magical beliefs that help us understand "good" and "bad" behavior. Unfortunately, we are still operating from the mind of a child.

Magical thinking helps us feel proud of our beliefs. Most religions have a magical belief that states, "My god is better than your god." This gives each a feeling of self-righteousness and superiority over others.

Magical thinking allows one to be dominated by something as innocuous as "faith." It is magically believed that our religious beliefs are directly handed down to us by our God and that the stronger our "faith" in these beliefs, the better the person we are. Those who follow the false beliefs and myths established by the ones in power have a strong "faith." Those who challenge or divert from the established beliefs are labeled as "lacking faith."

The notion of faith is magically believed to be like a deluge raining down on us from the sky. Rarely is this concept questioned as something more than a weak or strong conviction to a magical belief system. Whether one is considered to be Christian, Hindu or Muslim, it is the magical belief in faith emanating from a higher source that becomes the glue that solidifies a particular set of beliefs into a person's character.

Magical thinking is self-defensive in nature. We will protect and defend our magical beliefs to our death sometimes. The Christian doctrine insists that, "There shall be no false gods before me" to instill self-defense while the Muslim religion proclaims that "Allah is the one true God."

Most authoritarian systems that rely on false beliefs also have a built-in self-defense system. For instance, the Catholic Church relies on its disciples' rigid adherence to the rules. There is no questioning of the church's authority. Only those in power can change the rules.

Magical thinking is also very egocentric. This means that we see the world from only one perspective, and that is our own. Magical thinking allows us to make ourselves the "good guys" and those who are different the "bad guys." If you have white skin, magical thinking might tell you that cowboys are better than Indians, and white is better than black. When we think magically, we see the world through a very narrow viewfinder.

Magical thinking goes hand in hand with authoritarianism. When we think magically, we set ourselves up for abuse. We give our power away and do not confront our abusers because we magically believe that they are better than we are. People do not question the power and authority of others because it is magically believed that the power and authority were passed down from a higher source. This gives kings and rulers the right to do whatever they wish because the magical belief is that power is absolute and must be obeyed—because it comes directly from God. For example, the Council of Trent, by its position of authority, declared in 1563 that it had the sole right to interpret Catholic scriptures.

I can remember story after story of yoga teachers who have shamed, ridiculed, embarrassed and have even hit students. The teacher has claimed some god-like and elevated status in order to get away with this. Only the magical mind of the student would allow this to happen. The student might have magically believed that the teacher has a special power or knowledge that gives them the right to abusive behavior. This is the root of authoritarianism in action.

There hardly seems to be a culture unaffected by magical thinking. In the yoga tradition of India, a particular hatha yoga pose called the "scorpion" exemplifies this thinking. The participant is instructed to stand on his hands while lifting his legs above his head in a manner where he can touch his feet to his head. It is commonly believed that the head is where all our problems reside, so by kicking the head with the feet, psychological problems will be healed. Don Johnson writes in *Body,*

> *"The head which is the seat of knowledge and power is also the seat of pride, anger, hatred, jealousy, intolerance, and malice. These emotions are more deadly than the poison which the scorpion carries in its sting. The yogi, by stamping on his head with his feet, attempts to eradicate these self-destroying emotions and passions. By kicking his head he seeks to develop humility, calmness and tolerance and thus to be free of ego."*

Each one of us has our own personal mythology that we follow. We have magical ways in which we strive for love and survival. We might believe that no one will love us if we are not always perfect. We might create a fantasy that the only way to get attention is to do bad things. Besides our institutionalized beliefs, we also carry a host of individual magical beliefs.

In popular marriage rituals, a man often asks the father of the potential bride for permission to have his daughter's hand in marriage. The father is believed to be the owner of the daughter. It is usually the father of the bride who walks his daughter down the church aisle. The father then turns over his property (his daughter) to the groom in an exchange of goods. While most people in Western cultures would deny that they believe this ritual to be true they still continue to participate in this symbolic gesture during marriage ceremonies.

We remain a child when we remain locked in magical thinking. We get stuck in the world of fantasy and illusion. We base many important decisions about marriage or careers on our magical beliefs. We can demonize our enemy with magical thinking by insisting on our superiority. We are still baking mud pies in our imaginary ovens and building forts out of cardboard boxes. When we do not question our magical beliefs, we end up living in a world of fantasy.

Magical thinking is a way of viewing the world that does not correspond to the reality of nature. This leads to our Unnatural Stress Cycle. The magical stories created by our Cognitive Brain then become the catalyst for our body's stress reaction. In order to understand the damage that stress creates, it is important to grasp the beliefs that help initiate the stress response. Understanding stress and disease begins with learning how beliefs help to create a response in the body.

Magical thinking and false beliefs only take us further away from nature and our natural ability to be well. Healing happens when we drop deeper into our sensory and emotional experiences and leave our world of childhood illusion behind. The most significant healing begins when we can access our Emotional and Reptilian Brains. It is here that we are the closest to our natural origins.

Myths, Religion and Science

Through the growth and development of the Cognitive Brain, we have continued to seek answers to the questions about our world. Some times our answers are congruent with the reality in nature; often they are not.

Our own magical thinking concocts stories in our mind to help explain some of our dilemmas. These would be called personal mythologies. At other times, we carry collective or institutionalized mythologies shared by a group of people.

In the scope of our human history, there have been three primary belief systems created to help give our lives meaning and formulate our beliefs. These three belief systems are mythology, religion and science. While there are other belief systems that have shaped our lives, mythology, religion and science are among the top three. Sometimes these belief systems are aligned with our natural world. Most often, though, they have drawn us further away from nature. By exploring the role of our belief systems, we can better grasp the significance of the loss of our relationship with nature.

Mythology

Our earliest history of the development of our beliefs lies in the history of our mythologies. These mythologies are stories that we tell ourselves or are passed down to us by our tradition (the authority). These stories help give meaning to our lives. We now have a reason for why things happen. We have a sense of completion.

Much of the time, our mythologies are nothing more than the world of fantasy and make-believe. They derive from the mind of our childhood thinking. Most importantly, these stories often draw us further from our natural roots.

For instance, you are living some three thousand years ago. There is a violent lightning storm. You can only explain the lightning with the information that is available to you. All of your information comes *before* the creation of science. You create a belief that there is a god in the heavens who is throwing lightning bolts down on earth because he did not receive enough offerings. You name him Zeus. Your entire belief system is based on what you know at the time, which entails storytelling as a way to solve problems.

Based on what we know today about lightning, this belief is a false belief or mythology that was created according to the cosmology of the time. However well intentioned, it is not rooted in the reality of nature but in the storytelling of the mind.

Leonard Shlain writes in *The Goddess Versus the Alphabet*, "When Aborigines in Australia first saw an airplane over head, they accurately described it but imputed to the aircraft a preternatural spirit."

Our world has been inundated with many mythologies and stories that have helped give meaning and understanding to our lives and the world around us. Much has been written about the vast collection of mythologies that have been carried down through many generations. From Carl Jung to Joseph Campbell, our "hero's journey" and "maiden's plight" have become institutionalized within our culture. Unfortunately, Campbell and Jung might be considered part of the problem rather than part of the solution. These scholars' passionate study and perseverance in mythologies has only helped to keep people stuck in the world of illusion and magical thinking.

For many people, it is the age-old mythology that creates fear and shame around a menstruating woman. In some cultures, a common belief is that if a menstruating woman even touches or glances at a hunting tool, the hunt will be ruined. The hunters need to blame something for their failure to bring back dinner. This belief was very common in the past and is practiced in many parts of the world even to this day.

Using mythologies to help understand the world has been an important step in feeling safe. However, remaining attached to these mythologies can cause problems later on in our lives. When anchored in magical thinking and stories that are not rooted in nature, we ultimately lose our relationship with nature and our ability to be free of our cycle of stress.

Many of our false beliefs are not derived from our own personal experience but are passed down through many generations. Much of the time, we are handed mythologies that existed hundreds and thousands of years before, when the information that we had about ourselves came from a less developed reference point. Many of these false beliefs were handed down to us without our questioning, as if they were natural beliefs. Much of the time, our mythologies are not updated. We continue to follow belief systems that are no longer relevant, and we get stuck following outdated beliefs.

Most cultures adopt a creation mythology. Some believe that mankind emerged in a garden. Others believe that it was through the top of a volcano that was the source of human development. Still others believe that it was through the Sun god that the world came into existence. We all choose our own creation story based on our culture, surroundings and traditions. These stories that we create then become a large part of our belief systems.

In fact, much of the time these stories are not our own personal experience at all. We believe them to be natural beliefs when in fact they are false beliefs. The Greek and Roman myths are some examples of mythologies passed down for thousands of years. The stories in the Christian Bible, Talmud, Koran, Vedas, Cinderella and Snow White are also such magical stories. These are all stories with which we parent ourselves with when we have lost our relationship with nature.

The myth of Santa Claus is a classic example of a mythology that pervades our culture. Our authority figures (namely our parents, teachers and *the media*) keep perpetuating this myth. When we look up the chimney as children and shake our heads and say there is no way a fat man can fit through that tiny opening, our parents shame us by insisting that it is so. When we rationalize and insist that Santa Claus cannot possibly visit *every* household on Christmas Eve all across the globe, the media insists that it is so. News channels with their fancy radar machines even create an image of Santa's exact location. Children are handed down the myth of Santa Claus without being able to question its validity in a culture that wants them to "believe." We all then play our part as co-conspirators in accepting this myth as our reality.

Even the government is in on the myth. Children write letters to Santa Claus, addressed to the "North Pole." Instead of sending the letters back with an "undeliverable" or "no such address" stamp, the government files away these letters so that the child believes the letter was actually delivered. The government encourages the lie to continue.

Reparenting with Mythologies

When we are rooted in nature, we have a sense of what we are thinking and feeling. When we are lost from our natural source, we lose our ability to know the truth. We can no longer identify when we are hungry or tired. Instead we eat and rest according to the dictates of government law. We lose our ability to express our emotions and become numb instead.

Mythologies have been used to give us meaning and direction in our lives. They have been used to create an inner parent to help guide us. The mythology or story then becomes our truth. We lose ourselves when the mythology becomes more important than our own relationship with nature.

When we are immersed in our mythological thinking, we often trust our stories more than ourselves. Our stories become our inner guidance. We lose our ability to trust our feelings and desires because we do not want to let go of the story that we have used as our truth barometer. Once our self-trust is eroded, unnatural laws, or laws of the Cognitive Brain, now rule us.

We reparent ourselves with the words from a song or a story. A poem from our favorite book of literature or a popular cartoon fantasy becomes our role model of how we parent our self. A television hero or a rock star might become the parenting system we hold "near and dear." A set of fabricated rules or a centuries-old tradition surpasses our own feelings and intuition as our guide.

When we lose our relationship with nature, we relinquish our power to the saints and heroes we worship. Gurus, politicians, celebrities and sports stars become the means by which we attempt to reparent ourselves because we have lost our true self.

What is important to remember is that when we lose our self, we seek out authority figures to parent us. When we do not trust our self, we become prey to authoritarian systems used to control and manipulate us.

Personal and collective mythologies are not the only way that we are drawn away from nature. Out of mythologies grew religions. Religions are a form of institutionalized mythologies. Unfortunately, religions often are not guiding us closer toward our natural roots; instead, most religions tend to separate us from nature.

Religion

As we evolved from a mythology-based species, we soon formed religions. Religions were a way to develop rituals and shrines around our mythological beliefs. Religion offered us hope and understanding. The search for gods (such as gods of procreation, the harvest and the sun), gave our lives order and meaning.

We have continually questioned our existence here on Earth. Why were we born? What happens to us when we die? Why do people hurt each other? Religion came along with a systematic explanation. The explanations were based on the beliefs present at the time of the development of religion.

Christian mythology largely originates from a collection of stories gathered together in a book commonly referred to as the "Bible." The Bible was written by a handful of men who never even met any of the people about whom they supposedly wrote about. It was not until 30 to 110 years after Christ that the first works of the Bible appeared. It is these stories written by a handful of men that have become the parenting system for many. Ibn Warraq writes in *Why I Am Not a Muslim,*

"It is now recognized that the Gospels (Matthew, Mark, Luke, and John) were not written by the disciples of Jesus. They are not eyewitness accounts, and they were written by unknown authors some forty years after the supposed crucifixion of Christ. Matthew, Mark, and Luke are usually called synoptic Gospels because of the common subject matter and similarity of phrasing to be found in them."

Ibn Warraq then adds, "It now seems highly unlikely that any of the sayings attributed to Jesus in the Gospels were ever spoken by a historical figure."

Leonard Shlain writes about the creators of the Bible in *The Goddess Versus the Alphabet.* "Before the lights of literacy went out, the Christian Orthodox leaders—Paul, Tertullian, Jerome, and Augustine—had hammered together a religion whose central themes were sin, guilt, and suffering." Their words became the belief systems that others came to worship. According to Schlain, all of these writers had considerable difficulty with their own sexuality and a disdain for women. What they wrote only mirrored what they believed themselves to be true.

In fact, according to Schlain, it was the writings of Paul that formed the cornerstone of the Christian Bible. Paul originated the belief in the Holy Trinity. Shlain writes,

"After Paul converted the singular Yahweh into a nuclear Christian family, he was faced with the danger that Christianity was no longer a monotheistic religion. In one of the most complicated explanations ever contrived, Paul claimed that while Jesus was the Son of God, he was also God himself. In the centuries to come, people actually killed each other over the issue of the consubstantiality of Jesus and His Father. The problem has never been completely resolved.

Further adding to the polytheistic dilemma, Paul invoked a new entity to join the Son and Father pairing—the Holy Spirit."

Paul shaped the structure of the church and its major beliefs. Schlain writes, "In this sense it is not hyperbole to say that Paul invented the religion called Christianity." Another such example of mythology at work through the guise of religion occurs when we consider the ritual of circumcism.

To quote Genesis, Chapter 17, Verse 9;

"God also said to Abraham: "On your part, you and your descendants after you must keep my covenant throughout the ages. This is my covenant with you and your descendants after you that you must keep: every male among you must be circumcised. Circumcise the flesh of your foreskin, and that shall be the mark of the covenant between you and me. Throughout the ages, every male among you, when he is eight days old, shall be circumcised, including house born slaves and those acquired with money from any foreigner who is not of your blood. Yes, both the house born slaves and those acquired with money must be circumcised. Thus my covenant shall be in your flesh as an everlasting pact. If a male is uncircumcised, that is, if the flesh of the foreskin has not been cut away, such a one shall be cut off from his people; he has broken my covenant."

A story was written over two thousand years ago about a woman in a garden who ate an apple from a forbidden tree. She was forever banished from the garden while she, her mate and all of her descendants were cursed with a black mark on their souls. This is the story of Adam and Eve from the Bible's book of Genesis. This was a story created by one man or a group of men in positions of authority. Millions of people have been influenced by this one mythology.

The story achieved what it set out to achieve—to give meaning to people's lives. Now the magical mind could rest at ease as this story fulfilled an explanation about why there is pain and suffering in the world.

But the mythological story of The Garden of Eden has caused more problems than any that it could have solved. Many people who hold the story near and dear feel a sense of shame or worthlessness for having been born. Even those living thousands of years after the story was first introduced continue to experience this internalized shame. With the development and study of the mind and the creation of psychology, we have more clues about why we do what we do. The story of Adam and Eve, while well intentioned, is obsolete. Yet many believers still cling to this story as their own mythology.

We seek a solution for events that we cannot explain. Religion often offers us these answers. We create a story when the corn refuses to grow or there is a death in the village. "God must be punishing us," we reply. This gives our lives a sense of meaning. These same beliefs help to create our taboos and our rituals. A dance and a song are needed to insure the harvest in some cultures. The belief is that if the gods are not happy, punishment follows. A typical Christian belief is that people do bad things because they are born with original sin and are tempted by the devil. A common belief among Muslims is that Allah determines everything and they themselves are not responsible. Allah made them do it.

It has often been asked, "Why can't men control their sexuality?" A mythology was created in a religious context that gave an explanation. The explanation says something like this, "God made men weak and unable to control themselves." This gave the initiators of this belief a freedom from responsibility. God was now at fault if someone was always feeling sexual.

Many times, it is a person in authority, a parent or official, who either develops a false belief or passes it down to us. For instance, Don Hanlon Johnson writes in *Body, Spirit and Democracy*,

"Saint Paul encouraged people to be eunuchs for the sake of Christ. Origen, the great third-century theologian, castrated himself in a fit of Christian idealism. Until this century, it was castrati who had privilege of singing in the papal choir. Pope John Paul II to this day tells members of Roman Catholic religious orders that their celibate way of life is better than marriage and praises their decision to become 'eunuchs for the sake of the kingdom of heaven.'"

Many Catholics were raised to memorize the *Baltimore Catechism*. This conservative text influenced the lives of millions of people. For instance, Father McGuire, the author of the *Baltimore Catechism*, writes about the chief sources of actual sin. He states, "The chief sources of actual sin are: pride, covetousness, lust, anger, gluttony, envy, and sloth, and these are commonly called capital sins." Father McGuire proceeded to shame generations of young people for being human beings.

A child feels anger and along with this feels that he is a bad person because Father McGuire and the *Baltimore Catechism* said so. This book is a direct line to God, or so the magical belief goes. A child also feels sexual feelings and feels shame for having those feelings, based on Father

McGuire's proclamations. In adulthood, these false beliefs are often still very active in the lives of many people.

Each religion has its own set of false beliefs. For instance, the Eastern belief is that calmness or centeredness is the ideal state. This is one such example of a false belief. We were not born to be nice or calm and centered all of the time; we were born to allow our many feelings and experiences to flow through us.

Consider the following false belief from Paramahansa Yogananda, author of *Autobiography of a Yogi*. "Calmness is the ideal state in which we should receive all life's experiences." What this belief teaches is to repress all the feelings and experiences that are not calmness and centeredness. Human beings are shamed and considered "bad" if they have other feelings that are not "calmness."

Yogananda, by his sheer authoritarian position, declared that calmness is the ideal state in which we need to experience all of life's events. Have you ever seen a sky that was always calm? When was the last time you saw a child or a wild animal that was calm all of the time? Many would say that a person like this must have been very far removed from nature, from animals and from children. Yogananda may have even forgotten that he was once a child himself. Calmness is one state of consciousness, yet calmness is not the ideal state or the natural state.

If we look to nature for a role model, it is nature that continually changes. Storms roll in and out. Weather changes from calm to turbulent. The earth shakes to release excess energy in the form of earthquakes. Rivers flow to deposit storm run-off back into the ocean to be recycled for the next storm. Flow is the ideal state as described in nature.

By clinging to beliefs that are not in accordance with nature, we have managed to lose much of our natural flow. We hold back tears because our belief is that control is the ideal state. We direct our anger inside because we believe that we are sinning if we eventually express our anger outwardly. Having adopted beliefs that are opposed to our relationship with nature, we only end up hurting ourselves.

A clash began when religions appeared on the planet. This was a clash of beliefs. Religion-based mythologies began to conquer and subjugate nature-based mythologies. Wars, torture, murder and enslavement resulted. This conquering of people's beliefs was a result of the belief that "my god is better than your godless world." From the shores of South America to the missions of California, conquering others' beliefs has become normal and commonplace.

This behavior is commonly accepted as the work of missionaries and continues to persist under the cleverly disguised pursuit of helping cultures to feed themselves and become literate. Many missionaries are not sent to other cultures to actually help them; their primary role is to conquer their beliefs. Missionary proliferation by Jehovah's Witness, Catholics, Mormons and other groups is widespread today. While their roots began many years ago, conquering of others' beliefs remains commonplace today.

Witch hunts and holy wars happened for one reason—false beliefs. The ruling belief system considered witches, Jews and non-Christians as the enemy. The Crusades of the Middle Ages were instigated by Pope Innocent II in 1096 to win back the holy shrines of Palestine and defeat the "infidel" Muslims. This was all initiated by false beliefs.

For instance, a common Christian mythology states that one gets points later on if he can convert a "pagan" or non-believer to his Christian god. This is as if a Christian were to receive a sales commission for every convert to "Christendom." This mythology allows people to magically believe that they are saving another soul from limbo and will receive points for their efforts.

War and ideological skirmishes are common among groups associated with religion—based mythologies. It is a false belief that causes a Catholic to battle a Protestant and a Muslim to go to war against Hindus. Buddhists battle against Christians and Muslims wage war against Eastern Orthodox Christians. The Jewish struggle with the Muslims in the Middle East is nothing more than a war of false beliefs: my god is better than your god.

In-house fighting is also very common. Different sects of the same religion also have conflicts because of the differences in false beliefs. Conservative Jews battle with Orthodox and Reform Jews. The Eastern Orthodox Catholic Church has different beliefs than the Roman Catholic Church. The Theravada Buddhist and the Mahayana Buddhists many times have become bitter enemies because of the differences in their beliefs.

Our religion-based mythological beliefs may run unchecked for hundreds of years. We remain frozen in an old belief and forget to update our information. Circumcism of males and females is one such example. So are the Jewish Kosher laws. Leonard Shlain writes in *The Goddess Versus the Alphabet,*

"The new Israelite religion became very concerned with cleanliness, with an aversion to dirt and other "unclean" things. Pigs are smart, friendly animals that thoroughly enjoy wallowing in the dirt. Deuteronomy forbids

members of the Israelite faith from eating or keeping a pig, which is the first time in history a group had, using the force of religious doctrine, collectively condemned this member of the swine family. Apologists have claimed that the Old Testament was protecting the Israelites from eating an animal that commonly carried the trichinosis parasite, but the many other cultures that based their diet on pig meat did not suffer decline."

Two thousand years ago, when people may have gotten sick from eating foods that were not sanitized, these laws might have been appropriate. But today, even with our modern means of food preparation, the beliefs about what foods are clean and unclean still exist because the false beliefs have never been questioned. While the Jewish population still remains committed to condemning the pig, many cultures, like the Hawaiians and Polynesians, thrive on a steady diet of pig.

False beliefs come to dominate our lives. We are still rooted in magical thinking when we tell ourselves a magical story that is far removed from our natural reality. Religion-based mythologies are hardly the exception.

But magical thinking does not stop there. Religious mythologies, while still very popular throughout the world, have lost their reign as the dominant belief system. The new king of the hill is commonly referred to as the philosophy of science. Science has come to conquer religion just like religion conquered many nature-based mythologies. Science has become the premiere belief system throughout our Western world in hopes of giving greater meaning to our lives.

Science

A dramatic shift began to occur at the beginning of the sixteenth century. Up until this time, religion was the primary belief system responsible for providing answers to any relevant question. The leaders of the churches held supreme authoritative power.

But a bold astronomer named Nicolaus Copernicus came up with a startling new discovery. Copernicus proclaimed that the sun was at the center of the universe, not the earth. This conflicted sharply with the religious texts, which held the earth to be the center of the universe.

Thus, a long series of conflicts between science and religion began. There was a battle over beliefs. Each side was attempting to make sense of the world in which we lived. This battle waged over the centuries. While still maintaining a stronghold in many parts of the world, religion bowed to science as the dominant belief system for explaining our world.

In our modern era, it would seem that science "can do no harm." Science has absolute authority and the final say. The philosophy of science has become accepted by most as absolute, just as religion held a captive audience for centuries.

There is only one big problem. Science is not absolute. In fact, the mythology of science is often mistaken. Science is more often wrong than correct. Look at the myth of cholesterol. Years ago, scientists came up with a theory that said that fat is the cause of heart disease. We were told that we were eating too much fat. Then scientists changed their minds. There were now "good fats" and "bad fats." Peanut oil was considered "bad" while safflower oil was labeled "good." Then scientists changed their minds again. The determining factor was now the type of cholesterol in our blood, "good" cholesterol or "bad" cholesterol. So we all had our cholesterol monitored frequently. The scientists told us it was the bad cholesterol that was clogging our arteries. Scientists then created a substitute for butter called margarine. We were told that margarine was much better for us then the fats in butter. Soon we realized that hydrogenated oils like margarine that were made in laboratories by scientists were creating all sorts of health issues for us.

So it was recommended that we eat fish. That theory did not last long either. Some fish were loaded with "bad" oil. Scientists changed their minds again. We now could only eat certain types of fish. So after all of these panic attacks and scientific theories, science has been wrong more often than it has been correct. Who's to say that this latest theory isn't wrong as well? Time will tell.

Dr. Dean Ornish, author of *Dr. Dean Ornish's Program For Reversing Heart Disease,* concludes,

"The use of cholesterol-lowering drugs is based on the presumption that cholesterol is the primary determinant of atherosclerosis, whereas I am becoming increasingly convinced that other factors, including emotional stress, perceived isolation, lack of social support, hostility, cynicism, and low self-esteem, also play important roles . . ."

Donald Epstein further adds fuel to the fire in his book, *Healing Myths Healing Magic.* Epstein writes, "Recent clinical and laboratory studies have seriously questioned the validity of the theory that a blocked coronary artery is the primary cause of a heart attack."

If this wasn't compelling enough, Epstein concludes with the following. "Yet, an article appearing in the *Journal of the American Medical*

Association stated that tension, frustration, and sadness double the risk of a heart attack and permanent heart damage."

Science has prided itself on its exactness, yet the reality is that science itself is not an "exact science" and is instead loaded with hunches and guesswork. Recent findings indicate that the well-established practice of hormone replacement therapy for women going through menopause can be very dangerous and harmful. Science has had to swallow its pride once again. Many times science has misinterpreted our world and has led us away from nature. Robert O. Becker, M. D., and Gary Seldon sum this idea up in *The Body Electric.*

"Science is a bit like the ancient Egyptian religion, which never threw old gods away but only tacked them onto newer deities until a bizarre hodgepodge developed. For some strange reason, science is equally reluctant to discard worn-out theories . . ."

The authors further add, "I want lay people to understand that they cannot automatically accept scientists' pronouncements at face value, for too often they're self-serving and misleading."

Newtonian Theory Versus Quantum Theory

When we enter into a forest what do we see? That answer all depends on your perspective. If you are a lumberman, you might see how much lumber might be produced from the trees. If you are a land developer, you might see how many homes could be built on the land. If you are a naturalist, you might imagine how many acres could be protected.

When we take a look at our body and health, what we see also depends on our vantage point. How we view our wellness is determined by our beliefs. These beliefs stem from two primary theories about our world. These theories are called Newtonian and Quantum.

Newtonian Theory

In the early days of science, Isaac Newton and other prominent scientists theorized that the secret to our world could be found in breaking matter down into smaller parts. These smaller parts would give us an answer to our problems. This approach was called "reductionism" and this view of the world came to be known as "Newtonian."

For instance, if you want to find out how a wind-up watch works, you would take it apart and discover the function of each part. You would then create a theory about your discovery. By deduction and logic you would find your answer. This was an all-out attempt to utilize the Cortical Brain.

Scientists continued to use this reasoning to unravel the mystery of our universe. Microscopes and telescopes were developed. Measuring devices and scales all came into use. A cell was divided into molecules, and further divided into atoms. From these atoms came electrons and protons.

Through this Newtonian logic we have come to understand the world of genes. Under the scientific umbrella, the world is seen as a collection of particles. Genes are said to be responsible for everything from birth defects to addictions. It is the gene's fault if something goes wrong and our life can also be measured and quantified as a varying amount of chemicals.

Chemistry has become one of the offshoots of Newtonian theory. If it is deduced that the particles in your body are deficient, then a concoction of other particles is given to you to balance out the missing particles. The science of nutrition and pharmaceuticals is a product of this type of reasoning. In many cases, this theory works very well. For instance, if you have a life-threatening infection raging through your body, a doctor might give you penicillin or other antibiotics to help destroy the disease. In this manner, disease is identified as a chemical imbalance.

Often, this Newtonian view of ourselves works exceptionally well. If you were to be bitten by a poisonous rattlesnake, the most effective treatment might be to receive known anti-venom to reverse the toxic affects of the snakebite. Administered in a timely manner, this approach is usually very effective.

Scientists like Louis Pasteur helped to create this vision for the rest of us. Pasteur believed that our bodies are machines, so he advocated using mechanical approaches to treat the human machine. Under this theory, the health of the body occurs when the machine is functioning to its full capacity. The germ theory then evolved, which inferred that microbes equal disease.

Furthering the development of germ theory was a man named Abraham Flexner who was sent by the Carnegie Foundation in 1909 on a nationwide tour of all of the medical schools in the United States. Only those schools that adhered to surgery and drug therapy as the treatments of choice received generous grants. Other schools were forced to close due to lack of funding. According to Harvey and Marilyn Diamond, authors of *Fit For Life II*, "The now famous **Flexner Report of 1910** put the nails in the coffin of health care diversity in this country."

In the early days of scientific theory, chemical solutions became important in stopping the spread of infectious diseases. Smallpox, rubella and measles are some examples of this early success. These rules generally apply under particle or Newtonian theories.

However, the primary diseases of our time are not infectious diseases but degenerative diseases. Robert O. Becker, M.D., and Gary Seldon write in *The Body Electric,*

"Degenerative diseases—heart attacks, arteriosclerosis, cancer, stroke, arthritis, hypertension, ulcers, and the rest—have replaced infectious diseases as the major enemies of life and destroyers of its quality." These same authors add, *"Medical research, which has limited itself almost exclusively to drug therapy, might as well have been wearing blinders for the last thirty years."*

Science has been given free rein to categorize disease and illness. Yet much of our disease process has little to do with scientific or particle theory. Depression is one such example. Depression is first and foremost a disease of lack of energy flow outward. Feelings like anger and grief become stuffed within the body. Instead of flowing outward as nature would have intended, these feelings become lodged within the soft tissue of the body.

When this occurs, one feels compressed, lethargic and frozen. It feels like a giant vice is squeezing the head and spine together. If not released, the brain chemistry eventually begins to change. Science has only measured the change in chemicals in the brain and has failed to address the real problem. Depression is essentially a lack of feeling experience. One feels frozen in place and the natural flow of energy outward has become thwarted.

The answer to curing depression is not to alter the serotonin levels in the brain by administering an anti-depressant chemical. This is only a band-aid to help one not feel the symptoms. The answer lies in following depression to its source and attempting to release the frozen energy and emotions that are lodged in the muscles.

Science tends to create its own rules as it goes along. For instance, we all know the classic four seasons of nature's cycle. These seasons are referred to as Winter, Spring, Summer and Autumn. The world of molecules and science has added two more seasons. These new seasons are called "Flu Season" and "Hay Fever Season." We pay attention to these seasons when the scientific community reminds us that it is time to get our flu shot or purchase our hay fever medicine.

While science and Newtonian theory designed around dissecting individual molecules is a valid treatment when the disease is molecular-based, most diseases of our time are not. These new diseases, sometimes referred to as degenerative diseases, require other means of treatment. This new type of treatment is based on unraveling the blockage of energy that started the disease in the first place. This is called "Quantum Theory."

Quantum Theory

When we follow Quantum theory, we are much more likely to heal from the source. In many cases, healing will occur from our lower two brains, not from our Cognitive Brain as science wants us to believe.

The vision of our personal health cannot be limited to just a chemical or mechanical experience. Just like our vision as we enter the woods may have many aspects, so too does our wellness. This other vision holds more promise than the particle theory. Under Quantum theory, we are not reduced to particles or chemicals. The nature of who we are is energetic. Quantum theory honors the flow of energy that is based in nature.

When we see the world as energetic, we need to define what we mean by energy. This term is commonly used in eastern cultures, yet is very new in the West. Energy moves through all things, like an electric current. It is this current of energy that determines our health or wellness.

Nature inherently possesses an energetic flow. There are changing seasons. There are scores of fluctuating weather patterns. This flow of nature also resides in us because we are part of nature. Honoring this flow of nature only brings us more harmony and wellness. (Remember, it is our Cognitive Brain, the creator of rationalization and science, that wants us to believe that we are better than nature.)

Under Quantum theory, the laws of nature govern us. When we disregard the laws of nature, we begin to upset the natural cycle. Nature always holds true. Nature always wins. While science and Newtonian theory have brought us many life-saving treatments and formulas, we are primarily bound by Quantum theory, or the laws of energy.

Even die-hard scientists have broken rank and shifted over to the Quantum theory. Dr. Dean Ornish writes in *Love and Survival*, "Even Louis Pasteur changed his thinking later in life and believed that germs were only part of the picture and that other factors usually played an even more important role." Ornish recalls how Pasteur believed that the soil in which the microbe was growing held all of the answers, rather than the microbe itself. This soil is what we refer to as the body's own immune system.

The battle over beliefs can be best demonstrated using noted cellular biologist Bruce Lipton's analogy. Lipton says that the mission of science is an attempt to gain intellectual knowledge in order to conquer nature. If nature is predominantly the flow of energy, then science is attempting to conquer energy.

What better example of this idea than the latest scientific controversy? Scientists have now been able to genetically alter our food and everything else in our life. We can now eat food with pesticide genes already implanted within that food. Nature no longer is in charge of reproducing by itself. Scientists in laboratories have begun to conquer the reproductive rights of nature, from food to animals. The advent of human cloning is one short step away.

A scientist can modify the reproductive rights of a plant and then patent that idea with the government patent office. Under intellectual property rights, nobody else is allowed to reproduce that plant. This is one such example of scientific beliefs attempting to conquer nature.

While scientific theories and a Newtonian world view have become commonplace, it will only be through a shift in perception to a Quantum world view where many long-standing issues will be solved.

Beliefs About Children

The beliefs established by our rational Cognitive Brain are where science finds its home. While these beliefs have often helped to further our evolution, they have frequently only created more havoc. For instance, in the last fifty years or so, science (rather than nature), has been responsible for parenting us. Science took child rearing away from mothers who had always raised their children along natural guidelines. Our efforts to scientifically dominate nature have only created severe consequences.

Breast-feeding became taboo and laws were passed to abolish public breast-feeding of infants. Midwifes and doulas were ordered out of business as doctors and hospitals were the only ones allowed to birth children. Under the control of our emerging rational brain children have been raised as "laboratory experiments."

Elaine Morgan writes in *The Descent of the Child,*

"For hundreds of years doctors promoted an even more distancing assumption—that babies could not feel pain. Circumcisions could be carried out without anesthetic on the grounds that it doesn't really hurt them—they are not like us."

This rather callous belief initiated by the scientific mind has enabled medical authorities, parents and governments to poke at, prod, torture and experiment on babies because someone in an authority position created a belief that babies were not capable of feeling anything.

The issue of children and nighttime sleeping stirs up a lot of conflict. According to a cognitive approach children need to learn a stern self-reliance at an early age. Placing a child in a crib to sleep alone at night has become the modern protocol. A case in point stems from a book by Gladys West Hendrick called *My First 300 Babies.* Hendrick writes, "Wouldn't your child be stronger emotionally if he felt loved and safe in his own bed?"

This practice of isolating a newborn to its own crib has created dire societal problems. The first six months to a year in a child's life is a time when a child is developing beliefs about whether or not he feels safe in the world. Placing a child in a crib alone at night often leads a child to develop a belief that he is not wanted or that the world is not a safe place. This belief that the world is not a safe place is the core of where our stress issues derive from.

The first six months to a year is a time when real beliefs about our world are being created. Babette Rothschild writes in *The Body Remembers,* "At birth the brain is among the most immature of the body's organs." It is this first six months to a year when we are formulating our beliefs about whether we feel safe in the world or not. Any incidence of trauma becomes greatly magnified because of the immaturity of the newborn's brain.

An authoritarian figure practicing his own magical thinking might influence how we raise our children. For instance, many of us were raised with the beliefs created by Dr. Benjamin Spock, a well-known baby doctor. Dr. Spock has always recommended that children should sleep alone in a crib at night, even though this is against what has naturally been going on for millions of years.

In *Dr. Spock's Baby and Child Care*, Spock and Steven J. Parker, M.D. write,

"Children can sleep in a room by themselves from the time they are born, if convenient, as long as the parents are near enough to hear them when they cry or have an intercom in the bedroom. If they start sleeping in their parents' room, two or three months is a good age to move them."

Dr. Spock believed that a child should learn independence from his parents as early as possible. Most likely this is the kind of treatment that Spock received from his parents. What Dr. Spock did not realize is that his authoritarian rational emphasis has set many up for deeply rooted stress issues. Many people carry a belief that the world is not a safe place because they were left all alone at night.

This practice has done more damage to the Western psyche than almost any other practice. It is much more natural for a child to sleep with his parents for some time. This helps him to develop a belief that the world is a safe place and this is what nature would have intended. Through science and the straying away from nature, many of us have been forced to create false beliefs about whether we feel safe in the world or not.

Christiane Northrup, M.D., writes in *Women's Bodies, Women's Wisdom,* "No mammal leaves its children unattended and unsuckled the way humans do." In fact, only a left-brained scientific world view of children would allow this. When scientists started to raise children, our natural instincts were undermined. Most children instinctively want to crawl into bed with Mom and Dad. Northrup further adds, "Why should adults get to sleep with someone, while children have to sleep alone?"

Humans buy scores of stuffed animals and invite their cats and dogs to curl up in bed with them. Slumber parties for kids are common as children attempt to regain this natural instinct to fall asleep with others. All of this is an attempt to counter the beliefs created by being raised by scientific rationale. Science essentially negated the emotional life of the child in favor of a rational utilitarian view of the world. This shifting from a nature-based "feminine" way of birthing and raising children to a "patriarchal" scientific approach is at the heart of so many of our social and health problems.

A newborn child feels a wide range of feelings and sensations, from fear to wonder to pain. In fact, according to Joseph Chilton Pearce, a young child not only feels these emotions and sensations but *is* those sensations. She is nothing more than sensation; she does not stop and analyze these feelings. Soon our authoritarian and scientific systems begin to shame us for having these feelings and sensations. We start to believe that the authority (be it a book, document or person) is right and we are wrong. We begin to devalue our own experiences.

Scientists and Newtonian theory appeared on the scene as our gods and rescuers. But blinded by only chemical and mechanical beliefs, we remain ultimately frustrated. Looking at medical scientists as a group might shed some sad reminders of the danger of completely investing in left-brain thinking. As science has come to dominate our world view all of us have suffered the consequences, most particularly science-based medical doctors.

Dean Ornish, M.D., writes in *Dr. Dean Ornish's Program For Reversing Heart Disease,*

"We doctors don't set the best examples. Besides learning not to value or hear the emotional needs of our patients, we often learn to deny and split off our own feelings as part of our medical training. As a profession, we have among the highest rates of drug addiction and divorce of any identifiable group, and the average physician dies ten years prematurely. Each year, enough physicians commit suicide to equal a large medical school's entire graduating class. And that's just the known suicides. So it is not very surprising that many doctors do not believe that emotional distress or spiritual isolation can contribute to heart disease. It's easier not to."

Our beliefs become the cornerstone of our health. Our health is most often determined by what is happening in our mind. By aligning our beliefs with nature, we maintain our radiant health. Denying or trying to conquer nature only leads to more chaos and despair.

Our beliefs come from many sources. We carry false beliefs from our own personal experiences as well as from group mythologies. From our family systems to our neighborhood, we carry many beliefs with us. We also become rooted in institutionalized false beliefs like religion and scientific mythology.

Our Cognitive Brain has grown beyond the other parts of our brain. Often, in hopes of interpreting our world, this neo-cortex has only misinterpreted our world by trying to dominate nature. As a result of this wayward brain, we have many beliefs that are magical in nature. These magical or false beliefs are the lies that we tell ourselves every day.

The first step in healing means beginning to unravel the vastness of our beliefs. The goal is to discern the myths from nature's reality. Returning to nature first and foremost means returning to beliefs that follow the flow of nature. It is only when we recover our mind that this can happen.

Pillar Number One

Process Work

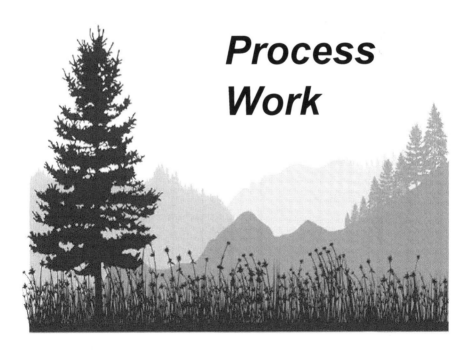

Recovery of the Mind

Our beliefs influence both wellness and disease. The mythologies that exist in our mind form the basis for the health or disease of our body. Much of the time, our beliefs are just stories that we create in order to resolve our conflicts about why things happen. So often our beliefs are not truths rooted in nature, but stories in our minds. This is the nature of our false beliefs.

When we return to nature, we begin to distinguish nature's reality from the magical fantasy created in our own mind. This work is called "process work." When we begin to understand our false beliefs and where they originate, we gain greater knowledge about how these beliefs affect our present reality.

The goal of our recovery is to learn how to relax. Relaxation is the opposite of stress. When our minds activate a false belief, we often enter the Unnatural Stress Cycle. These false beliefs come from several sources including personal mythologies, authority figures, and peers. They keep us locked in our stress cycle, preventing us from entering into the state of relaxation.

There are two components of process work: 1) intellectual process, and 2) developing emotional wisdom. The goal of intellectual process work is to identify the story that shapes our beliefs. We do this by looking at family history, major life events and significant losses. Sensory and emotional process work involves learning how to access emotions and sensory experiences. Both are required to fully process our conflicts.

Intellectual Process Work

There are many ways to recover our mind. Process work involves identifying the triggers to our stress cycle. The first step is to begin to unravel where your beliefs come from in the first place. From here, you move into working with these beliefs.

We parent ourselves with the many tapes playing in our mind. These tapes lie at the root of much of our disease process. We may parent ourselves with songs or television shows. Books or religious messages might be the parental tapes that get lodged within the mind.

The beliefs that we have stored within our mind often lead to stress later on in life. Most of the time, these beliefs are unconscious to us. We proceed throughout our day without ever questioning our beliefs or their source. When we begin to examine our beliefs, we take the courageous first step toward recovery.

Step Number One: Identifying the Story

Our beliefs lie within our brain like a stack of records in a jukebox. We constantly play these beliefs out. Some beliefs get played more often than others. We cannot begin to change anything until we first recognize what it is that causes our uneasiness.

We all have a voice in our head. This voice is a collection of tapes based on our life experiences that we play over and over. Most of the tapes we have stockpiled have been recorded from a very young age, perhaps age two or younger. Some of the tapes that we listen to can even originate from our experience in the womb.

These tapes are survival tapes. They are messages we *believe we need* in order to keep us alive. The messages are based on painful experiences that we thought were going to kill us or were passed down to us by authority figures.

A very simple way to begin the healing process is to state the following;

I believe that I will die if . . .

Fill in the blank. There may be more than one false belief, but there is usually one primary belief that guides your life. It may be helpful to recall all the instances in your life that caused the most pain. This will help to identify a pattern that was based on your false beliefs.

For example, if you experience tremendous pain every time a relationship ends, your false belief might be, "I believe I will die if I am rejected or abandoned." If you experience what feels like life-threatening pain when you are by yourself, your false belief might state, "I feel like I will die if I am alone." This belief might have been created by a single traumatic episode or by a repetitive pattern over time.

When we have no knowledge or understanding about the pain in our life, we develop coping or survival skills to prevent us from feeling that pain again. The original pain may have felt like death, so we develop a tape in our brain to avoid that pain again. When we do not know why the pain message is speaking, we learn ways to avoid it altogether.

Take for instance a child who grows up with parents who seldom meet her infancy needs. She does not get the tenderness and caring that a child deserves. There is alcohol abuse and frequent violence within the household. Sexual abuse is the norm for this child. She experiences much pain from her childhood.

As a result of this pain, she develops belief systems in order to survive. These belief systems become her own personal mythology. She develops the false belief that in order to survive in the world she needs to always be in control and never let go. If she lets go and loses control, she falsely believes that she will die. This is how she lives her life. Any conflict that arises in her life as an adult usually centers on her false belief about losing control. This belief then becomes the voice that keeps playing in her head. The tape says, "Don't lose control or you will die."

Our false beliefs can be anything from, "I feel like I will die if I let go" to "I feel like I will die if I do not have someone to manipulate." "I will die if I have to trust someone" might be one person's belief system that runs his life, while another person might be guided by the false belief, "I will die if I am not perfect."

As previously mentioned the beliefs we carry originate from four primary sources: inner wisdom, personal mythologies, authority figures and peers. Inner wisdom is when we are rooted in nature and follow what our physical and emotional needs might be. It is the other three methods where we begin to lose our relationship with what is natural. Starting with personal mythologies we will explore the nature of our beliefs and how these beliefs draw us away from nature and into our Unnatural Stress Cycle.

Personal Mythologies

As we go through life, we move through common stages of development. If we live a long life, we will experience infancy, adolescence, adulthood and old age. We share stages of development in our learning process as well. When we learn to walk, we first learn to scoot, then to crawl. From here we begin to make it upright with the help of a coffee table or chair. After a while we are free to take on the world from an upright position, and off we go. It takes many steps to learn how to walk. We all go through these stages as we learn how to stand on our own two feet.

There are also stages of development that help to establish our beliefs. These stages are critical in establishing the belief systems within us. When we become wounded or traumatized within a particular stage, we formulate a false belief that corresponds to this period in our life.

The first belief we acquire is that the world is either a safe or hostile place. This belief becomes fixed between the time of conception and about one year old. A child, either in utero or living in the adult world, needs to feel safe. She is neither able to satisfy her own needs nor protect herself from danger. She relies on adults to do this for her.

The primary way a child learns to feel safe in the world is to have constant body contact with a trusted human being, hear a familiar voice, smell a familiar smell or see a familiar and trusted face. When these elements are present, a child will develop a belief that she is safe in the world. These elements need to be in place around the clock for a year or more to create a belief that the child is safe. Creating a belief for the child that the world is a safe place is much less effective if these elements are only present when it is convenient for the adults, like only in waking hours, between nine and five.

Without these consistent elements or through a significant event that disrupts these elements, a child might develop a belief that she is not safe in the world. Alexander Lowen refers to this element as the "Schizoid" complex.

Being placed in a crib at night reinforces a child's belief that he is not safe. He has to go it all alone and to fend off danger by himself. He does not have constant warmth and safe body contact to enable him to relax and let go. He tightens up at night in order to feel safe. His fragile brain does not understand that the adults are just down the hallway. he believes that he has been abandoned and must go at life all alone.

Many of us continue to ignore or neglect this basic need of infants. A child needs to be held to feel safe, yet many times we push the child away because we are tired or distracted. If a mother and child do not bond, the child will develop the belief of not feeling safe in the world. Rejection by the mother is a common way for a child to establish a belief that the world is not a safe place. A girl may grow up into adulthood believing that she belongs on another planet. She feels unsafe wherever she goes. She is always a bit paranoid and has difficulty trusting anyone completely. This is the result of not getting the constant bonding and physical contact required to establish a belief that she is safe.

One single event could also shape this belief. Imagine that your parents decide they need to take a vacation by themselves. You are six months old. You are still not quite sure if the world is safe. Your beliefs are not developed yet. You are left with a grandparent whom you do not fully trust. This single event could traumatize you and help to establish a belief that the world is not safe.

Here is how our beliefs are contrasted. We often see a parent pushing a stroller with a young infant in it. Frequently the child is crying ferociously.

The scientific mind has taught parents that a child needs stimulation. Hence, most strollers are designed with the child facing forward and the parent pushing behind. The young infant might not be able to comprehend that the parent is still behind pushing the stroller. In a child's mind, when a parent goes out of visual view, they are gone forever.

But a young does not need this kind of stimulation. This action has broken the basic rule of nature. A child needs to first and foremost feel safe. Someone who was rooted in nature would understand this. When the child opens his eyes from sleeping he must be able to see or hear mom or dad. This instills in the child the reminder that the world is a safe place so that this belief can be imprinted. A more appropriately designed stroller would be one where the child faces backward, always having eye contact with the parent.

The next stage in our development occurs at age one to two years old. This is when we are meant to have bonded with our primary care giver (usually the mother but not always). We feel attached to this person. We believe we are one and the same. If we are not allowed to complete this stage of our development, we often acquire a belief that we have been abandoned. We develop an abandonment complex. Alexander Lowen refers to this as the "oral" stage of development.

Let's say that Mom and Dad left you at the mall accidentally when they were shopping. They just forgot about you. You looked around and found yourself alone in the world. It is very likely that at this moment you went through a traumatic experience and formulated a belief in your mind that you had been abandoned. This belief became lodged in your brain because of the energy of terror that surrounded the event. Throughout your life this belief often rises up. All of this is the result of a single event.

Later we encounter other stages of development that seek to find completion in our young lives. We seek out control over our lives. Then we learn ways to be in our power or to give it away. Finding our autonomous selves is another stage that seeks a sense of completion.

Whether they are issues of safety or control, power or abandonment, we formulate beliefs about our world that come to be called our own personal mythologies. Much of the time, these mythologies are not real or based in nature. Our magical mind has come into play. These mythologies are just the stories that we tell ourselves based on our experience of our world and our interpretation of the events around us.

Authority Figures

Just as our beliefs are shaped by the personal stories we tell ourselves, another source of our beliefs is our authority figures. The authority can be a real person, like a government or religious figure. The authority can also be a dogma from a written text or oral tradition.

When we lose the ability to trust ourselves, we connect with authority figures to establish our beliefs. While sometime being rooted in nature, often they are not. Because we have lost our ability to question the authority and the story itself, we accept the story as truth.

For instance, many boys were raised by parents who insisted that "big boys do not cry." These boys were handed a false belief that they needed to hold back all of the tears in order to get love in their family. This is not nature's way. These parents, being the authority, created this belief. A boy's inability to challenge this belief at a young age helped to cement this belief into his consciousness.

As an adult you may still find it difficult to cry because this false belief continues to be a large part of your identity. You may still believe that crying or letting go of emotions is equated with weakness or disappointing Mom or Dad. Unless this belief is challenged, it will continue to affect your life.

Peers

Our peers are also a strong influence on our belief systems. Peers are those whom we regard as equals. A peer can be a friend, business associate, spouse or relative.

Let's say you are twelve years old and you live in a tough neighborhood. You continue to hear many messages about what a real man is like. Your biggest influence is your friends who have lived in a gang culture their entire lives.

Your peers believe that being a man means joining a gang and proving your courage by going out and hurting or killing someone. Since you respect the beliefs of your peers, you begin to accept and take on these same beliefs. You then begin to believe that manhood means being tough, mean and willing to create an outrageous act of violence in order to be accepted by your peers. Your peers have helped to shape your beliefs.

When we do not question the beliefs of our peers, their influence over our own beliefs is strong. We trust their view of the world as absolute truth and end up taking on our peers' distorted view of the world. We continue to remain removed from nature.

The Columbus Theory

In order to heal from our false beliefs, we need to challenge them. This will help us know if they are based in nature or someone else's fantasy mind talking. Just as Christopher Columbus did not believe that the world was flat and set sail to prove his theory, we too can challenge the authority figures who placed false beliefs upon us. We can either set sail to dismantle our false beliefs ourselves, or we can believe other authority figures that have a different opinion. Once we gather more information, we can judge for ourselves.

Once you have identified a false belief, then you are ready to go on to step number two. This step involves your willingness to grow or your willingness to protect your pain.

Exercise: Understanding Your Story

Where did your beliefs originate? Who were the authority figures that helped to shape your beliefs? Were you influenced more by your peers or your parents? Did religious leaders or school teachers help to shape your primary beliefs?

Step Number Two: Dialoguing with the Behavior

Once you have identified your false beliefs, you can begin to change them. Change takes a commitment to work from the inside out. Our beliefs can be altered by re-recording the tapes in our head.

Let's look at the case of a man named Andrew. Andrew has a false belief that in order to get love he must always be perfect. He strives for perfection in everything he does. His yoga practice is perfect. His clothes are arranged perfectly. His house is in perfect order. He spends most of his life wrapped up in striving for perfection.

This belief has become the source of his stress response. He is almost always engaged in a stress reaction due to this belief. In order to begin the necessary changes, Andrew must first recognize the extent to which this belief controls his life. He must then begin to dialogue with this behavior to instill a new belief.

If Andrew falsely believes that perfection equals love, he must begin an inner dialogue that attempts to dissipate this pattern. He must start to repattern this belief with a new belief, which might sound something like the following. "I do not have to be perfect all the time in order to get love."

This work is sometimes called Inner Child work or Reparenting work. When we begin to do this Inner Child work, it is as if there is an adult talking to the young child. It is the child who is holding onto the false belief. The adult part of us needs to reassure the child that this belief is not valid. When we can begin this task and learn these skills, we are moving forward in our recovery.

When we lose our self at a young age, we lose our inner dialogue. We lose our ability to trust ourselves and come to rely on outside authoritarian figures for guidance. Without a supportive inner dialogue, we quickly become prey to easy manipulation and abuse. We do not know how to question, say "no" or judge for ourselves. We can reclaim these abilities by recovering our inner dialogue.

Reparenting

Inner Child work begins with learning to create a little you, sometimes symbolized by a doll or teddy bear. You then learn to dialogue and find out about your true feelings and needs. This is the core of reparenting work. You learn to be your own parent. You know what you need. You know that your feelings will not kill you, no matter how horrible they might feel at the time. You learn to have a healthy inner dialogue with yourself.

Margaret Paul, author of *Healing Your Aloneness*, has been a pioneer of reparenting techniques. One helpful technique that she uses is the Inner Child/Inner Adult dialogue. A person actually spends time talking to himself from an adult perspective and asking the Inner Child within what he wants and needs.

Margaret Paul states, "All the problems in our society stem from the internal disconnection between the Adult and the Child. All unloving acts toward others and toward the planet are manifestations of the internal disconnection and abandonment, which is handed down from one generation to the next."

Step Number Three: Identifying Your Commitment

When we develop a false belief at a young age, we also make a commitment to follow that belief system. We become fiercely loyal to our false beliefs. We will do almost anything in order to avoid confronting or changing our belief systems. We protect and defend our beliefs with severe intensity.

Recovery means being willing to make a commitment to confront your false beliefs. Making this commitment means committing to facing our pain, no matter how long it takes. This might seem like a very unnatural process. When we spend our entire life attempting to avoid pain, why would we suddenly want to invite pain into our life? Yet, that is exactly what is needed in order to recover from false beliefs. It needs to be normal to feel our pain so that it can be released. Your body needs to learn that you will not die from pain. You need to experience being alone or out of control many times to *know that you will not die from this*. In this way, you will be recreating a new tape, a healthier message and healthier voice within you.

Your mind truly believes that you will die if you have to experience the pain of rejection, being out of control, being powerless or being alone. Every cell in your body is trying to keep you away from that pain. In order to recover, you must change your experience of "normal." Your mind needs to remember what it feels like so that it can recreate a new message. Every time that you feel this pain, your mind registers that you did not die.

Step Number Four: Changing the Behavior Associated with the Belief

The beliefs we harbor inside us ultimately lead to our stress and discomfort. After we have recognized which beliefs we have acquired, we can begin to change the behavior associated with this belief. The types of false beliefs that we carry within us are varied and may include the following:

- I am bad if I make mistakes (shame).
- I don't belong here in the world.
- Nobody will love me if I am fat.
- I will die if I am abandoned.
- I am a failure if I stop and rest.
- It is not safe to let someone get close to me.
- I will die if I stop rescuing others.
- Nobody is to be trusted.
- I will die if I am rejected.
- I will die if I am not perfect.
- My world will end if I am out of control.

The first step of process work is to identify the issue. In Andrew's case, he knows that he errantly believes that he will die if he is not always perfect. This false belief is now at the core of his stress response.

In order to change, Andrew must first begin to practice not being perfect all the time. He must do something different. If his house is always perfectly neat, he must practice being a little messy. He must surrender his state of control by practicing imperfection. If what he is doing is not working, he must try something else so he can learn that imperfection is not the enemy.

His mind does not differentiate between his false belief and fighting a war because his false belief is really an imaginary threat. His need to be perfect becomes an imaginary tiger chasing after him. When Andrew can begin to realize that the threat is only imaginary, he can change his behavior more quickly.

He must teach his mind and body that he can survive when being less than perfect. He may have learned in his family that the only way anyone in the family received love or attention was to be perfect. He now begins to change the behavior to teach himself that he can receive love without always having to be perfect.

The more Andrew practices this new behavior, the more natural it becomes. After a while he feels normal not always having to be perfect. He feels less pressure now. With time and practice he now has changed a false belief into a natural belief.

Step Number Five: Seeking Support

Nobody can do this work alone; a solid support system is necessary. In my own practice I will not take someone into their deep emotional work unless I am certain they have already developed a strong support system to guide them through their pain. Those who are in recovery might need someone to lean on from time to time as they enter into a state of chaos in the process of rebuilding parts of their life.

A support system can consist of friends who will be there for you 24-hours a day for as long as it takes to feel and release your pain. It may take weeks, months or years to recover the lost pieces of yourself. When choosing people to serve as your support system, shy away from those who may abandon you when the road gets rough. Choose people with good listening skills, a willingness to experience their own pain, and a desire to support you in the most difficult of times.

A support system can also be a professional therapist or group. Availability is important. If professional support is only available from nine to five on weekdays, and you only get to speak with her if you are in her office for fifty-five minutes once a week, then you may need additional support. Support needs to be ongoing and around the clock.

Working with a professional therapist might help you gain the support and confidence you need to continue your process work. A skilled professional facilitator can help you sort out not just the events in your life causing conflict, but also the underlying roots of the beliefs associated with them. You may also wish to join a support group. You will not feel so alone in your struggle to change your beliefs and behavior.

A healthy support system is an important and vital step along the road to recovery. Your support system must be willing to be there for you and let you experience your own pain so that you can release it. Knowing that there is someone there for you makes the letting go much easier.

Grieving the Old Belief

A step often missed in our recovery work is grieving the old belief. You cannot just tape over an old belief with a new belief. The old belief will still be there, only now you have to remain on guard so that it does not pop up unexpectedly.

Grieving is about letting go. When we can grieve, we make room for something new. In a culture that places emphasis on holding on, grieving is not always a simple or easy task. However, it is important.

Just as we need to grieve the loss of a loved one, we also have to grieve the beliefs that no longer serve us. When we grieve these false beliefs, we let them go for good. If we just cover them up with new beliefs, they will still remain. They may be buried underground, but they are still present.

Grieving requires actually feeling the emotion of grief. Some people feel most comfortable working through grief in a group with the helpful support of others. Others prefer grieving alone. The essential ingredient to grief work is to contact the emotion of grief while identifying the belief that you are grieving. Tears and full body waves of contractions are part of the grief experience. We are not supposed to be in control when we grieve. Being out of control with our grief is the natural way.

Developing Emotional Wisdom

For centuries now, a common goal for many cultures has been to "educate" the masses. Bringing literacy to every household has been a worldwide campaign. Along with literacy came the pressure to excel in math, science and many other intellectual pursuits.

These are all cognitive activities and have their valuable time and place. The problem arises when our rationalization and reasoning activate the Unnatural Stress Cycle. Our attempt to educate the world has turned many of us into information addicts and kept us frozen in our Cognitive Brain. We often neglect the many other aspects of our human existence.

There are many types of intelligences of which we are capable, such as academic, creative, intuitive, kinesthetic, sensory, emotional, relational, and many more. Unfortunately, we have created a culture where intellectual intelligence is where we measure our value.

Our spelling bees and academic decathlons have become our intelligence measuring rods. Our merit system is based on report cards and grade point averages. Scholarships and admissions to the most highly acclaimed colleges and universities honor those who receive the highest intellectual scores. The most highly respected colleges admit students with a high degree of academic intelligence and employ professors who are highly efficient at communicating and teaching their academic knowledge to their students. Some of the highest paying jobs in American society go to those with a good deal of academic intelligence—doctors, lawyers and MBA graduates.

We continue to grade ourselves on our "intellectual" scores. First we compare ourselves to the scores from previous years. Then we attempt to wager one region against another. Finally, we compete globally against other countries. Through this ongoing process, the U.S. has become a nation of intellectual addicts while sacrificing our emotional, creative and sensory intelligence.

The IQ test was first developed by a Stanford psychologist named Lewis Terman just after World War Two. Daniel Goleman explains in *Emotional Intelligence,*

"That people are either smart or not, are born that way, that there's nothing much you can do about it, and that tests can tell you if you are one of the smart ones or not. The SAT test for college admissions is based on the same notion of a single kind of aptitude that determines your future. This way of thinking permeates society."

We are rarely taught or encouraged to pursue any type of emotional or sensory intelligence. In fact, we might know more about our cars and the stock market than we do about our emotions or our own bodies. We can send a man safely to the moon, yet we are not able to feel our own aloneness. We can invent a nuclear bomb with all of our cognitive brainpower, yet we do not know how to grieve.

Most of us seldom know what it is that we are feeling. We spend so much time with numbers, words and computer software, but we are untrained in expressing our feelings. We do not know if we are tired or sad. Our depression might be deeply held anger. Feeling "low" might really be fear, but we do not know the difference. We might not know if we are angry or are feeling disappointed. An expression like, "I just had my heart broken" might really be, "I feel abandoned."

We have little or no knowledge of the emotions that dictate our lives because we are rarely allowed to express them or receive training in how to feel them. Nobody wants to see a presidential candidate cry in public. This is a death sentence for the election campaign. It is front-page news when an athlete displays deep emotion. Emotions that pop up from time to time are regarded as an alien incursion.

We spend a great amount of time attempting to control, repress or hold back our emotions. This is the kind of society that we have created. Most of us walk around numb, not recognizing how we are feeling. We are sensory and emotionally illiterate.

We are bombarded with messages from authorities that attempt to invalidate our feeling experiences. These left-brain dominated sources continue to fear emotions, so they label them as "bad" or "weak." We have many role models when it comes to academic achievements, but we have few role models for practical emotional wisdom. It would seem that we are still leaving our emotional life up to our Cognitive Brain dominated scientists.

These scientific role models often show up in disguised forms. Religious and spiritual leaders often deny our emotional wisdom. Even many psychotherapists approach emotions from a rational perspective and do us more emotional harm.

One such example of the cognitive analysis and denigration of the emotional world comes to us from the Church of Scientology. Developed by L. Ron Hubbard, Scientology teaches that the brain is either in its "analytical" mind or its "reactive mind." The analytical mind refers to a fully conscious person. The Scientologist refers to a person feeling strong emotions as "unconscious" and in his "reactive" mind.

This is another attempt by the Cognitive Brain to analyze and minimize our feeling experiences. The Cognitive Brain is suspicious of emotion. As a result, this part of our brain attempts to label these emotions as useless or bad. Under the Church of Scientology doctrine, consciousness is equated with control.

Our intellectual achievements have become the standard by which we have measured our success. Yet this is only a tiny part of our full being. Daniel Goleman writes in *Emotional Intelligence*, "At best I.Q. contributes about 20 percent to the factors that determine life success, which leaves 80 percent to other forces."

It is these "other" factors that help to determine how happy and well adjusted we become in our lives. We often spend so little time actually learning how to enhance and develop them. Our religions and business organizations continue to minimize or outlaw our emotional experiences.

For instance, Scientology regards all emotions as a lie and states that the real solution to any problem is to rationalize everything. But recovering our mind requires gaining emotional intelligence. Learning to feel our feelings and move through them is the goal of our recovery process. When we can honor the sensory and emotional experiences that shape our lives, we live in a more fruitful and healthful state.

What would it be like if "emotional intelligence" courses were taught in school, along with literature and science? What if, along with our annual national science competition, we had an annual emotional or sensory awareness week? Or perhaps, what would it be like if our families turned off the television for awhile and had weekly or daily "weather reports," where each person were allowed to express his feelings?

At this point, our only barometer for our child's development is the quarterly report card, which states a lot about his intellectual achievement, but very little about what is really going on inside of him. We do not have a grading system to report these "other" factors of our emotional life. Imagine what it would be like to actually have workshops on how to express anger in a healthy fashion. Think of the possibilities if we actually taught a "communication" class in school that had nothing to do with television and film.

When I work with clients, I first determine their level of feeling by asking several questions. Is she able to feel and accept pain in her life? Does she know what anxiety feels like? Does she have a wide range of feeling experiences, or is she rather numb? We all have a different level of feeling based on our level of emotional intelligence. One person might feel on a level eight out of a possible ten, while another might feel on a level two. Their experiences would be quite different.

A feeling must be felt in its entire intensity in order to be released. If you have resistance to getting in touch with your anger, you may want to bypass the anger and go right to forgiveness. This does not help the release of emotions but only prolongs the repression. A feeling must be felt and released in the order that it appears.

All emotions have a purpose. We are meant to grieve when we experience loss. We leap for joy when we celebrate victory and we explode with our entire body when driven to anger. Every emotion requires a skillful full-body expression. Analyzing our feelings from our head does very little to actually express them.

Take anger for instance. Anger is a call to set a boundary and requires saying "No!" which we need to express with our entire body. There are three stages to expressing anger. First identify the feeling and notice where you store anger in your body. Second, dialogue with the feeling. Contact a professional therapist or friend, write in a journal or talk to your own "inner child." Finally, you must release the energy of anger from your body by expression. Kicking your legs or hitting a pillow with your fists are good ways to release the energy of anger.

We must begin to allow our children to feel their feelings. For example, if you are in a supermarket and your child is upset because you will not buy him his favorite breakfast cereal, it isimportant to honor his feelings rather than shame him for feeling the way he does. Whether in the market, outside, in the car or at home, that child needs to have his temper tantrum and grieve the loss and disappointment of not getting what he so desperately wants. Grieving and temper tantrums are just a few ways of cleansing our bodies of hurtful feelings.

If the child is not allowed to express his feelings, he will bottle them up inside and will learn that he is not allowed to express emotions in his family or culture. Those bottled up feelings will remain in his body and he will find addictions to avoid feeling the pain that has been created. We begin to heal when we start teaching our children how to feel and express themselves more fully. We come into alignment with nature when we allow our emotions to flow through us.

Classroom education about drug use is not enough. We must be a positive "feeling" role model for our children. We must first teach ourselves how to sit with our feelings and then pass that information on to our children. We spend hours each week with our children and their intellectual homework, but how much attention do we give to their emotional world? We must ask ourselves, "What is the role of education?" Do we continue to produce machines that can perform a task at will or further enhance our full range of development as human beings?

Our feelings need to be supported at the workplace. When making money is not our primary goal, then our emotional needs will take a larger priority. We might be allowed a certain number of "emotional health" days off—days that give us time to be with our feelings.

Throughout our lives we will experience trauma and wounds. The shape, size and duration of our wounding are less important than how we deal with the wound. If we are allowed to grieve and let go of our pain, we will be much better off than if we hold on to it.

We begin to separate from our true selves if we don't allow ourselves to feel our pain fully, grieve this pain and then release it. Have you ever wondered how a small child moves through several different emotions in a very short time period? This is because she has not yet lost her self and still knows how to feel. She has not yet learned what society wants her to learn—i.e., to stay in control and repress what she is feeling inside. The energy of her feelings just passes right through her and she quickly releases it.

In order to learn how to feel, we must become like children again and be spontaneous with our feelings. We must learn to not repress our feelings or to stuff them inside because they are "inappropriate" at the time.

A simple alternative to the Inner Child program is to ask yourself twenty times per day, "What am I feeling now?" This needs to be an ongoing effort to become in touch with what your feelings are and to stay alert to them. There is no need to try to change those feelings. Simply accepting your feelings and acknowledging them is enough. This way you become present with your feelings. If we keep checking in with our feelings and spend more time feeling rather than numbing them out, they will become normal to feel.

As you awaken in the morning, a valuable first question to yourself might be, "What am I feeling now?" rather than, "Where's the coffee and morning newspaper?" Throughout the day you might keep reminding yourself to check in frequently. A simple note in key places around your home or office usually is a good reminder. A symbol or colored dot might help to remind you of your commitment to keep checking in with your feelings frequently. As you lie down for bed at night, you might once again ask yourself, "What am I feeling now?"

Our belief systems have continued to guide us away from our natural means of expressing our emotions. In some cultures, anger is a sin and grief is a sign of weakness. These are both examples of false beliefs continuing to be passed down through the authoritarian systems.

Emotions are not a disease, as some would want us to believe. Emotions are nature's way of allowing us expression and health. Learning emotional intelligence is just another step in learning to be responsible for our own wellness.

Recovery means being willing to experience your feelings, as intense as they might be, and learn from them. It is not necessary to try to change these feelings; simply accepting them is enough. When we can just feel our feelings, as uncomfortable as they might seem to us, our body learns that we will not die from them. Our feelings will seem overwhelming at times, but it is important to ride them out nonetheless. It may feel as if you are swimming upstream when you first begin. After awhile, it will become much easier and a normal part of your life.

Conclusion

Process work involves both intellectual and emotional process work. We must recognize the beliefs that we carry within us. We must work to develop a relationship with our emotions to clear these beliefs.

Learning how to feel means consciously placing ourselves in situations where we intend to learn about our pain. Rather than attempting to avoid certain situations that bring up intense feelings, we seek out these situations in order to learn about our pain. This will become part of our newfound commitment.

Recovery work is not something that one does when it is convenient. Making the commitment to grow and to feel pain is a 24-hours a day, seven days a week job. There are no holidays off. There are no timeouts.

Recovering our mind means being willing to identify the false beliefs that distance us from our natural roots. The next step is to change these beliefs and their associated behaviors. Getting out of our head and developing emotional intelligence becomes an important ingredient through this process.

As we begin to unravel the mythologies that we carry, we begin to understand how we became removed from nature. Challenging our authority-created beliefs is one step. Examining our own personal mythologies is another method. In addition, getting in touch with our emotions and learning to have a full emotional life becomes a vital step in this process.

Exercise: Learning How to Feel

- What are the most difficult emotions for you to feel?
- Where did you learn about your emotions?
- How does your present culture and environment continue to undermine your emotions?
- Who were your role models, and what did they teach you about your emotions?

PART TWO

LOSING
YOUR BODY

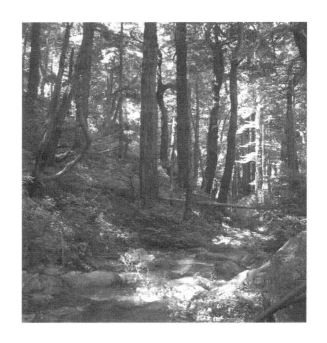

I. The Nature of Stress

Your body tells a story about your physical and emotional history which traces back to the point of your conception. Your particular story becomes locked within your tissues. Every cell in your body tells this story.

Your story is reflected in your posture, the wrinkles on your face, the way you walk, your aches and pains, your frequency of illness, and how you move and breathe. The fact that you may wear eyeglasses may be part of this story. A surgery or a stay in the hospital will certainly be included in your body story.

Your health or illnesses are not just random acts handed out like candy. These illnesses are the stories that have been developing in your body over many years. What goes on in your mind affects your body. The beliefs that you carry will ultimately determine the state of your health or disease. The effects of your life events will end up residing in your body.

When you live in harmony with nature, your body reflects a story that flows with nature. When you fight nature or attempt to ignore it, your body responds entirely differently. Nature teaches us about flow.

Science has attempted to attribute age, genetics and nutrition to our illness and disease. While these factors do play a role in our health, they are only minor influences. When we ignore the forces of nature, we subject ourselves to the negative effects of stress, repression and physical trauma. These stressors compress and contract us, hardening our tissues and stiffening our joints.

What Is Natural?

When you live in alignment with nature, you follow natural principles. You follow the flow of energy and seasons, rest when tired, respond when threatened, and move as nature intended.

When you are threatened by a real danger, either a wild animal or a natural occurring phenomenon (like a hurricane or an earthquake), your body responds naturally to this danger to help keep you alive. This real danger activates your body to call it to action. You are able to defend yourself in the situation or move away to safety. This is called your **Fight or Flight Response**.

You do not have to think about this process because it happens automatically. Natural responses are rooted in your primal brain. Some people would call these natural instincts. You do not debate your body's reaction. You just move out of danger's way or defend yourself.

When the danger has passed, you return to your natural state of relaxation. You let down your guard and take a deep breath. You are no longer hyper-alert because you feel safe. This reaction is called the **Relaxation Response**.

The Myth of Stress

Many of us want to believe that stress is a virus that gets lodged in our bodies. We have been told that stress is a foreign invader that takes us over. We want to blame stress for traffic, the unstable stock market or our difficult relationship. Actually, stress is none of that. Stress is not something that we can blame although we are tempted to do so. Stress is not a poor job nor busy city life. Stress is not a mutant bug that was picked up in some dense and tropical rain forest. Stress is nothing more than an interpretation. Stress is an interpretation of an event that we perceive to be life-threatening. We create most of our own stress based on our real and false beliefs that we carry with us.

Debbie Shapiro writes in *The Bodymind Workbook*, "Stress is our psychological reaction to an event; it is not the event itself." We often wish to blame external circumstances, but stress is only our response to the events in our lives.

Stress is a feeling that states," "I do not feel safe." First and foremost, stress is an emotional and energetic experience. Although there are qualities to stress that can be measured and quantified, stress is not scientific; it is emotional.

"I don't feel safe" is an emotion. There is nothing in a laboratory that a scientist can give you to cure this problem. Only when you begin to follow nature's guidelines will you begin to heal from the effects of stress. One of the primary means by which you lose your body is the effect of stress. In order to recover your body, you must begin to address how the "Stress Response" manifests itself in the body.

The word "stress" is a very misunderstood word. We have heard a lot in the last few decades about the effects of stress on the body. This word has become a household term that we throw around. Phrases like "stressed,"

"stressed out," and "over-stressed" are all too familiar to the vast majority of us. We seem to accept stress as something that goes along with living in a modern age, but we seldom know what it is that we are actually talking about.

Researcher Dr. Hans Selye first popularized the term "stress" in the 1930s. Dr. Selye was an Austrian-Hungarian-born endocrinologist and medical researcher who spent most of his time in the laboratory. As a research scientist, he employed the tools by which he was trained—left brain analytical reductionism. His perspective emerged from Newtonian thinking. The answers he deduced were found in molecules. He based his findings on what he could see in a microscope or test tube.

We have come a long way in our understanding of stress and its effects on our bodies. This understanding is how the long-term effects of stress can be extremely damaging to the body. Most people would not disagree with this in the least. At the time Hans Selye was a pioneer. His work was revolutionary. However, since this discovery it seems that stress has *not* become better in our lives, but much worse. The reason that stress has not been cured is that Dr. Selye misdiagnosed the cause of stress. While there are certainly chemical implications of stress, these chemicals are not the cause of stress.

The cause of stress is an emotion. This naturally occurring emotion is, "I do not feel safe." It is an energetic and emotional reason. A research scientist in a laboratory is unable to determine this because the tools he uses could never measure emotions. The body responds energetically and emotionally to a stimulus first. Chemical changes take place later.

Identifying the root cause of stress begins to change how we heal. If you are still labeling stress as a chemical experience, you will look for a remedy in a bottle or in a tonic. When stress is interpreted as an emotional experience first and foremost, then and only then will you begin to shift how this reaction is ultimately healed. Working from an emotional and energetic perspective aligns us more closely with our natural roots.

Identifying the Stages of Stress

Stress begins as an emotion of not feeling safe. The stress reaction is based on the beliefs in your mind. These beliefs quickly determine a course of action to protect yourself and instill a sense of safety back into you.

The stress response was meant to be a momentary response to get you out of a life-threatening situation. When a wild boar approaches, you react in a way that helps you survive. You either prepare to meet the attacker head on or gather all of your strength and run like crazy in the other direction. You did not need to think about this. It just happened. It was an instantaneous reaction that you were not even conscious of.

Stress was designed to save you from *actual life-threatening* events, (like a wild animal, a tornado or an attacker). These *actual life-threatening* events were the result of a primitive brain that registered death if we did not protect ourselves from such an event. Reactions to *actual life-threatening* events were based on *real beliefs* that were imprinted in our primitive brain—a brain that knew to protect one from danger. This was how stress was designed to function—responses triggered by *actual life-threatening* events based on real beliefs. These real life events then activated our Fight or Flight Response designed by nature to prepare us for action and keep us safe.

Something has since changed. That change, which has allowed us to evolve at such a rapid rate in the most recent part of our history, is the unparalleled expansion in the growth of our brain. This growth is not just in size, but also in its function.

The brain is now able to create imaginary life-threatening events for you due to your ability to use your expanded thinking brain. Very rarely is your stress response triggered by an actual life-threatening event anymore. (Yes, it does happen from time to time). Most of your stress response is triggered by imaginary life-threatening events that are based on false beliefs that you have about yourself. It is these false beliefs that help to create your imaginary life-threatening events that trigger your stress response.

For instance, in the world that many of us live in today, you do not fear being awakened by a ferocious saber-toothed tiger. However, many have a fear of financial failure, or you hang on to your relationships so tightly for the fear of being alone. These are not real life-threatening events. These are imaginary events based on your false beliefs about yourself. You believe that financial failure will kill you because you have a false belief that says that you are a failure if you lose your money. You might believe that you will not survive a relationship breakup because you believe that to be left or abandoned is the same as dying.

These false beliefs were created in your early childhood as you experienced what felt like death when a similar event occurred. Thus, you created a false belief about the experience, and later on in life these false beliefs cause your stress response to be triggered by your imaginary life-threatening events.

Arthur Janov writes in *The New Primal Scream,*

"Most of us can function on a day-to-day basis when we only have to deal with the pain of our past stress. We do it with smoking, drinking, tranquilizers, and so on. But when something devastating in the present resonates with something in our past, we suffer from the 'stress syndrome.'"

Your mind does not know the difference between imaginary and real life-threatening events. Your body still believes that grief or sadness will kill you. You might enter into the stress response the same way as if the danger to you were real. You are preparing for battle, only this time the war is within you. Even though this is an imaginary experience, your mind still believes it to be real. In fact, most of your conflicts come from within yourself, rather than from the outside world around you.

The author of *The Body in Recovery*, John P. Conger, writes,

"The body cannot distinguish the truth from the lies we tell it. If we imagine a terrible threat to us, even though we are walking down a safe street, our body cowers and sweat drips suddenly from our armpits. A pretended life creates stress and ill health."

This is similar to going to the movies. You might scream, cry or be frightened out of your wits because someone is projecting an imaginary story onto a large screen. Your palms become sweaty and your breath becomes shallow as you feel this tension. Your body does not know the difference. Jon Kabat-Zinn, Ph.D., writes in *Full Catastrophe Living*, "Much of our stress comes from threats, real or imagined, to our social status, not to our lives."

For many people, the stress response is no longer just a momentary escape from danger. The stress response can be constantly activated when your body reacts to imaginary life-threatening events. For instance, you might have a false belief that you will die if you fail. Every day you go to a regular job that might keep triggering this imaginary life-threatening event in your life. This job may give you reason to worry. Some people nearly always remain in their stress response and are never quite relaxed. Their imaginary life-threatening events continue to be with them since they have created these false beliefs with their newly evolved brain.

You might claim to "love" your job, but it might be your job that is the imagined life-threatening event that is killing you. You might feel so "in love" within your relationship, but it might be this relationship that activates your stress response. Your relationship may very well be your enemy. Many times the people or situations in which we are the most involved trigger our stress response.

The real life-threatening events that trigger your stress response might occur when you are hanging off a cliff and have only moments until you fall to your death. Severe heat from a flame can cause real life-threatening pain. The problem lies in the fact that your brain does not know the difference between these real and imagined life-threatening events.

Your imaginary life-threatening events might be both very tangible and physical or something in your own head. For instance, a dream, thought or sudden memory of a painful event might be enough for the Fight or Flight Response to be triggered. Post-Traumatic Stress Disorder (PTSD) is one of these occurrences.

A seemingly peaceful person could be walking down the street when a memory of war emerges in his head. This memory becomes the trigger that creates an imaginary life-threatening event, which then leads to the very physical Fight or Flight Response. He might "freak out" because he perceives that he is being attacked. The whole event may occur in his head but translates to real symptoms.

This experience is very common even if you have never been to war. A thought of not having enough time or not being good enough can be the internal trigger that sets off your Fight or Flight Response. Any memory or thought can be enough to stimulate a stress response.

The following are examples of imaginary life-threatening events that can cause a stress response:

1. Emotional Stress—All uncomfortable feelings. Thoughts that anger, grief or sadness might kill you.

2. Mental Stress—Long hours studying for an exam might create mental stress and can be perceived by the brain as an enemy to the brain, thereby activating the stress response. The false belief that—"I need to be perfect" might trigger the imagined life-threatening event "mental fatigue."

3. Physical Stress—Overexertion of the body might be an imagined life threatening event; e.g., shoveling dirt for too many hours without a rest.

4. Stress Related to Changes—Too many changes too quickly. For example, you change your job, relationship and move to a new city all at the same time. This might be an imagined life-threatening event.

5. Financial Stress—Too many bills and not enough income.

6. Stress Related to Over Stimulation—Noise, people and decision-making can overload your system, throwing you into your stress response and causing you to feel as if you will die.

7. Relationship Stress—Conflicts, death, abandonment and trust issues can trigger the brain and create an imagined life-threatening event based on your false beliefs.

8. Health Stress—Non-life-threatening physical pain can be interpreted as an imaginary life-threatening event based on a false belief that "all pain is bad." This type of pain might be something like a minor burn, backache or headache. Many cultures teach an aversion to pain, so it might be common to grow up believing that pain is "evil."

9. Work Stress—The thought that—"I hate my job" can be enough to trigger your stress response.

10. Time Stress—You either have too much time or not enough time on your hands. This can be perceived as an imaginary life-threatening event.

There are many more instances in your life that your brain may perceive as imaginary life-threatening events, causing you to react with your biologically implanted stress response. This is just a small sampling. In the modern world, these events are the equivalent of the mountain lion and the saber-toothed tiger chasing after you. The important part to remember is that these events would not have the impact that they do unless you had already developed false beliefs that will trigger them. It is not the event that is the root of stress, but the fact that we have developed a belief that the world is an unsafe place and these events just trigger that belief.

Stress Is Just an Interpretation

"Stress *begins* in the mind and *ends* in the body," writes Dr. Archibald D. Hart in *Adrenaline and Stress*. This is very true. It is the mind that creates most of your stress response for you by its *interpretation* of the events in your life as life-threatening or not. These interpretations are all based on your individual belief systems.

For instance, some people feel that standing in a crowded room is an event that their body interprets as life-threatening and causes them to react as if it were being attacked. Others would feel excited and energized in this same room full of loud noises and lots of people. Why does one person react one way and another person react another way? Your reactions and interpretations of what is life-threatening are based on your childhood experiences and the beliefs that you have developed.

A person who reacts with a stress response in a crowded room most likely experienced a traumatic event as a child while being exposed to many people. Perhaps he was separated from his parents for a short time and this felt like death. He might have developed a false belief that crowded rooms were scary places to be in because he was not in control. The person who feels excitement in a crowded room might not have had the same experiences. She might get all of the attention that she so desperately seeks. For this person, the opposite might be true. Aloneness might be her greatest fear.

I can remember being at a crowded major league baseball game as a child. When the game was over, I was hit in the elbow by a smoker's pipe that someone had thrown from high above. I was shocked and stunned. I can remember imprinting a belief that crowded places were not a safe place for me to be. I had experienced pain in a crowd, and my false belief told me to stay away from crowds.

We all have our own interpretation of a life-threatening event. Some might be more comfortable out in the woods alone, sailing alone in the middle of the ocean on their boat, or racing down a mountainside at high speed on their mountain bike. This is where they find their peace. For others, these events might feel like a death experience and cause them to enter into the stress response.

We all interpret stress differently. It is not necessarily the fault of the stressor, which causes us to react, but our *interpretation* based on our false beliefs that we have developed. This is why it does little good to blame the traffic or our boss when we feel so irritable. These external cues are not the cause. Debbie Shapiro writes in *The Bodymind Workbook*, "In other words, the situations in our lives are neither negative nor positive—they just are. It is our personal reaction or response to them that labels them as one thing or another." One person's pleasure might be another's stress response.

It does not matter whether you are experiencing what you would consider a positive or a negative event. Your body might not be able to tell the difference. Dr. Archibald D. Hart writes in *Adrenaline and Stress*, "The excitement of getting married or watching the home team play a winning game can produce as much stress as struggling to meet a publisher's deadline or facing an angry boss." Dr. Hart adds, "I would venture to say that the positive, pleasant stresses in life are *more* likely to lead to stress disease. This is one thing that makes stress disease so mysterious and dangerous."

To reiterate, it does not matter whether you experience an event in your life as positive or negative. Your body will respond if it feels that the event is life-threatening. Even what would seem to be the most positive relationships, the most wonderful vacations or the most incredible experiences in your life may be causing you the most harm.

Since *we all* develop false beliefs that trigger our stress response, *we all* suffer from the effects of stress. There is a popular myth that only people who live in cities or western cultures are affected by stress. This is not so. A nomadic tribesman feels the same stress response as a CEO of a large corporation. The imagined life-threatening events that triggered the stress response might be different, but the end result is the same.

For instance, a business executive might feel as if he is going to die, and thus his stress response is triggered, if he is late for a meeting. The nomadic tribesman enters into his stress response if there is no rain to provide water for his thirsty camels. Both are external events and both create the same reaction in the human body. In this way it is easy to see how we might be reacting to our external events most of our lives.

Stress Begins in the Womb

We all want to survive. This survival instinct is something that is built into our brain. When you experience something that you interpret as life-threatening (pain, discomfort or attack), you automatically protect yourself by activating your Fight or Flight Response. The Fight or Flight Response is something that you first learn while in the womb and in early infancy. Later on as an adult you keep repeating the same patterns of either fleeing or contracting your body in response to a threat to your survival.

Arthur Janov, author of *The New Primal Scream*, writes, "Abnormality starts in the womb when the mother is stressed and transmits this stress to the fetus, which then gears up to handle the input, changes functions, and increases its stress hormone levels. There is altered thyroid function, immune efficiency, etc. Thus the stage is set for abnormality; the baby is already abnormal before it has seen the light of day."

Take for instance an infant who is left in a crib alone at night. The darkness and aloneness might be interpreted as an imaginary life-threatening event that continually causes the child to activate his Fight or Flight Response. He might tighten up the muscles around his eyes as a way to protect himself. While this might seem very benign at the time, it will lead to problems down the road. As an adolescent, his vision might begin to fail because every time he feels threatened by an imaginary life-threatening event, he will contract the muscles around his eyes, (there are six of them for each eye), and the shape of his eyeball will be distorted. This will throw off his focal point and his vision will blur.

Dr. Arthur Janov talks about an incident in *The New Primal Scream* in which an adult is plagued by severe migraine headaches because the oxygen was cut off to his brain while he was being born, and he interpreted birth as a life-threatening event. He contracted his muscles as a way to protect himself from the trauma he was experiencing. As an adult he continually faces migraine headaches on a regular basis whenever he feels stress (his interpretation of imaginary life-threatening events). His job and the pressure that he puts on himself is enough to cause these stress patterns to continue. He contracts the muscles in his neck and scalp without noticing it, thus cutting off the blood flow and leading to the migraine attacks.

Stress patterns are learned responses that attempt to protect us. Once learned, they do not go away easily by themselves. The problem that makes these patterns so challenging to navigate through is that they are wired into your nervous system.

Let's take the case of Jason. Jason noticed that when he was interpreting something as life-threatening, he would tighten up the back of his neck. This might be a near-accident on the freeway or just not enough time to get all the things done that he had planned. It does not matter what the external event might be. His brain and nervous system have already set up a neural pathway to tell which muscles to tighten up for him under his times of stress. This is a well-grooved pattern that is *"resistant to change."* He even noticed that while practicing yoga (which he enjoyed very much), his neck would tighten up. It seems that placing his body in a strenuous position is often interpreted by his brain as a life-threatening event. Even the things that we enjoy the most can be interpreted as life-threatening events.

Experiences that induce your stress response early on are imprinted in your memory. It might not even seem to be something that one would think of as being "traumatic." For instance, a one year old who is dropped by her mother might become so traumatized by the experience that she may go through life never being able to trust anyone. Peter Levine says in *Waking the Tiger*, "Being left alone in a cold room can be totally overwhelming to an infant, frightening to a toddler, distressing to a ten-year old, and only mildly uncomfortable to an adolescent or adult." We all imprint events differently. One's mild discomfort of an event is another's terror.

It is this stress response that can harbor in your body for years to come without your even being aware of it. Peter Levine says,

"Traumatic effects are not always apparent immediately following the incidents that caused them. Symptoms can remain dormant, accumulating over years or even decades. Then, during a stressful period, or as the result of another incident, they can show up without warning."

The "Emotionality" of Stress

Stress is first and foremost an emotional experience. "I do not feel safe" can be translated as "I feel afraid." As an emotional experience, this can only be healed by an emotional response. Whether the stress trigger is real or imagined, the response is still the same. Not feeling safe becomes the emotional reaction.

Hans Selye, a scientist and the first to coin the term "stress," had no way of knowing this. He had no tools or experiments to measure an emotional reaction. He just measured chemical changes in the body. For decades we have been told that stress is about the changes in our biochemistry. Now it is clear that chemicals have nothing to do with the cause of stress.

It is your emotional response that begins the healing of stress. In a natural world when you are afraid you might grieve. You might curl into a fetal position and grieve the experience. Whether real or imagined, you still grieve it.

As a child who is suddenly awakened by a "bad" dream, you might let your whole body cry and grieve the experience. You might run to the safety of mom and dad's arms to be held. You do not hold back or try to maintain a strong position. You let the energy of emotion flow out. Even though the adults might sheepishly explain that, "it is only a dream and dreams cannot hurt you," as a child you are not so sure. Your stress response has still been triggered.

Not yet ingrained in the control mechanisms of a modern culture, the body of a young child will grieve the experience. He just cries until there are no more tears. His stress response is very emotional. When he is finished crying, his body returns to a state of relaxation because he is able to release the emotion.

Adults are no different. Your thoughts, dreams, and memories many times help to initiate your stress response. The only difference is that most adults have developed many false beliefs about their emotions. Many believe that it is not okay to cry and express their emotions. They do not let themselves feel the fear that has risen. They push down every emotion and find another way to numb it out. Tight muscles and a hoard of addictions become the most logical ways that many use not to feel emotions.

A rational-based culture accustomed to analytical thought responds with reason and addictions. In contrast, nature's response to the stress response is through the release of emotional energy. It may not always be safe to respond with emotions right away. You might need to respond emotionally when it is safe to let your guard down.

If you are busy battling a wild lion that has wandered into your camp, an emotional response at this time might kill you. You cannot have the alertness of the stress response and the relaxation of the emotional letting go simultaneously. In this case the time to let down your guard and have an emotional response is when the lion is no longer a threat. The outer world must feel safe before you can begin to address the inner world.

Calmness Is Not Relaxation: The Myth of Meditation

You can either experience relaxation or stress. You cannot have both at the same time. Relaxation is when you are the most at ease and when you can drop your guard. You do not have to be hyper-alert or under constant vigilance. Your body has surrendered to minimize internal and external stimuli. There are no threats, either real or imagined.

Stress is about being on guard and under constant vigilance. You are alert and constantly aware. You are suspicious of attack, either real or imagined. You are in constant check of your thoughts and surroundings. You are in control.

The world of meditation came to us from the Cognitive Brain or cortex. Meditation is essentially a thinking process of watching and analyzing thoughts. It is most often performed from a position of control and erectness. Meditation tends to intellectualize our emotional and energetic experiences. Stress and meditation teach us the same thing—that we have to constantly pay attention and stay in control.

Meditation comes to us from a time and a culture when there were not many pain medications. For many, meditation has become the way to be medicated from any pain, either internal or external pain.

Calmness and relaxation are not the same thing. Calmness is about control and occurs from the head up. When we are calm we are almost always in our stress response; the body is often still at war. Relaxation, on the other hand, is a full body experience. Calmness is about alertness and being on guard. Relaxation is about letting go and surrendering.

Congruence is a vital aspect in our healing. Do your mind and body believe the same thing? In the yoga world, we are taught that relaxation is about meditation and controlling our thoughts. This is not relaxation at all.

Nature teaches us to have all of our experiences, not just a chosen few. When removed from nature, control and calmness become our idealized reference points. This is very different than the world of relaxation. When relaxed, your whole body and mind surrender. There is no threat internally or externally. When you live with the belief that calmness is the ideal state, anything that is not calm becomes the enemy to be on guard against. Being off-center is considered failure or defeat, often resulting in the activation of the stress response.

Meditation teaches us about calmness and control. Occasionally these might be desired states of consciousness, but they are not the ideal states to achieve at all times. While meditation might be a short-term solution to perform stress reduction, it is not the answer to heal from stress itself. Stress reduction, which is one use for meditation, does not heal you from stress. If stress is an emotional experience that can only be healed by an emotional release, meditation and calmness fall far short of achieving this goal. Stress reduction techniques only help you to not feel the effects of stress.

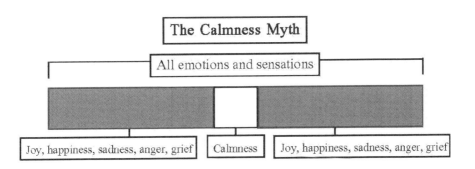

Stress is an emotional and energetic experience first and foremost. Most often stress is triggered from the beliefs in your Cognitive Brain. If the Cognitive Brain is responsible for most of your stress, why would more Cognitive Brain activity be the solution? A child living close to nature would not calm his mind nor control his thoughts. He would grieve his fearful experiences and let the energy of emotion pass through him. Only a rational dominant culture would try to negate the natural instincts of a child and, consequently, nature itself.

The body has a language all to its own. A body that is relaxed demonstrates this in its posture and its musculature. A body under stress is a body under control. A calm mind from the head up almost always equals a controlled or "stressed" body from the neck downward. There is very little congruence between the mind and body.

As a body worker for many years I would often hear from clients how their meditation has created a sense of calmness and relaxation in them. But when I would first place my hands on these clients, an entirely different scenario would unfold. I would often discover a hardened and stiff body stuck in distress. The Cognitive Brain had created a magical story; the body was telling the truth though. This person was not really relaxed at all.

When watching the body language of a child, he curls into a fetal position or wraps himself around an adult for comfort and safety. There is a surrendering of everything—body, mind and emotions. The child is out of control. He has abandoned reason and intellect. He is immersed in waves of emotions and is following nature's way.

When we remain constantly calm, we are afraid of every other state or emotion that is not calmness. We remain hyper-vigilant to avoid falling off center and losing control. Failure to remain calm or in control becomes equated with a wild bear knocking down your door. You must remain poised and on guard for attack. You are still in your stress response.

Another common false belief promoted by meditation advocates is that thoughts are the enemy. This is what the experts have labeled as the "monkey mind." Unfortunately, it is not your thoughts that are creating your stress; it is your beliefs. Meditation does very little to address these beliefs or address ways to heal from them. Meditation tends to act like a painkiller and suppresses the symptoms of your pain. The issues are still there; they are just numbed out.

The Cognitive Brain has labeled your emotions as a disease or the enemy. When you are unable or unwilling to express the energy of your emotions, you often find an addiction of your choice as a way to repress these emotions. Many times your thoughts are your greatest addiction. By meditating your thoughts away, you have done very little to address the roots of your stress conflict—the beliefs you have about your emotions. This is like a food addict who learns to control his food but does very little to address the emotions behind his disease process. He is still addicted; this time, he is addicted to control itself.

Whether it is anger, relaxation, depression, or calmness, the body has a position for each state of consciousness. When you are in your calm state you are still in control, still hyper-alert, and most often still in your stress response. Only when you can surrender to the entirety of your experience and seek safety do you enter into your relaxation response.

Nature teaches us about flow. Rivers flow downhill to oceans and lakes. Storms flow in and out. Seasons flow with great regularity each and every year. We are taught to expect flow when we live close to nature.

A mind removed from nature loses the ability to flow. This includes your states of consciousness and your emotions as well. A mind removed from nature is like a stagnating river that has been dammed. One single emotion or state of consciousness is not nature's way. This includes calmness. When your states of consciousness do not flow, you get stuck in a state of trance. Being in a state of trance is not always a healthy or healing state.

The body does not lie. A client of mine named Steve was an avid meditator. Steve would meditate twice a day on average. Steve also suffered from significant grinding of his teeth at night. This condition was equated with his need to stay in constant control of every aspect of his life.

Steve went away for a ten-day silent vipassana meditation retreat where he meditated for several hours each day. When he returned home, his jaw was equally as tight, if not more so. His meditation retreat had only taught Steve how to reinforce his need for control in his life. His body responded by tightening up even more. It appears that Steve was really addicted to control, and by practicing meditation frequently, he was actually engaging in his addiction.

The body has a language to it. Calmness and control can be exhibited through the body some of the time. However, when you deliberately place calmness and control as the priority, your body often suffers the consequences.

Meditation is not "good" or "bad." This is just another behavior. Meditation can be compared to the debate over gun ownership. Guns are not "good" or "bad." They just exist. How guns are used, though, becomes a judgment of being "good" or "bad." In the same respects, how meditation is used could be labeled as being "good" or "bad."

Unfortunately, most people use meditation to reinforce an already ingrained addictive pattern of control. Many people end up hiding, repressing their emotions, or leaving their body through meditation. For many people, meditation becomes a way to escape and numb out. Meditation teaches you how to go inside and observe your thoughts. Unfortunately, observing your thoughts often distances you from your feelings. Rather than experiencing your own story, you become its narrator.

When you can sit with whatever state you are experiencing in the moment, you are aligned with nature. Your body reflects this congruence, and relaxation becomes the end result. The relaxation response becomes apparent when you can let your guard down, including your vigilance to your emotional states. Like a child who honors nature, emotional release is the pathway to freedom from the stress response. Calmness and control have their place in our lives but not as a response to stress.

We Have Forgotten How to Relax

Most Westerners have forgotten how to relax. The stress cycle keeps you hyper-alert and on guard. You constantly remain focused and aroused. In a natural world, you enter into a state of relaxation when the danger is gone. This occurs when you can let down your guard and decrease your alertness.

When stress is created by false beliefs, the danger seldom goes away. You remain on guard and alert. You seldom get a chance to enter into your relaxation cycle. Instead, you remain frozen in fear and create many addictions as a way to numb this cycle. The energy of fear does not have a chance to dissipate, but remains stored within you.

There are many messages given to us about relaxation which are often very distorted and unnatural. For some people the message that they were given is that relaxation is the same as laziness. It is believed that if you are not producing something or learning something, then you are wasting time. Wasting time in many cultures is a social taboo.

Others have received the message that relaxation is a sin. This is translated from the Judeo-Christian tradition that one of the seven deadly sins is "sloth." The word "sloth" can be translated as laziness. People engaged in a state of relaxation are often considered lazy by others. According to the Judeo-Christian tradition, the devil is reported to inhabit the body of a lazy or "slothful" person.

Because our worth is often measured by our productivity, the stress cycle seldom comes to completion. You very rarely complete the stress cycle and enter into relaxation because this state in many cultures has been labeled as "bad" or "negative." You are not encouraged to be in the relaxation state on a regular basis. It is only on rare occasions, such as a day at the spa or a weeklong retreat, where you actually can begin to allow your relaxation response to take hold.

Making relaxation a priority is one way to initiate change in your behavior. Instead of doing business at lunchtime, you can remove yourself from work activity while you eat. In the high tech culture we are far removed from our "Gone Fishing" and "Out to Lunch" signs. For many, cellular phones and pagers remain with us at all times. This practice only creates more stimulation and ultimately continues to engage the stress response.

While convenient at times, these devices are a reminder of most people's inability to relax. Technological devices are like invaders or enemies in your castle, always tracking you down and finding you. Your castle is no longer safe from invasion as long as you let technology continue to intrude upon you and keep you hyper-alert.

BODY LANGUAGE

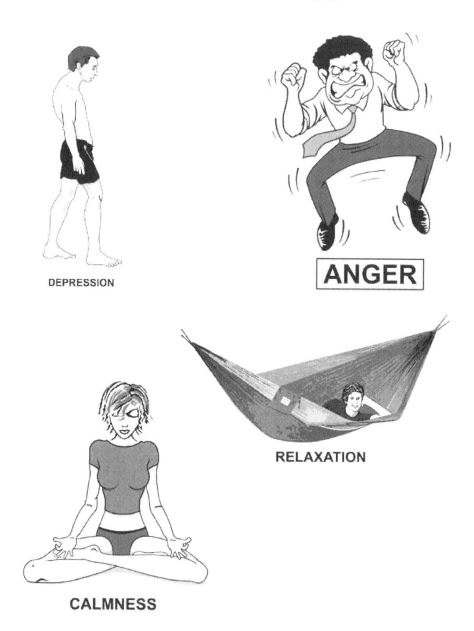

The Physiology of Stress
(The Fight or Flight Response)

Stress is primarily an emotional experience. By allowing the energy of emotion to pass through us, we will ultimately heal from the stress cycle. As Hans Selye pointed out, there are some physiological signs of stress as well. These are scientific biochemical reactions that you can actually measure.

When you perceive a life-threatening event, whether real or imagined, your body prepares for battle. You enter into your stress response, which has become popularly known as the Fight or Flight Response. It is this Fight or Flight Response that causes so many problems.

With regard to the stress response, you have two nervous systems. These two different neurological pathways are the Sympathetic Nervous System and the Parasympathetic Nervous System. The Sympathetic Nervous System speeds you up and is activated when the Fight or Flight Response is triggered. The Parasympathetic Nervous System slows you down, resulting in relaxation. In order for your Parasympathetic Nervous System to operate, there needs to be no threat to your survival, either real or imagined. This is when we feel the most relaxed.

When your Fight or Flight Response is triggered you react in one of three ways. You either enter into 1. Fight, 2. Flight (Internal Escape), or 3. Flight (External Escape). In whichever manner you react, you are still attempting to combat a potential enemy. You have learned throughout your childhood how to best protect yourself. Some people would call the Fight or Flight Response a defense mechanism for avoiding total annihilation. The brain believes that if you don't defend yourself, you will be destroyed.

The three interpretations of the Fight or Flight Response are a way of dealing with your fear of total annihilation. You might use one or all of the Fight or Flight Responses. It is rare to find an individual who just uses the Fight Response and neither of the Flight Responses. The following is a more in-depth look at each of these Fight or Flight Responses.

1. Fight—The Body Is Preparing to Take Its Attacker Head-On
During the Fight aspect of the Stress Response, the body prepares to take its attacker head-on. Imagine a scenario where you are out on a

mountain trail and all of a sudden a grizzly bear appears out of nowhere and starts charging straight toward you. You grab your walking stick and hold it tightly like a sword. All of your muscles tighten. Adrenaline races through your body. You are hyper-alert as blood rushes to your head. You feel as if you have suddenly acquired three times the strength as you had just moments before. Your body knows this will be your last stand if you do not do something. You are now in the Fight Response.

There are many changes that occur in the body in a relatively short time period. The pituitary gland in the brain, sometimes referred to as the "Master Gland," releases a chemical called adrenocorticotrophic hormone (ACTH). ACTH travels directly to the adrenal glands located just above the kidneys. What ACTH does is multifold. The cortex of the adrenal glands is stimulated, which in turn release cortisol and cortisone. These two hormones then travel to other parts of the body to do the following: fight inflammation, increase muscle tension, free fatty acids and increase blood sugar.

At the core of the adrenal glands, ACTH has another job to do. ACTH assists in the release of adrenaline and noradrenalin. These two hormones activate the heart muscle, increase the use of cholesterol, give the muscle more glucose, increase blood pressure and speed up the heart rate. In essence, your body is preparing to go to war.

Your heart races and your muscles are rigid and engorged with blood. Blood vessels constrict in some areas to allow blood to flow where it is needed the most (the large muscles and the brain). Your digestion is slowed down as blood is moved away from the abdominal area to go to the brain and large muscles. Non-vital functions are slowed down to move the glucose to where it is needed the most. Because of the cortisol and cortisone released, there is a decreased sensitivity to pain (in case you were to become injured). You shorten your breath to conserve movement.

This is the Fight Response. It is about contraction and hyper-vigilance, about holding on and building a suit of armor around you to defend against attackers. You become a warrior. The Fight Response is like a turtle with a tough outer shell that pulls his head in for protection. We shorten our muscles and hence our entire body as a way to defend ourselves. We shorten and contract just like the turtle's head being pulled inside in order to feel safe. The only problem is that most of the time we cannot recognize the enemy. Most often it is not a real grizzly bear that turns on our Fight Response but an imaginary-life threatening scenario.

2. Flight (Internal Escape)
"You Can Have My Physical Body But You Cannot Have Me"

Many learn to protect themselves by leaving their body. This is a very effective tool that we have devised in order to avoid the threat of death. This is called Flight—the Internal Escape. When you see that grizzly bear running toward you, many times you might just give up. You do not tighten your muscles as in the Fight Response. You become even more relaxed in your musculature. You do not plan an outer defense. You just surrender. You play dead. You go inside. You leave. You surrender your body as you take your consciousness someplace else.

This internal escape happens to many of us in childhood. When you experience pain, physical and sexual abuse, or imaginary life-threatening events, often you learn to defend yourself from these events by splitting off. You develop different personalities when you do this. You might be so good at splitting off that you live your life as one of these other fantasy personalities. You seldom are your true self but some split-off personality that you develop in order to protect yourself from what your brain thinks is the enemy.

Many people associate the personalities of the internal escape of the Flight Response to be associated with traumas suffered in childhood like sexual abuse or torture. These are just the tip of the iceberg. In my work as a Body-Mind therapist, I have never found anyone who did not split off in some way or another. Any experience of pain or threat of death during early development can produce personalities that split off in order to protect you from the threat of annihilation.

For instance, the obvious method that a young child might use to defend herself against sexual abuse from a stronger, more powerful adult is to surrender to the imagined life-threatening event and mentally disappear while it is happening. This often begins an ingrained pattern. Whenever there is stress (or more precisely, an interpretation of a real or an imagined life-threatening event), she splits off into this other place. This world of "make believe" then becomes her home where she feels the most comfortable and safe. She is seldom fully present.

For example, if she feels the pressure of having to study for a test as a teenager, she might consider this to be an imagined life-threatening event and go into her head as a way to defend herself from what her brain thinks is an attacker. From here she leaves her body just as if she were cornered by a real grizzly bear and this were her only hope of survival.

Her nervous system still believes she is being sexually abused again. Any perceived threat to her survival, either real or imagined, might initiate the internal flight mechanism.

A child who grows up alone with few friends and siblings might learn to split off into the world of make believe. This begins to create a pattern where, when under stress as an adult, she flees inside or responds with the internal escape mechanism of the Fight or Flight Response. She does not just create this; she has learned how to survive her loneliness by going inside.

Noted trauma specialist and author of *Waking the Tiger*, Peter Levine explains about how the body reacts during times of stress. He says,

"Similarly, the body reacts profoundly in trauma. It tenses in readiness, braces in fear, and freezes and collapses in helpless terror. When the mind's protective reaction to overwhelm returns to normal, the body's response is also meant to normalize after the event. When this restorative process is thwarted, the effects of trauma become fixated and the person becomes traumatized."

We all have instances when we split off as children. We all experience moments of pain that we do not know how to process. Fantasies about being a sports star or an adventurer might be one way that you split off and leave your body when you experience perceived life-threatening events, real or imagined. This is commonly referred to as daydreaming. Those who daydream are usually trying to avoid some form of pain by leaving their body. This defense strategy has already been developed due to one's early childhood experiences. You do not have to be sexually mistreated or tortured in order to develop this internal escape response to stress. Anyone can learn how to flee inside as a means of attempting to stay safe.

It is not only the occasional societal misfit or homeless person who has learned how to split off. This condition is very common in our culture, even among very successful and fully functioning individuals. Peter Levine writes in *Waking the Tiger,*

"It must be emphasized that, since primal wounding and splitting are so commonplace, the survival mode is the starting place for all of us. Survival personality is not merely a one-dimensional facade, an empty shell devoid of depth and richness. Quite the contrary, this mode can often allow

a functioning well above the average level, commanding truly impressive talents and abilities."

We have all known someone who has split off as a way to escape pain. These people often demonstrate an absence or vacantness. They seldom know what they like or what they want because they are rarely present. Often, people who seem to have everything together can be operating from their split-off selves. They spend most of their time in a different world. They may also seem very creative, spiritual or eccentric. These people are seldom in their bodies and seem to be on another planet.

Recent research has been conducted on the Internal Flight mechanism of the Fight or Flight Response. Peter Levine has dubbed the Internal Flight response as "freezing" and writes in *Waking the Tiger:*

"Universal and primitive defensive behaviors are called the "fight or flight" strategies. If the situation calls for aggression, a threatened creature will fight. If the threatened animal is likely to lose the fight, it will run if it can. These choices aren't thought out; they are instinctually orchestrated by the reptilian and limbic brains. When neither fight or flight will ensure the animal's safety, there is another line of defense: immobility (freezing), which is just as universal and basic to survival. For inexplicable reasons, this defense strategy is rarely given equal billing in texts on biology and psychology. Yet, it is an equally viable survival strategy in threatening situations. In many situations, it is the best choice."

It is this freezing that has caused many problems in humans. We learn how to run inside our heads to stay safe. This is like "playing possum" where no pain is felt. We learn to disassociate and go inside of ourselves. We split off into other personalities because of this freezing response. What one is saying in a traumatic situation is that "the enemy can have my body but cannot have me. I have left and have gone away." This way no pain is felt.

This is the fantasy world of children. Sometimes this state of mind is considered the place of creativity. Much of the time, it is not a creative place but a magical world where no pain is felt. As adults this split-off place becomes a normal aspect of the adult life. Peter Levine writes in *Waking the Tiger*, "Individuals who have been repeatedly traumatized as young children often adopt dissociation as a preferred mode of being in the world. They dissociate readily and habitually without being aware of it."

The authors of *The Primal Wound,* John Firman and Ann Gila, write about this magical world, recalling a story from Pia Mellody:

"One way such children may escape the pain of severe abandonment by the parents is to fantasize about being rescued by a hero of some kind. Little girls may imagine a knight in shining armor who has loving feelings for her and who does things that demonstrate this love by connecting with her, finally giving her life meaning and vitality. The fantasy is often very much like the fairy tale Sleeping Beauty, *in which Sleeping Beauty lies asleep, out of touch with herself and her surroundings, until the life-giving kiss of Prince Charming awakens her. Children spend so much time in this fantasy world because it creates a state of euphoria. I spent hours as a child daydreaming about my knight in shining armor. If I felt bad I could play out this fantasy in my mind, get high, in about ten minutes, and stay there for at least two or three hours. I think that when we put a pleasurable picture in our minds and think about it, we can stimulate an emotional response to it that may lead to the release of endorphins into our system. Endorphins literally relieve emotional pain and create varying degrees of euphoria."*

The freezing response manifests itself in much of our lives. Much of the time we do not even realize that we have gone away. Peter Levine says, "Spaciness and forgetfulness are among the more obvious symptoms that evolve from dissociation." For many, this mode might be the normal way of being in the world—split off, numb and frozen. Peter Levine continues to explain, "The best way to define dissociation is through the experience of it. In its mildest forms, it manifests as a kind of spaciness. At the other end of the spectrum, it can develop into so-called multiple personality syndrome."

For some, this numbing out by going inside can be a real detriment. Many children with Attention Deficit Disorder (ADD) or other learning difficulties live in another world. They have learned how to split off to avoid their pain. How can you expect a child to remember something when he is constantly splitting off into a world of fantasy within his head in order to avoid his pain? These children then are labeled with having a disease (ADD or ADHD) and often are placed on medication when the reality is that they have just split off into the dissociation part of the Fight or Flight Response. In other words, at their core they do not feel safe and by "leaving their body" they are practicing a very real survival technique.

When we escape from our pain into our head, we are entering into our world of "magical thinking." This is the world where Prince Charming and Santa Claus reside. This magical place is where we are always hoping to win the lottery or hoping that some hero will come rescue us from our pain.

The world of magical thinking stems from this disassociation with reality. You might leave in order to avoid what feels like life-threatening pain. This is the same technique that a child uses to turn a mud ball into a pizza or a piece of wood into a battleship. You might laugh and think it's cute when a child does this. Many continue to split off into the world of magical thinking, even as adults.

What is important to remember is that your methods of protecting you from pain have a purpose. They have helped you to survive. If you want to continue to evolve, you must identify your false beliefs, your perceived imaginary life-threatening events, and learn to be present with yourself. Leaving your body behind, no matter how mystical it might seem, is not a tool for health or for recovery. When you do this you are still running from an imaginary enemy and still engaging your stress response. Learning to recover your self means learning to drop your armor. Splitting off, going inside and living in a world of "magical thinking" are just another way to be armored.

3. Flight (External Escape)
"A Moving Target Is Much Harder to Hit"

The third aspect of the Fight or Flight Response to perceived life-threatening events is the external escape component. This is the part of you that immediately kicks in to high gear and tries to outrun your potential enemy. If you were faced with that grizzly bear rushing towards you, immediately you would turn and run as fast as you could in the other direction without thinking about it. You would not attempt to confront the bear or freeze and play dead. You have already decided ahead of time that your best defense is to outpace the potential attacker. Your body instinctually knows how to respond. You have been preparing for this moment for quite some time. You know how to run. Running is your best defense.

This is how the External Flight Response would manifest itself in a real-life emergency. What happens when your threats are only imaginary? Your body keeps responding in the same way. You continue to run away.

A person who uses the External Flight Response for his survival will be the person who is always busy and on the move. There is nothing that is constant. Everything is always changing. Boredom equals death. Movement gives one hope. There is never any predictability.

You can recognize this person right away. She needs to own the newest car, always has a new boyfriend, and changes her living address often. Stagnation means death for her. She needs to keep moving and is always on the go. She constantly talks on her cell phone. Six months is as long as she can last at any job. She falsely believes that if she keeps moving, she will not be caught and will not die.

In this day and age when imaginary life-threatening events are the primary enemy, your body continues to react the same way as if the enemy were real. A person who is in her stress response with her external escape mechanism activated may not even know what her enemy is or what she is running from. All she believes is that if she stops running, her life will end. There is busyness and urgency about everything. She seldom takes time to relax. Even her vacations are filled with busyness, as she tries to see and do as much as possible. Drama and excitement fill her life.

The External Flight Response to a perceived threat is the third aspect of the stress response. Running, moving and staying busy are key elements in this attempt to ward off danger. Understanding how you respond to perceived threats will be a good first step to help bring you back to your relaxation response.

The Long-Term Effects of Stress

Stress is a naturally occurring reaction to a stimulus that we interpret as life-threatening. Your body will naturally enter into the stress response if, for example, you are being chased by a mountain lion. Essentially, your body goes into contraction, your heart speeds up, and large doses of adrenaline are pumped into your blood stream. You are preparing to do battle. It is nature's gift to you for your survival.

The stress response is a natural protection mechanism for most mammals. As we evolved, the stress response has helped people overcome some formidable encounters. Real life and death battles with wild animals and fierce elements of nature have been won with help from the stress response. Our human species has been able to overcome many obstacles that might have ended our existence if it were not for the stress response.

The stress response was designed by nature to be a momentary and short-lived experience. After the danger has passed, you would go back to your Relaxation Response. But as our brain has continued to evolve, our experience with stress has changed. Since the brain has created most of your enemies, you now falsely believe that you are almost always under attack. You feel as if you need to be defended constantly. Having to stay on guard and in your stress response will always take a tremendous toll on your body. The following are some of the long-term effects of the stress response.

1. Emotional Repression

First and foremost, stress is an emotional experience. Emotions are forms of energy. The most profound effects that we experience due to long-term Fight or Flight engagement are energetic in nature. Repression of our emotional energy leads to many physiological changes in the body. This topic will be discussed in detail later in the chapter on *Repression*.

2. Proliferation of Stress Hormones

When your body enters into the stress response, you are bombarded with hormones to ensure your survival. These hormones are released to perform a certain task *for a short period of time*. The problem is that these hormones have long-lasting detrimental consequences when they remain within you for long periods of time. Essentially, you are killing yourself with your own hormones that were designed to save you.

Adrenaline is one of these hormones. Over time, adrenaline begins to wear you down. Your heart rate remains increased. Your breath is shallow. Blood pressure remains elevated as blood vessels continue to be constricted. As a result, the tendency for plaque to be deposited on the vascular walls is increased. Strokes and coronary occlusions are some of the results.

Adrenaline surges can also account for unhealthy eating habits, restlessness and poor sleeping habits. Dr. Archibald D. Hart writes in *Adrenaline and Stress,*

"However, since an elevated adrenaline level can also give a person a heightened sense of well-being, increased energy, reduced need for sleep, and feelings of excitement or even euphoria, we are often completely unaware this destruction is taking place. It is easy to see why many become addicted to this state of arousal. The feelings of security it provides can give one a dangerously false sense of well-being."

Cortisol and cortisone are painkillers and anti-inflammatories. These chemicals are also released into the bloodstream when you enter the stress response. Over long periods of time, your sensitivity to pain is diminished, causing you to go numb. When you go numb, you lose your ability to feel anything good or bad. Other chronic problems often develop because of lack of sensitivity in your sensory awareness system.

Deane Juhan, author of *Job's Body*, writes about the sustained effects of cortisone in the body.

"From the adrenal cortex comes an important hormone, cortisone, which has an effect upon connective tissue quite the reverse of that of somatotrophin: cortisone inhibits the activity of fibroblasts, the very sources of connective tissue. Prolonged application of cortisone to the skin markedly reduces the number of fibroblasts, and the ones remaining are smaller than normal.

"This effect of cortisone has been used pharmaceutically in the treatment of fibrosis—dense connective tissue deposits created in the muscle bellies by repeated strain. This hormone also acts as an anti-inflammatory substance, and as such has been applied to inflammations of all kinds to reduce the swelling and discomforts they create. However, the negative effects of continued exposure to cortisone have revealed themselves to be substantially greater than the positive effects in the long run.

"Anything that depresses fibroblast activity obviously interferes with the normal healing of wounds, bruises, fractures, and the like, no matter how effectively it reduces swelling associated with these injuries. Nor has cortisone proved to be useful in the treatment of infections and inflammatory allergic reactions as was once hoped; it simply removes discomforting symptoms, without affecting either the basic mechanism or the course of the infection. In fact, since it weakens the connective tissue, it has been shown to actually facilitate the spread of infection from previously localized areas."

3. Stress and the Immune System

It is often said that most illness is stress related. You help to create many of your own illnesses because you are in your Fight or Flight Response. Your immune system was designed to ward off most major and minor invaders, from the common cold to bacterial infections, and is generally very effective at protecting you. However, there are times when even a healthy immune system can be overwhelmed with trying to protect you from a lethal invader.

Illness is a multi-level experience. Sometimes your genetic dispositions are involved, as in the case of sickle cell anemia. At other times you are subject to environmental factors, as in cases where large doses of radiation are leaked into the environment. Your depleted immune system appears to be a major part of the illness process as well.

The problem is that most people do not have healthy immune systems because the stress response is nearly always activated. The adrenal glands continue to produce anti-inflammatory hormones like cortisol and cortisone, which destroy the body's immune system over time by destroying the cells that were meant to protect you. White blood cells and T-cells are affected by elevated levels of these hormones in the body. Most autoimmune diseases can be linked to the inability of the depleted immune system to protect the body. The following are a few example of this process.

Debbie Shapiro writes in *The Bodymind Workbook*, "Rheumatoid Arthritis: This is where the immune system starts attacking itself, attacking the collagen, which is the connective tissue in the joints, as if it were an invading antigen." She goes on to add, "Meningitis: This is infection of the cerebral fluid, resulting in inflammation of the membrane covering the brain or spinal cord, and is usually caused by bacteria or a virus. Infection implies a weakness in the immune system and an inability to protect ourselves." Time and again, much of your illness process can be traced back to your weakened immune system caused by the stress response.

4. Shortening of Muscles

When you remain in your fight response for a long duration, your muscles will stay contracted and chronically shortened. Over months or years, this contraction of your musculature can result in the deterioration of your movement, along with many aches and pains. Your posture will suffer as well as you might become compressed and rigid. As the stress response remains active, one's muscles will have a difficult time letting go.

There are many reasons why muscles contract. Muscles contract to display or withhold emotion, to lift a load, to provide movement or to respond to a cold stimulus by causing you to shake in order to provide warmth. Muscles also contract in response to fear, either real or imagined.

Muscles have two functions—to either relax or contract. Muscles were designed to be the mechanical aspect of our human experience to allow us to be mobile. When a muscle remains contracted over time, a number of things often happen. First off, the muscle loses the ability to receive nutrients like oxygen and to remove waste products like lactic acid. A healthy muscle is smooth and has a fair degree of tone. An unhealthy muscle feels like a piece of gristly meat. When this happens, the muscle becomes dried out and weakened while lacking vitality.

As muscles stay chronically contracted, they also tend to bond or become glued together because of the pressure and lack of movement. This is a process called "Hydrogen Bonding," in which the hydrogen molecules grab on and attach to the oxygen molecules. When Hydrogen Bonding occurs, muscles do not function efficiently and independently. Over time, everything becomes glued together. You do not have to be a "little old lady" for this to happen. Most people who adopt the fight response to counter their stress will tighten their muscles and develop this pattern to one degree or another.

After awhile it hurts to move, so most people stop moving, making the problem even worse. Muscles were designed to contract and relax at regular intervals and to glide across each other. Chronic stress will cause one's musculature to become dried out, glued together and weakened. This is just another aspect of the long-term effects of the stress response.

Rosie Spiegel writes in *Bodies, Health, and Consciousness,*

"Muscles that have been shortened and made tense through the years have lost their elasticity and their natural fluid content. Dehydration of the muscle tissue is a by-product of chronic tension and immobilization. This can occur in the matrix of blood-rich muscle tissue, and in connective tissue, and the abundant variety of tendons and ligaments that are ubiquitous in your body's structure. Several words describe this phenomenon: calcification, fibrosis, adhesions, fixations, and contractions. In this situation, soft tissue hardens, compresses, and becomes less pliable. Associated with these occurrences are joint stiffness, muscular tightness, limited range of motion, pain, discomfort, low energy, and chronic fatigue. Certain psychological conditions, such as chronic depression, are also related to fixations in the body's structural patterns."

In response to a perceived stressful situation, contracting the musculature is a common option. You pull yourself in tighter and shorten your muscles, forming a suit of armor around yourself. You become hard and rigid as a way to protect yourself. You actually become smaller as the muscles around your spine contract and pull you down.

This was not how nature designed your muscles to be used in the long-term. Muscles are chiefly designed for locomotion purposes. They help you to pick things up and move around, or move your rib cage to help you breathe. The effects of a long-term Fight Response create muscles that can no longer move. As this process continues, you become more and more frozen within your own body.

When muscles are shortened, they initially fatigue. This causes discomfort at first. When you continue to remain contracted, your discomfort can lead to pain. Eventually, the body cannot handle this painful stimulus for too long so it has another defense. It goes numb. The body will shut off the painful stimulus because this has now become normal. You may still be in a state of contraction even though your body has numbed out the sensations so you do not have to feel anything.

This is what happens to many people when receiving a massage. As the therapist kneads through a tender area the receiver of the massage often replies, "But I didn't feel sore in that spot." What most of us do is numb out many painful sensations, and eventually the body shuts off the sensation. The contraction has not gone away, only the sensation of pain.

Many people report that they do not feel "stressed." They do not feel their muscles tightened and contracted all of the time. This is because the body has shut down the sensations of contraction and pain. There is no healthy reference point for comparison; you only know what contraction feels like, and contraction feels normal to you. Those who remain unaware that their muscles are under constant contraction live with reduced sensory awareness. It is commonly believed that it is those "other" people who have stress. It is rarely us.

As the muscles remain shortened the joints are often affected as well. Joints were designed to have a full range of motion, and chronically shortened muscles do not allow joints to move freely. Without adequate movement and hydration, your joints begin to stiffen and harden. This often leads to irregular patterns, such as arthritis. This is not necessarily the result of aging but the result of a prolonged stress reaction pulling muscles tighter and joints closer together.

5. Hardening of Fascia

Connective tissue is an important part of the body and plays an even more important role in your wellness or disease states. There are many different types of connective tissue in the body. For instance, blood, bones, tendons and cartilage are all forms of connective tissue. There is also a type of connective tissue called "fascia" that is instrumental in your well-being.

Connective tissue consists of cells and fiber imbedded in a "matrix" or "ground substance." This ground substance is like a gelatin. A bone would have a small amount of ground substance, few cells, many fibers, and mineral deposits. This is what makes a bone harder to the touch. On the other hand, fascia has a large portion of ground substance, medium amount of cells, and medium amount of fiber. This makes fascia a much more pliable and liquid material than bone.

Fascia is a material that travels throughout the entire body. Every muscle fiber is surrounded by fascia, as are nerves and blood vessels. Fascia encapsulates fat cells and travels throughout the body like a dense sweater. All organs and glands are embedded with fascia. If you were to cut open an orange and look inside, you would see a good example of what fascia looks like in your body. All of the hard white substance in the orange resembles your body's fascia. Imagine squeezing the juice out of an orange. The remaining white material would be like the fascia in your body. If you were to magically dissolve all of the muscles in the body, what you would have left would be a honeycomb of fascia.

Fascia has many functions. One such function is that fascia supports the body in its uprightness as it supplies tensile strength, like guy wires holding up a radio antenna. Your body is not a series of columns stacked on top of each other, as many were taught to believe in science and anatomy class. If you were made of columns, you would not be able to move. Rather, you are a series of guy wires pulling in all directions that allow you to be lifted up in the field of gravity. Fascia does this for you.

Fascia also compartmentalizes all of your organs and cells. Before you can have a heart, you have to have a layer that will contain the heart cells. This is called the "myocardium." Fascia that surrounds the bones is called the "periostium." In fact, fascia cells were the first cells to develop as your young organism was forming. It was the fascia cells that gave you form. Fascia gives you structure and form while helping you remain upright in your posture.

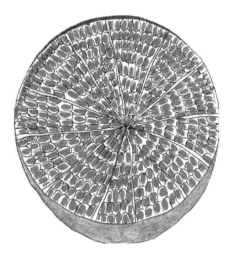

Fascia is like the white substance inside of an orange.

A muscle belly can be dissected into smaller parts called muscle fibers. The muscle fibers are then made up of many myofibrils, which are tiny strands of muscle and are wrapped in a thin layer of fascia. Fascia does not just form a container for the muscle belly; it travels through the muscle belly.

There are three types of muscle tissue: cardiac, smooth and skeletal. The heart is made of cardiac muscle. The internal organs and blood vessels consist of smooth muscle. External muscles are made of skeletal muscle.

Fascia wraps around every fiber of every type of muscle. This includes the heart and organs. When stress causes muscles to contract, those muscles pull the fascia tighter and also contract the organs, blood vessels, and glands.

Fascia also has a very important quality. Fascia allows energy to travel through your body. The "life force" or "chi" that regulates your livelihood travels through your vast network of fascia like electricity that energizes every cell in your body. Fascia acts like a copper wire that conducts energy throughout the body. While not able to be measured scientifically, nearly every nature-based culture has a keen sense of "chi" or "life-force energy."

Joseph Heller and William A. Henkin talk about these energetic properties in *Bodywise,*

"The fasciae are extremely important . . . because, as the most pervasive tissues in the body, they are believed to be the means whereby CHI is distributed along acupuncture routes. Research has shown that the least resistance to the flow of bioelectric energy in the body occurs between fascial sheaths and that when these routes have been charted, they have found to correspond to classical acupuncture channels—Mantak and Maneewan Chia, Iron Shirt Chi Kung 1"

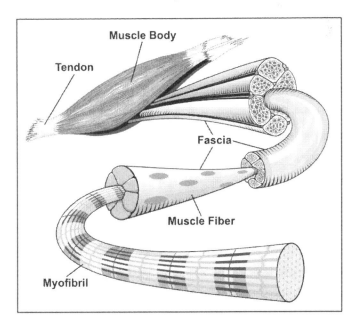

Why is fascia important? Fascia is a critical link in understanding the nature of stress, disease, addictions and impaired energetic flow. Your muscles shorten in response to stress, repression and physical trauma. Covering your muscles are sheets of fascia that carry energy through your body, compartmentalizing each cell and organ, and giving you structure. Over time your muscles lose their ability to relax and end up in a chronically shortened state.

Fascia moves with muscles like a latex glove worn over a hand. The fascia relaxes if the muscle relaxes. If a muscle is chronically shortened, the fascia also shortens, dries out and becomes very brittle. Fascia has the ability to change shape under the right conditions, for the positive or the negative. Shortening and reduced blood flow cause fascia to glue together, (Hydrogen Bonding), and lose its elasticity. This is what happens to most people who *age poorly*. The fascia loses its ability to carry the necessary energy and then becomes a poor conductor of energy flow at this point. The cells do not get nourished, resulting in a breeding ground for illness and disease.

What most people do not realize is that fascia should be considered is an organ. While not traditionally recognized by medical science as such, fascia is the most abundant tissue in the body with a specific nature and cellular component that distinguishes it from other tissues. It has a specific purpose beyond being "waste material" that a surgeon scrapes off when operating on a person's body. Fascia is instrumental in the conduction of energy throughout the body as well. Without fascia we could not exist.

Decades of tightened muscles due to the Fight Response cause contraction and pull the fascia even tighter. The fascia then loses its elastic shape and ability to carry energy, resulting in pain and illness. Most of our modern day stress is due to the false beliefs in our mind. The tightening and hardening of our fascia corresponds directly to these beliefs.

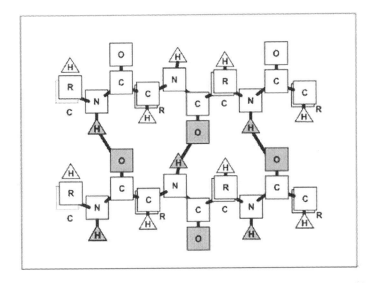

"Hydrogen Bonding"

Degenerative Disease

There are two primary types of diseases: molecular and energetic. The Western medical system is primarily concerned about molecular diseases. This approach is based on Newtonian thinking, which breaks matter down into smaller pieces (reductionism). In many cases this type of thinking is very effective in treating a health crisis, especially molecular-based illnesses. Treating the biochemistry of the body has been very helpful in eliminating many of the contagious diseases of the past. These might include small pox, rubella, influenza or plague. However, most diseases of our modern Western age are not molecule-based. Rather, they are energy-based or degenerative in nature.

Degenerative diseases, including Parkinson's syndrome, multiple sclerosis, arthritis, cancer, and heart disease all have to do with the body's constant reaction to the stress response. As the Fight or Flight response remains turned on as a result of perceived real or imaginary danger, the body will ultimately pay the price.

Stress weakens fascia and contributes to the onset of degenerative diseases. This happens in several ways. First, the tightening of your muscles over time causes the fascia covering to tighten and harden. The fascia loses its ability to transfer energy throughout the body. Energy blockages result and this later translates into physiological damage to the tissues.

The second way in which stress weakens the fascia is through the release of stress hormones in your body. The hormones that are released into the body as a result of the stress response lead to the direct degeneration of your connective tissue or fascia. Deane Juhan writes in *Job's Body*, "Individuals who are chronically stressed or disturbed in any way weaken their entire connective tissue network over a period of time, exposing it to pathological invasions of all kinds." Deane Juhan explains that healthy connective tissue that is not overwhelmed by stress hormones will contain a disease so that the body can best heal it, while weakened connective tissue will help to spread the disease.

Deane Juhan explains,

"The many compartments of fascia throughout the body are of great assistance in the prevention of the spreading of infections, disease, and tumors. Each separate compartment tends to contain the destructive agent, and prevent its spilling into adjacent compartments. This is accomplished partly by the fibrous walls of the compartments, and partly by specific chemical barriers in the fluid ground substance. Of course, this means that weakness in the fibers or disturbances of the protective chemicals in the ground substance contribute directly to the spread of infections and diseases from compartment to compartment."

Deane Juhan goes on to add how weakened connective tissue can help in the spread of some cancers.

"The connective tissues surrounding some types of tumors—including cancerous ones—are particularly illustrative of this point. When these tumors are in remission or are growing very slowly, the surrounding connective tissue is dense and fibrotic, with a viscous ground substance. In contrast, the connective tissue around rapidly growing tumors is much looser and softer, and the ground substance is much more watery."

As Juhan emphasizes, the chemical consistency of the connective tissue itself is very important in the role of the immune system. The chemicals of the stress response can have a very negative effect on the condition of not only your connective tissue but also your entire immune system.

Stress is responsible for many of your diseases and illnesses. If we could take accurate measurements of it, stress would show up as the leading cause of death in the Western world. Most often your stress response is rooted in your mind and corresponds to your false beliefs. As you examine the role of stress, you might begin to realize the devastating impact that it can have on your life.

As you unravel the mystery of your own stress, begin to empower yourself with new information and a brand new commitment in order to heal. Stress is one way that we lose our body. Now we will begin to explore the second manner—Repression.

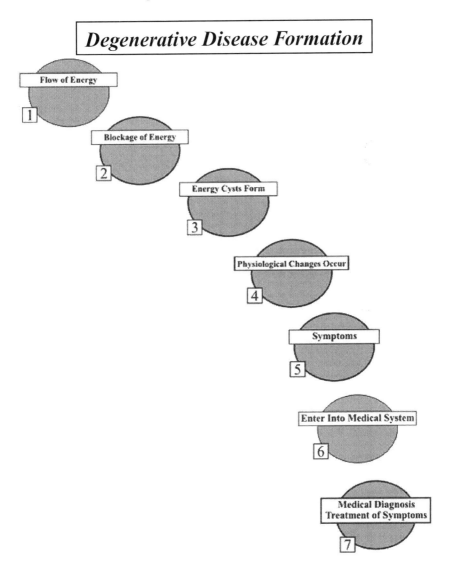

Degenerative Disease Formation

Flow of Energy
1

Blockage of Energy
2

Energy Cysts Form
3

Physiological Changes Occur
4

Symptoms
5

Enter Into Medical System
6

Medical Diagnosis
Treatment of Symptoms
7

II. The Nature of Repression

What Is Repression?

Underneath your fancy clothes and educated minds you are pure energy. In a healthy state, a stream of energy flows through you. However, many of your beliefs about who you are prevent this flow from happening. The second of the primary forces in your life that undermine your health is that of "repression." Repression is somewhat different than stress, even though they are both based on the flow of energy. However, repression is just as deadly as the effects of stress.

Nature intended there to be a flow of energy throughout your body. When you do not allow this energy to flow, you block what is natural. Repression creates a pattern of stopping the flow of energy and emotions over a long period of time. When not allowed to flow out, the energy of emotions becomes stuck within your own tissues. This process usually forms a well-reinforced pattern over time. It is your beliefs once again that lead you into repression.

You have muscles in your body for several reasons. Muscles are used to help you lift a load and create movement in your life. You breathe because of the muscles of respiration. Your heart muscle pumps blood throughout your body. Muscles act as pulleys to hold you upright. Muscles are even used to keep you warm. This occurs when your body shivers involuntarily in the cold.

Muscles are also used in the expression of emotions. Without muscles you would not be able to express your joy or deepest grief. You would have a blank expression on your face in times of emotional experiences if you did not have muscles to express those emotions. Your muscles enable your body to fully feel and release the energy of emotions. Through your own vast muscle network, you are able to express the energy of emotion and release that energy.

Muscles are also used to hold back the energy of emotion. This is called *repression*. It is natural to cry when you feel like it. It is natural to be out of control from time to time. It is natural to feel anger, sadness and joy whenever these feelings arise.

Feeling and expressing emotions is as natural as the seasons or the swelling of the tides. Your body has a rhythm and a pace all to itself. The nature of energy is to want to flow. When your beliefs engage your muscles to prevent this flow of energy, you have now entered into the state of repression.

The repression of energy is like placing a brick on a small garden plant and expecting the plant to grow. The plant will never have a chance. You do the same thing in your life when you repress your natural emotions. You stunt your growth and create most of your own problems. You build up walls to ward off feelings and sensations, just like the brick that impedes the plant from growing.

Repression is about holding on inside as if someone were winding a crank to tighten you up a little bit more and more each day. After a couple of days, you might not be able to see a big difference. After a lifetime of repression, the affects however, are quite dramatic.

There is a common myth that only some people have emotions some of the time. The left-brained rational world wants you to believe that it is the rare few who are "moody" and have emotions. Nature's reality is that we are all emotional energy. Emotions are not just something that some people experience from time to time. Expressing emotions is a big part of the human experience.

Repression begins in the womb, is apparent through the birth process and continues on into your childhood. A child in a mother's belly who has to constantly hear his parents fighting learns to repress any noise and negative energy. A mother who is feeling her own stress creates stress hormones that are passed into the womb where the child experiences them. In *The New Primal Scream*, Dr. Arthur Janov writes about the effects of repression on a child still in the womb. He says, "A baby who needs has no alternative but to either feel continuous agony or shut off. He can't get to the store for cigarettes or phone a pal to see a movie. He represses." As an adult, you might use your thinking brain to repress all pain by rationalizing frequently. An infant in the womb cannot do this yet. The way the infant represses is to tighten her muscles, and as Arthur Janov says, to "tune out."

A child in the womb is essentially one and the same with the mother. The child experiences what the mother feels. If the mother feels stress (fear) her body releases stress hormones and her muscles tighten up. The child may experience this response over and over. He interprets this as being under attack. He has nowhere to go to escape, so he represses the pain and holds on for dear life. He tightens his muscles in order to not feel the terror.

Repression seems to happen at critical time periods when the child needs comfort and does not get it. This explains why we all do not repress at the same time in the same manner. Timing is very important when you learn to repress. When you have a need that is not fulfilled and you cannot fulfill it for yourself, most often you repress that pain. It is these acts of repression that have established patterns that continually plague you as an adult.

What Is Natural?

The body has natural ways to release energy. Shedding tears is one of those ways. Tears are like a faucet that releases the pressure from a bursting plumbing system. Shaking, sweating or other body movements are other ways to release energy.

I have witnessed some clients sweating profusely in one localized area or throughout their entire body after a bodywork session. This is one way the body sheds excess energy. Other clients have spontaneously begun to shake uncontrollably to release this internal awakening of energy. A temper tantrum is a perfectly normal way for a child to release energy from her body by rolling around in a fit, screaming and yelling. Her whole body is used to express the energy of her emotions.

After facing trauma, an animal will stand up and shake itself out. This shaking helps to release energy rather than allow the energy to settle back into the body. Moving your muscles involuntary through shaking, vomiting or sweating are ways nature intended for you to release excess energy.

As an adult in a highly controlled society, you are trained to hold on. Message after message encourages you to keep it all together and not demonstrate emotion. After a traumatic event you have a tendency to hold still, which ends up freezing the energy within you. You then repress the energy which becomes part of your muscular pattern.

For instance, if you grew up in a family where you were told that big boys do not cry, you might have learned how to repress your tears over time. Holding back the tears in one incident usually does not create a pattern of repression, but frequent acts of repression will cause a definite pattern. As an adult, when tears begin to well up, you automatically repress them and store the sadness inside. You constrict the muscles of expression to hold back this emotion. You are now storing energy, little by little.

Repression of emotions and sensations is a reoccurring theme in most lives. A Catholic priest, told by superiors and dogma that to engage in his sexuality is a sin, will need to repress his sexual desires or go underground with it if he chooses to remain faithful to his order. He will use the muscles of his pelvis to repress or hold back any sexual energy that wants to be released. This is the act of repression. Repression is a behavior that evolves over time. Is there any wonder why there is a significant amount of prostate cancer among celibate Catholic priests?

A study of 1,400 Catholic priests indicated a strong relationship between prostate cancer and repression. Larry Clapp, Ph.D., J.D., writes in *Prostate Health in 90 Days*, "The celibate priests were found to have a high incidence of prostate cancer and significantly increased risk of dying from prostate cancer, as compared to age-adjusted controls."

Repression is a pattern that evolves over time and is reinforced with each occurrence. This pattern then becomes the norm. When we block the flow of energy that nature intended, we create a pattern of repression. Repression is another way you lose your body.

The Evolution of Energy

Throughout history we have continued to evolve and change as a species. We ascended out of the water to dry land and came out of the trees to our uprightness. We have passed on genetic material from one generation to another along the way. We have also passed on child-rearing techniques and hunting skills. This is the nature of evolution.

There is another interesting component of our evolutionary history. For thousands of years we have continued to pass on the energy of the last generation. In essence, beyond any genetic material, your energy has evolved down through the ages until the present moment. This is something that is passed down within your cells from one generation to the next.

How does this work? An analogy that I like to use is the one of the Olympic torch. Several months before the winter or summer Olympics, a torch is lit in Athens, the birthplace of the Olympic Games. The flame from that torch is then carried from runner to runner, from boats to countrysides, to towns and cities, until the flame reaches the destination of the next Olympic Games. Each runner runs one to five miles with the flame in his torch, passing on the flame by lighting the next runner's torch. This continues until the flame reaches its final destination.

The evolution of our energy is similar. An egg and sperm meet and create a new being filled with life-force energy. The next generation creates more eggs and sperm that carry the energy down to the following generation. This is just like the Olympic flame. The flame is never extinguished. It just passes from one person to the next. Your energy moves through a different body every generation, but it remains the same energy. This energy keeps us all connected to the past and the future, just like carrying the same flame for a few miles connects all the Olympic runners.

Through your body, your energy has continued to evolve. Your cells, genes and biology have been the receptacle in which that energy has been stored. Each generation has been a vessel to move that energy on to the next generation. This is the story of the evolution of energy.

Denial of Feeling

In an ideal world, your energy moves freely without blockage, like a stream of water cascading over a cliff into a waterfall. Unfortunately, you do not live in an ideal world.

Energy has been repressed over the course of human existence. You have attempted to block its flow on many occasions. Educational systems, religious beliefs, parenting practices and governmental policies have been instrumental in creating blockage in the free flowing energy systems. Once again, it is your false beliefs that lead to blocking the flow of feelings in your body.

For instance, an educational system which emphasizes academic intelligence over other types of intelligence (such as emotional or creative intelligence) attempts to block the energetic flow of the human being. Sitting still, memorizing data and incessant use of the Cognitive Brain leads one to establish beliefs that negate or deny emotional experience. Rational thought is favored in these instances over natural wisdom. Most people throughout their schooling history have received thousands of hours of intellectual training. Little or no emotional training is common, though.

Parenting systems are often not much better. Prohibiting a child to speak up or have a will of her own is a system that attempts to repress a child's energetic flow. Telling a child that it is not okay to cry or feel sad blocks an energetic system that hungers for the release of energy.

How did you lose your self anyway? How did you learn not to feel? When did this all begin?

Repression of feelings and sensory information is actually not new. This behavior has been going on for quite some time now. For instance, the practice of making war has been a tradition for a very long time. Tribes battled other tribes. Regions squared off against other regions. City-states dueled for territory. It has been a long-standing tradition for different religions and cultural groups to wage war against each other. Nations and groups of nations have come to create mega-wars, or world wars. Recently, corporations have covertly hijacked governments and manipulated those governments to wage war for the security of assets and corporate profiteering.

Soldiers are required for war to be waged. Usually (but not always) this position is reserved for men because men have historically been linked to the warrior role. To be successful, the art of making war requires disciplined soldiers. Disciplined soldiers are not allowed to cry or show deep feelings. This would indicate a sign of weakness.

How can a soldier live a natural emotional life if he is trained to be a killer? He might not be able to perform his duties as a soldier if he expresses his feelings. He might feel some remorse or sadness concerning his violent acts, perhaps affecting his performance and threatening his survival and that of his fellow soldiers. (After all, it is much easier to kill another human being if you can objectify him as evil and not become emotionally involved.)

As long as the human species has been attempting to resolve its conflicts by means of war and violence, we have been continuing the tradition of repression of emotions. If a little boy wants to grow up to be a good soldier, he must learn early on how to control his emotions. Now that women are allowed to be soldiers, the same process is taking place.

Another example of repression of feelings might occur in an athletic competition. Contact sports, boxing, martial arts and highly competitive athletic pursuits require a great deal of repression of emotions to be successful. Could you imagine a boxer who cried every time that he was hit by a punch? It might seem that the most successful athletes are those who can perform well, act like machines and leave their deepest feelings out of their performance.

Many tend to numb out their sensory experiences the same way. If you are feeling hungry, tired or physically hurt, you might ignore the message that there is something wrong. You might choose an addiction to kill your body's painful message. The message might be saying, "Stop and rest" or "Slow down so that I can repair myself." Pain is there for a reason. When you choose to ignore the message, you pick an addiction to numb it out.

The repression of feelings and sensory information happens in all societies and all cultures. It is a practice as old as time. Perhaps at one time it helped our species to survive. I like to think of the repression of emotions as a very primitive and tribal custom.

For instance, what would happen if you were living in a tribe and one day you experienced a bad "emotional day?" Living in the environment where your daily survival needs are your priority might not allow you the chance to experience and release your feelings. You might not be able to perform vital societal functions such as hunting, fishing or caring for the children. Can you imagine a woman saying," "I can't feed my children today because I am feeling very upset and need to take time for myself"? Another example might be of a young adolescent male rejected by a young female. He doesn't want to go on the hunt to supply food for the tribe because he needs to be alone and process his feelings.

In times when your survival needs are a priority, the repression of feelings and painful stimuli might be useful. This practice has helped us to survive. In essence, the practice of repressing feelings and sensations is very much a part of tribal belief systems. Tribal thinking states, "The needs of the tribe come before the needs of the individual."

A modern day version of the tribal system comes in the form of corporate life. You are often taught (not naturally, but stemming from false beliefs), that the business is more important than your own personal life and health. This is commonly referred to as "professionalism."

The work place has become the modern equivalent of the military. A "professional" does not bring her emotions to work. A "professional" continues to perform her job despite physical pain or relentless emotional upheaval. Even when she is tired or upset, she is expected to carry on. Learning how to control her emotions is how she has "disciplined" herself to be a "good soldier" in the work place.

If you are at work and are feeling sad because there is a conflict in your personal relationship, your eyes might tear as you fight back the sadness. A co-worker approaches and mutters, "What's wrong?" as if experiencing an emotion were a capital offense. In a business and professional environment, expression of emotion often evokes suspicion and distain.

Losing control of your emotions at work is a sign of weakness or failure. You might become undependable and less likely to be respected by your peers if you display emotion. You are not as likely to get the promotion. When you display deep emotion, you are said to experience a "breakdown." Nobody stands up and cheers as you express your pain. You are rushed outside in a hush of embarrassment. Not only your businesses, but your schools, churches and families continue to encourage similar repression and control of your feelings and bodily sensations.

Learning how to repress your emotional experiences stems from many different sources. Another common source is the legal system. You are admonished by the courtroom judge to leave your emotions outside. As a juror, you are told to examine the evidence and reach a verdict with rational thought alone. The courtroom, you are told, is no place for emotions.

While many people still spend their days and nights attempting to meet their survival needs, much of the world's population has moved beyond this point. While repression of pain (either emotional or sensory) is relevant in a culture where basic survival needs are a priority, it is irrelevant in a "modern" culture. It is as if you are playing a new game with the same set of rules. You are still practicing the repression of sensory and emotional experiences because that is how it has always been done.

When you learn to repress your feelings, you soon develop false beliefs about your feelings. You come to believe that your anger will kill you. Loss of control becomes the evil that is lurking behind the corner. You are on guard for a new enemy—your own emotions.

To reclaim your body, you must make a major shift in consciousness. You have to begin to acknowledge and express your feelings rather than continue to stuff them deep inside yourself. You need to begin to listen to your sensory pain and the messages that are presenting themselves.

Not only do you tend to repress those emotions that feel bad, but many times you end up repressing your joy and your happiness also. Take for instance the case of "survivor's guilt." Someone you care about is suffering or has died. You feel that you cannot truly be yourself and express any joy because there is or was no joy in the other person's life. They are in pain or have suffered and you will feel guilty or shameful if you feel good. You repress or deny any good feelings. This is one way in which you have learned to repress that which feels good.

There are other ways to repress your good feelings as well. Many times you might get hooked into believing the mythologies from religious books that condemn you for feeling good. A common belief among Christians is that only the poor, stoic and sufferers will enter into heaven. The Baltimore Catechism, a classic handbook for many Catholics, states that "pride" and "envy" are two of the seven capital sins. In the Catholic tradition, it is a sin to have too much or feel too good about yourself. This would make you want to repress any good feelings that you might be experiencing.

Religion is not the only source of emotional repression, but it certainly comes close to the top of the list. It is common to look at the heroic feats of religion, such as setting up soup kitchens and hospitals, yet many refuse to look at the horrible damage that religion causes. It is almost like the story of the pyromaniac who lights the house on fire only to run in and save the cat. We want to decorate him for his heroism, yet the pain and suffering that he has caused is far greater than any good deed that he performs. Religion has this influence as well.

Religious systems that claim to put a restriction on which feelings are acceptable are attempting to dam up the river of natural energy that desires to be released. Anger, lust and sadness are just a few of these blockages immortalized by religious systems. When you try to hold back your anger or grief because of the religious beliefs demanded of you, the natural flow and release of energy is curtailed.

Unfortunately, these systems have been in place for many generations, longer than history even has accurate record of them. We have been creating systems to repress energy for a very long time now. In fact, these repressive systems have become normal for us. Most cultures are now accustomed to the repressive way of life. Everything from staying in control to holding it all in are normal behaviors.

Repression of energy is a cross-cultural practice. Western cultures are extremely repressive, telling us that anger is a sin and that your body is evil and inhabited by the devil. The way to heaven, we are told, is to be good all of the time and hold yourself together. Turn the other cheek and don't express how you are really feeling.

Eastern cultures can be equally as repressive, if not more so. Control of the senses is encouraged in order to attain the magical state of "enlightenment." The message "sexuality is for the unenlightened" is conveyed.

The intention of energy is to naturally flow through us. Emotions are just one form of energy. When not allowed to flow freely, we develop blockages in this flow. It is these blockages that affect the physical body.

The Consequences of Repression

Repression of feelings and sensory experiences leads to many problems down the road. Pain, illness and addictions are the end result of the energy stored within the body. As one learns how to hold back his emotions, his physical body will ultimately pay the price.

Repression is a practice where you use your own muscles to hold back and not express the energy of your emotions. Many people are encouraged to be strong, stoic and calm all of the time. This practice does not allow the emotional energy to be released. Energy has to go someplace if it is not expressed and released. Where does it go? This energy goes into your body and forms what some refer to as "energy cysts." This is a term made famous by John Upledger, a pioneer in Cranial Sacral Therapy.

Energy cysts are blockages in energy that bundle up or pool in places where the muscles have been particularly active in withholding expression. Remember, you can have expression or repression, but it is difficult to have both at the same time. High levels of stored energy are found in places where muscles dam up the flow of energy.

For instance, if you have a difficult time expressing emotions in the area around your eyes, you might use the muscles of this area to hold back emotion. There might be tightness or a discoloration associated with the area around your eyes. There might also be significant sensation, such as pain or discomfort, or no sensation at all (numbness). Temperature changes or other visual or kinesthetic landmarks might also be present when attempting to locate areas of energy cysts.

If muscles remain contracted long enough and the energy cyst persists over time, the physical bodily tissues begin to change. A muscle that is chronically shortened will begin to lose its elasticity and liquid nature. This muscle will dry up. Muscle tissue will also begin to form hardened or "gristly" areas.

Muscles are like tiny motors. When contracted in exact patterns, these muscles allow you your mobility and coordination. Muscles that lose their ability to function fully will cause you to limp or to become imbalanced in your movement.

Muscles are also attached to bones. When muscles remain chronically shortened over time, your bones are pulled closer together. This can cause shortening of the spine or compression of a joint, perhaps in the knee or hip area.

Repression of energy is one of the prime factors in the occurrence of degenerative diseases. Degenerative diseases are unique in the respect that science has not been able to cure them because they are energy-based rather than molecule-based.

One such example of the scientific community's frustration with identifying the nature of degenerative diseases comes to us from the authors of *Alternative Medicine: The Definitive Guide*. The many medical doctors writing this book conclude the following response.

"The medical establishment generally contends that there is 'no known cause' for MS [multiple sclerosis], yet billions of dollars have been spent researching potential causes and cures."

In fact, this statement is a common thread in all degenerative diseases. The scientific community spends billions of dollars looking for a cure for these types of diseases under a microscope. Unfortunately, that is not where the answer lies. The answer lies in your energetic and emotional worlds. Even the nineteenth-century French chemist Louis Pasteur, the recognized father of the germ theory, stated just before his death that instead of condemning parasites, bacteria and viruses as the culprits in disease, it is important to attend to the environment. "The germ is nothing," he said, "The soil is everything." The environment is your own energy flow.

Another puzzling disease for medical scientists is scoliosis. Time after time, medical professionals wish to blame hereditary patterns or genetics for most cases of scoliosis. Repression of emotions is a much more realistic answer as to the source of scoliosis. Scoliosis develops most often in young girls about the time that they are going through puberty. As nature is pushing a young person into adulthood, this person may not be ready for this change.

In the case of young girls, nature is creating hips and breasts. As nature is pushing her up and out, her mind might want to hold her back down. She uses her own muscles to try to stay small. She may not be emotionally ready for womanhood yet. Her spine has to go somewhere, so it begins to bend due to nature's forces pushing against it.

Melanie is a prime example of how scoliosis becomes a pattern of repression that begins in the mind. Melanie was a very competitive gymnast as a young girl. When puberty arrived, Melanie was not happy. She fought these changes. Having hips and breasts were not favorable in the competitive gymnastic community. Melanie's balance was thrown off. She was losing her competitive edge due to having to adjust to a new body.

Melanie recalls trying to make herself smaller. She did not want to grow up; she was not ready for womanhood. Melanie tightened up and repressed the energy that nature was bringing forth. As a result, a curve in her spine developed, not to mention a significant tightness in her neck and shoulders.

Jamie is another example of repression leading to scoliosis. Jamie was tall for her age. She stood out among all of the other girls. When passing through puberty, she developed large breasts for her age. Being tall and having large breasts was not comfortable for Jamie. She suddenly attracted a lot of attention (especially from men).

As a result, Jamie subconsciously repressed the energy of nature and tried to shorten her body. She tried to hide by tightening up. She rolled her shoulders forward to try to hide her breasts. As nature was pushing her up and out, her mind was pulling her in and down using her own muscles. As a result, she began to develop a curve in her spine. This pattern persisted for forty years until coming to treatment.

Repression of what is natural will ultimately show up someplace in your body. Coming back to nature means learning to release those areas that have a history of holding on and pulling in. The antidote for repression is expression.

Emotional Body Language

Emotions are energy. If you experience a situation that causes you to be angry and you do not allow yourself to be angry, there is a good chance that the anger will become trapped within your body. Perhaps your eyes will store the anger or your lower back will block the energy of anger like a beaver dam plugging up a wilderness stream. Your energy will cease to flow.

How does this happen? Young children are freer in allowing their emotions to move through them. When they are upset they have a temper tantrum, which releases the energy of their feelings. They kick their feet, hit their hands on the floor, roll around and scream at the top of their lungs until their voice is hoarse. When they cry, their whole body lurches up and down. They do not spare anything and feel their feelings with every inch of their bodies, releasing them and moving on.

When you are socialized into the world, that soon changes. The flow of emotions is plugged up as you learn to stay in control. You are taught that there is no place in the world for out of control children or adults. Unfortunately, your families, work environment, cultural messages and religious influences often teach you how to repress your anger and other emotions. Since you are taught to not feel certain emotions, the energy of these emotions becomes stored in the body.

Those feelings do not just dissipate. They are somaticized, meaning they become a part of your physical structure, if you do not release them. Those trapped feelings keep building up and creating more and more pockets of dammed up energy. These feelings are like little balls of energetic mass that are frozen within your muscle tissue. Every time you hold back your anger or sadness and refuse to express and release it, these emotions become stored within you. Those tight shoulders might be caused by something more than just your work. Your unexpressed anger at your parents may be trapped in your trapezius muscle at the base of your neck. Your resentment of your boss might be the reason your lower back hurts so much. Cancer of the colon might really be your unexpressed grief surrounding the death of your sister.

A tremendous amount of energy is required to keep repressing what wants to flow out of you. You may be frequently tired because you are using all of your energy to hold everything in and pushing it down even further. Muscles conditioned to repress emotional energy need a constant supply of nutrients to hold on tightly at all times. Of course you will feel tired when so much bodily nutrition is going to hold on tightly. Your muscles are almost always working. These muscles are not working to lift you up or move you across a room; they are working to prevent the release of emotion.

Here is an example of how this process works. Steve gets migraine headaches quite frequently. He experiences intense pain around his left eye and left temple region. He cannot function when he is experiencing a migraine episode. What happens to Steve is the following.

Steve has learned for a long time to repress his anger. It was not acceptable in his home while growing up to express anger. He learned early on that in order to get his needs met in his home, he had to learn to repress his anger. He was told that little boys who were out of control with anger were punished or were not loved.

As an adult, after many years of practicing this repression of anger, his body is beginning to feel the effects. Steve, rather unconsciously, tightens up his neck muscles every time he feels anger. A "stressful" day at the office or at home might elicit this response frequently. Once the neck and scalp muscles tighten up, the blood to the temporal artery and adjoining areas is cut off. Over time, the connective tissue, which surrounds the muscles and arteries, tends to harden like cement, preventing the muscle from relaxing at all. Constant and intense pain is the result of this persistent pressure placed on the muscle and artery.

After years of pain, Steve has resorted to accepting this as "normal" and has become addicted to prescription pills, alcohol and sex in order to numb out his frequent pain. If Steve were to just learn how to express his anger, then all of this would change. Steve is not alone in his repression cycle. What Steve experiences is a very common event in many lives.

Referring to this energy blockage, Candace Pert says in *Molecules of Emotion*, "Another healer I respect tremendously is John Upledger, creator of craniosacral therapy, a modality that aims to balance the cerebrospinal fluid through gentle manipulations of the cranium. He talks about 'somato-emotional cysts,' pockets of blocked emotion held in the body, causing a breakdown in the energy flow and general health."

Candace Pert continues in *Molecules of Emotion,*

"Can suppressed anger or other 'negative' emotions cause cancer? In addition to the recent studies by various researchers like David Spiegel of Stanford who have convincingly shown that being able to express emotions like anger and grief can improve survival rates in cancer patients, we now have a theoretical model to explain why this might be so. Since emotional expression is always tied to a specific flow of peptides in the body, the chronic suppression of emotions results in a massive disturbance of the psychosomatic network."

Pert continues with the following statement,

"More recent, 1980s studies by Lydia Temoshok, a psychologist then at UCSF, showed that cancer patients who kept emotions such as anger under the surface, remaining ignorant of their existence, had slower recovery rates than patients who were more expressive. Another trait common to these patients was self-denial, stemming from an unawareness of their own basic emotional needs. The immune systems were stronger and tumors smaller for those in touch with their emotions."

Joseph Heller and William A. Henkin write in *Bodywise,*

"Although we are supposed to learn about control as we become socialized, the social view of control is pronouncedly immature, emphasizing restrictions rather than motivations, so that we learn to dam our energies up rather than use them in ways that might benefit both ourselves and others. Instead of learning to expand ourselves to embrace the world, we learn to close ourselves down and close the world out."

Candace Pert recalls her own personal struggle during some very difficult times. She says, "I had only intuited that suppressing my emotions was dangerous and might lead to cancer, but now I had amassed enough hard scientific data to convince me that I needed to heal my emotions if I wanted to pull through this difficult time—alive and healthy."

Eventually over time, stuck emotions contribute to disease and illness. Dr. Arthur Janov believes that even something as simple as loneliness can affect your immune system if repressed. The body will begin to break down because you have learned to not feel and release your feelings.

Once the flow of emotional energy is blocked, your body then absorbs this energy like a sponge. Candace Pert writes,

"Anger, fear, and sadness, the so-called negative emotions, are as healthy as peace, courage, and joy. To repress these emotions and not let them flow freely is to set up a dis-integrity in the system, causing it to act at cross-purposes rather than as a unified whole. The stress this creates, which takes the form of blockages and insufficient flow of peptide signals to maintain function at the cellular level, is what sets up the weakened conditions that can lead to disease. All honest emotions are positive emotions."

Dr. Arthur Janov adds in *The New Primal Scream*, "Clearly, repression is carcinogenic."

I recently heard a well-known psychologist give his daily radio address on the foolishness of the child's temper tantrum and the ways this behavior should be repressed as soon as possible. I could not disagree any stronger. The temper tantrum is a natural way for a child to release pent up energy of disappointment or anger. The energy must come out through kicking the floor, rolling around, screaming and crying. Nobody teaches a child how to have a temper tantrum. Only a repressed, left-brained rational world teaches a child how to repress the energy of a temper tantrum and control behavior. In my workshops, I make it a special point to teach adults how to recover the temper tantrum and to skillfully express their anger and frustration by kicking and hitting pillows and cushions with their arms and legs. Expression leads to freedom; repression leads to death.

Alexander Lowen writes in *Pleasure: A Creative Approach to Life:*

"A muscle becomes tense only under stress. When a body is moving easily, it feels no strain. Stresses are of two kinds, physical and emotional. Supporting a heavy weight is a physical stress, as is the continuation of a movement or activity when a muscle is tired. Feeling the pain of the tension, the person stops the activity or drops the weight. If, however, there is no way to remove the stress, the muscle will go into spasm. An emotional stress is just like a physical one; the muscles are charged with a feeling that they cannot release. They contract to hold or contain the feeling just as they do

to support a weight, and if the feeling persists long enough, the muscle will go into spasm because it cannot get rid of the tension.

"Any emotion which cannot be released is a stress for the muscles. This is true because an emotion is a charge which presses outward for release. A few examples will illustrate these ideas. Sadness or hurt feelings are released through crying. If the crying is inhibited because of parental objections or for other reasons, the muscles which normally react in crying become tense. These are the muscles of the mouth, throat, chest, and abdomen. If the feeling which cannot be released is one of anger, the muscles of the back and shoulders become tense. Inhibited biting impulses lead to jaw tensions, inhibited kicking impulses to leg tensions. The correlation between muscle tension and inhibition is so exact that one can tell what impulses or feelings are inhibited in a person from a study of his muscular tensions."

Heller and Henkin comment on what happens when you hold back your emotional energy.

"As with other physical holding, one occasion or two or a dozen is unlikely to damage the body. But if repression becomes a repetitive pattern, the muscles accumulate a little more tension and then a little more in addition to that, until the rib cage, chest, and diaphragm become set, and the child's torso becomes chronically tight. Then he breathes less and eventually develops a physical inability to express sadness or even to be aware of feeling the emotion—by crying."

It is these early moments when the repressive patterns set in. These events will later plague you if you do nothing to free up the repression. Dr. Arthur Janov writes in *The New Primal Scream*, "Holding in (feelings) and the development of cancer as a repressive disease are part of the same syndrome, emanating from the identical early event."

Much of the problem lies in how you were taught to repress your emotions. When you were young, your emotions came very naturally. Within a ten-minute period you could express eight or ten different feelings. You could go from anger to grief to joy within a very short period of time. When you began to be socialized, you learned that it was not okay to express certain emotions. You soon learned which emotions society calls the "positive" emotions and which ones are the "negative" ones. You had better not make any mistakes. This is almost like another lesson from your grammar book. While not publicly spoken about, you are taught to seek out the positive emotions and stay away from the negative ones. For some, even an elevated expression of any emotion is sometimes very threatening. Many learn to hold *even* their joy and happiness back.

Most have had their emotions bottled up inside of them for a long time. Heller and Henkin write in *Bodywise,*

"Fear: excitement without breath. As education instills this attitude in our children they spend a lot of their adult lives (we spend a lot of our adult lives, because this is what happened to most of us) holding. We hold our bodies tense: We hold onto our limbs and bones, not with our hands but with our musculature: we hold fast to our feelings and thoughts and beliefs and to the very bodily attitudes that in some ways engendered them in the first place."

Candace Pert writes in *Molecules of Emotion,*

"If the immune system can be altered by conscious intervention, what does this mean for the treatment of major diseases such as cancer? The idea that emotions are linked to cancer has been around for a while. In the 1940s, Wilhelm Reich proposed the then heretical idea that cancer is a result of failure to express emotions. Reich was not only ridiculed by the medical and scientific establishment, he was actually persecuted. It was perhaps the only time in history that the government of the United States held an official book burning, calling for all available copies of Reich's life's work to be rounded up by the FDA and incinerated."

The Repression of Pain

Human beings are a unique species because we have learned how to suppress pain. Most other species have not yet evolved to this level. This difference separates us from other creatures, large and small. Humans have evolved to such a degree that we can now mask much of the pain that pervades our lives. While this might seem like a positive step in our evolution, it has some very dire consequences. In the process of learning how to eliminate pain, we have abandoned nature's way.

Pain is present to tell us something. Most people have decided to kill the messenger rather than to listen to the message. Many have become very clever at finding new ways to kill those painful messages.

Pain shows up in many forms. Sometimes this pain is a stabbing, knifelike pain, indicating that your heart is not happy with how you have lived your life. Other times, the pain manifests as a depressed and contracted core that makes you feel tired and withdrawn all the time. The pain can also come from a sensory experience (like cutting oneself with a knife) or an emotional experience (like grieving at a funeral for a loved one).

Regardless of the way pain appears, there is a reason for it being there. Pain is a message from someplace else within us. There is something out of balance or injured that is begging for attention. However, the evolutionary process has perfected the art of numbing out the message, and many refuse to address the message.

The irony is that nature gave us pain so that we could continue to evolve as a species and to protect us from further injury. Arthur Janov writes in *The New Primal Scream* "Repression got the species to be where it is, made us into human beings, and helped us to develop a cerebral cortex with all of its logic and rational abilities."

Pain is not a disease, nor is it an aberration without purpose or merit. Pain is a messenger meant to be listened to since it is only a symptom of a deeper imbalance. Whether it is from a splinter in the bottom of your foot or the achiness of the flu, pain is there to tell you something. The message is advising you to stop and rest or take this splinter out of your foot before it causes more damage. Pain is nature's way of warning you and protecting you from your own demise. Pain is part of nature's survival tools handed down to you and can be seen as a part of nature's gifts to further your evolution. Without it, you would not know to take your foot out of the hot fire or to cover your wound so as to not bleed to death.

Control and Surrender

When experiencing physical trauma, there is almost always some pain involved. Pain is a bodily sensation. This pain has a message for us. By grieving the pain and expressing your hurt, you enter into the state of surrender. This state allows your muscles to soften and allows the energy of the physical trauma to move out of you more easily.

When you cry or enter into your surrender state, you are letting go. When you acknowledge the sensation of pain and grieve this sensation, you begin to heal. Becoming vulnerable allows your muscles to stay soft and the energy of physical trauma to pass through you more easily. Surrender and vulnerability lead to a healthier body. When you can surrender and express your pain, you stay open in your physical body.

Many people are taught to be strong at all times. You will not allow yourself to be vulnerable. You will not let yourself cry when in pain. You equate vulnerability with weakness. Now you are engaged in an active role of repressing the sensation of pain. You are in control.

Being in control of your sensations and emotions requires you to utilize your own muscles to hold back the energy of expression. Holding on and being strong only activates your muscles to catch this energy. The body then becomes like a sponge that absorbs and holds onto the energy. Once locked in your body, it is very difficult to get out. This energy settles into your muscles and fascia, resulting in hardened tissues.

If you can grieve your hurts, you will ultimately follow nature's guidelines and work to heal. This means to grieve the hurt and pain that you experience and acknowledge your hurt. Seeking comfort and safety will soften you to let go of this energy. Isolation and holding on will only store this trauma within your body.

You were created to experience the entire spectrum of emotions, including sadness, anger, and grief. It is not more mature to learn how to control certain emotions; it is downright foolish. You are only hurting yourself. When you begin to allow yourself to experience all of your feelings, you will stop storing the energy of your emotions and start healing.

III. The Nature of Physical Trauma

There are several forces that affect your body. Not only are you subjected to stress and repression, but you are also affected by physical trauma. The long-term effects of physical trauma are the third aspect of how you lose your body.

From the moment of conception to the present, your body reveals a road map of where you have been and what you have been through. Most accidents, surgeries, falls and collisions are reflected in the body. Even many seemingly insignificant or minor incidents are still seen in your body. The story of your body goes back even farther than your mind wants to remember.

The body is like the metal door panels in a car. Every time you bump your car into a stationary object, the metal is dented. Every time someone else opens his car door into the side of your car, there is a tiny scratch and the paint is chipped. Minor incursions from parking lot bangs to golf ball size hail pelting your roof will reflect the story of your car. Those dents don't just go away by themselves. Unless your car is taken in for repairs, you are hopelessly stuck with multiple dents.

Major car crashes add even more to the dismantling of your car. A head-on collision can severely damage your car while a rollover can destroy your car beyond repair. Major traffic accidents and acts of nature can render your car useless.

Your body remembers its physical trauma as well. A skiing accident when you hurt your hip might be forgotten in your mind, but your body still remembers. A fall on an icy sidewalk is stored in your elbow. Years of collisions while playing competitive high school sports have not just disappeared. These assaults still reside in your body.

The body is like a sponge. In this case, the body is like an energy sponge. Your body has the capacity to store energy or release energy. Most physical assaults to the body end up storing the energy of that experience. Physical trauma occurs when a large amount of energy enters the body in a short period of time.

This is based on a simple principle first outlined by Albert Einstein, $E=MV2$. This formula states that the faster an object is moving and the more an object weighs, the more energy it carries with it. If you fell off a three-story building, you would be more likely to have more serious injuries than if you fell off a one-story building. This is due to the longer distance and faster speed. The faster an object travels, the more energy is produced.

Being hit by a feather pillow most likely would not cause you much harm. There is very little weight or energy behind the impact. Being struck by a 3,000-pound car traveling at 20 miles per hour is another story. This is because there is more weight, thus more energy entering into your body. An object the size of a marble usually would have little impact if it hit you. However, a bullet, about the same size as a marble, being fired from a gun could kill you. This again is because there is a tremendous amount of speed (thus energy) behind the bullet.

Can you remember back to your childhood years growing up? Can you remember some of the times when you were hurt? Every time a baseball hit you in the side or a hockey puck slapped against your forearm, the energy of impact traveled directly into your body. A fall off a skateboard or a body check on the basketball court has also stayed with you. The pounding of an off-road motorcycle race or the collisions of a rugby match all are stored within your body. Your body records every fall out of a tree and every punch by the neighborhood bully.

Imagine taking a hammer and pounding the side of your house. One stroke starts to make a small hole. You raise the hammer up again and strike it against the wall. Again and again you strike until there is a very large hole in the wall. The wall has absorbed the energy of the hammer. The bigger the hammer, the greater amount of energy released and the bigger the hole becomes.

The body is no different. The bigger the impact, the more energy your body absorbs. The faster the collision occurs the more energy of impact is absorbed. Single physical assaults on the body are one way the body stores energy. Continuous assaults that are repeated are also ways for energy to be absorbed. Playing football one day might not be significant. Imagine all of the impacts from playing football in high school, in college and then professionally. Every practice and game adds to the body's trauma.

This impact trauma might be the equivalent of running as fast as you can and throwing yourself at your garage door. Try doing this 30 times a day, every day, for years on end. That impact will surely begin to be felt in your body.

It is no wonder that many professional athletes find it difficult to walk after retirement. Surveys show that the life expectancy for an ex-professional football player is much less than the average person. Current statistics show that the average life expectancy for a retired professional football player is fifty-five years of age—fifty-two if he were a lineman. These former players also suffer from a host of other major maladies—such as depression or Alzheimer's disease.

Many want to blame arthritis for their knee pain. Back stiffness is commonly attributed to old age. This is not nature's reality. In many cases, your sponge of a body has absorbed as much impact energy as it can store. Physical symptoms eventually begin to manifest themselves. Physical trauma has taken its toll and is still alive in your body.

Your Body's Story

What is the story of your body? What kind of physical traumas have you been through? Your body tells a story if you were only to listen. Most people do not just throw their back out one day. Their back has been wound very tightly from years of holding and by a history of physical trauma that has never let go. When a back does go out, it is like the last straw that breaks the camel's back. Reaching for a can of soup high on the shelf is not the culprit. Perhaps a whole history of physical trauma is to blame. A body wound so tight by impact requires only a tiny twist to set it off into complete spasm.

Your memories may be short in your mind but not so in your body. The body remembers and tells your entire story. Hips that do not swivel might reflect an old trauma. A slight limp or difficulty getting up out of a chair may have more to do with an auto accident that occurred twenty years earlier than you might imagine.

Begin to identify your body story by drawing a timeline of the most important physical events that you can remember. You will be surprised at what you remember. There might be single past events, such as a car crash, or repeated assaults on your body from competitive high school sports.

Whiplashes and skiing accidents do not just go away by themselves. Your falls and accidents become ways in which your body stores the energy of the impact, like the hammer hitting the wall. Just because you may not be able to see the wound all of the time does not mean that there is not any damage.

When we are treated for an injury, we are most often treated by a medical system versed in Newtonian philosophy. Wounds are cleaned to prevent bacteria from harboring. Broken bones are splinted. Severe bleeding is stopped and arteries are sewn back together.

However, this is only the beginning of the healing. Unfortunately, most people are unaware of the long-term effects of physical trauma once the bleeding stops and the bones are set in place. Now it is important to follow the guidelines of nature and heal the energy dynamics of your physical trauma. In the present Western medical system, this is seldom attempted. Once the bandages are taken off, most people falsely believe that they are healed and back to normal. Unfortunately, they are mistaken.

Look at your body as a metaphor. You may feel as if there were a knife in your back, a flame in your hip or a noose around your neck. Perhaps there is so much pressure in your head that you feel like you are wearing a helmet that is too tight. Draw a picture of your body story to get a clearer picture of what is going on.

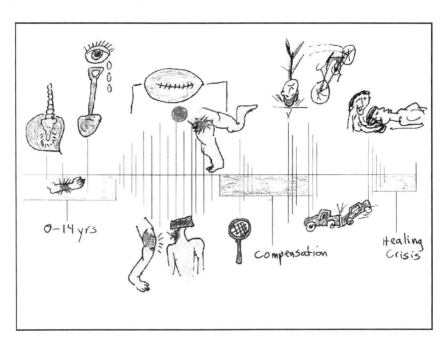

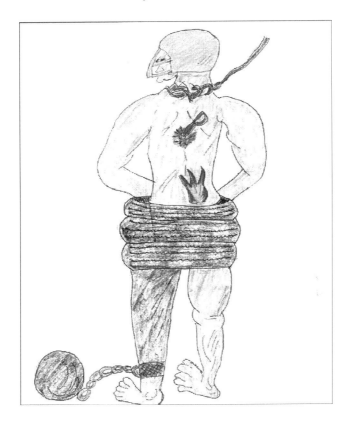

Michael's Story

Michael was a very active child. He played all kinds of sports growing up. He fell off his bicycle from time to time. He bumped into trees. He slipped in the wet street while playing touch football. By the time he was ten years old, his young body, like a sponge, had absorbed many assaults to several different areas of his body. In those areas, Michael had stored a tremendous amount of energy from physical trauma.

The chief energy intrusion occurred when Michael was a junior in high school. He was a star basketball player on the varsity squad. One day, while reaching up to grab a rebound in a game, an opponent unknowingly was positioned underneath him. As Michael came down with the rebound, he was "low-bridged." Michael's feet never hit the floor. The first part of his body to contact the floor was Michael's back and left hip.

A gasp went through the crowd followed by an uneasy silence. Everyone wondered if Michael was all right. He lay on the floor without moving. You could see the grimace on his face. The coaches and trainers rushed over to his aid. He lay there for a few minutes, obviously in agony. Soon he was helped off the court. The fans cheered, thinking he must be fine since he was walking.

Michael missed the next week of practice and the following three games. The medical doctors examined him and told him that he had only suffered a bruised hip. There was no other damage that showed up on the x-ray. He was relieved that he would be able to play soon.

Michael's game never completely returned to top form. He was a little hesitant to extend his body out fully. In fact, this was just the beginning of a whole series of major injuries that plagued Michael for many years to come. Despite the clean bill of health from his medical doctors, Michael had experienced a significant physical trauma to his body.

Just because nothing was broken did not necessarily mean there was no damage. Michael's left hip remained in spasm. The fascia tissue began to shorten and harden around this area. This is a process that takes many years. The sensation of pain had been numbed, so Michael did not feel the hardening of fascia. The connecting fascia around his left knee had additional strain on it. In fact, Michael later began to have problems around his left knee. He sprained his left ankle several times before his basketball career was finished. This was only the beginning.

At age 30, Michael began to feel old. His back went out for the first time. Michael assumed that he was just not getting enough exercise, but that was not the case. The muscles on the left side of his body, from his ankle to his neck, had been shortened. The surrounding fascia had hardened and was glued together. He was twisted from the inside out. Michael could not get out of bed without grimacing and felt frustrated and angry that his body had given out on him. He blamed everyone and everything, including his doctors.

This traumatic fall during a basketball game is still alive and well in Michael's body. Over time, a series of compensations had been made to adjust to the many spasms created. There were some areas of significant energy storage where the energy cysts remained. The point of impact during his fall spread out like octopus tentacles throughout his body. With traditional Western medicine and therapy, he would be condemned to live with this physical trauma. This is because a Newtonian view of the world, which the Western medical system is based on, does not address how energy is stored in the body. Only a system based in nature can help to heal Michael.

How to Heal with Nature

After any accident, it is important to rule out any life-threatening damage. This includes severed arteries, broken bones, head trauma and serrated nerves. A molecule-based medical system does this best.

However, after any life-threatening condition has been stabilized, it is important to begin to heal with nature. The energy of impact remains with you long after the bruises disappear. There is a memory of injury that may persist for your entire lifetime. If you watch animals in nature, you will get a better grasp on how to heal.

After an animal experiences physical trauma, it usually shakes or wiggles itself out. This is a way to begin to disperse the energy of impact. Watch a dog run around in the back yard. If it slips and falls down, it will immediately get up and shake itself out before it continues to run around.

The secret is to activate the muscles associated with physical trauma as soon as possible after the trauma occurs. This is what animals do. Remember that your body is like a sponge and absorbs and stores energy in your soft tissue. By activating the muscles of impact soon after a trauma, you are preventing these muscles from storing a memory of trauma.

Muscles need to feel safe to work properly. When you experience physical trauma, your brain and nervous system do not believe that it is safe to move. They transfer this message to the muscles themselves, indefinitely freezing the muscles and nervous system.

If you can move the area of impact gently as soon as possible after the trauma, you start to teach the nervous system and the muscles that it is safe to move. The muscles do not have to hold on. Moving in a gentle and conscious manner will start to release the memory of impact.

When immobilized for long periods of time, you begin to lose sensation to an area. The brain and nervous system cut off nerve sensation to the frozen areas. H. David Coulter writes in *Anatomy of Hatha Yoga,* "Without movement, the awareness of touch disappears."

Notice a modern low speed car bumper made out of high-tech plastics. When bumped by another car at low speed, there will be no damage. The bumper will bounce back to nearly perfect shape. The energy of impact has been released. This is what you should be doing with your own body.

Because of the training of medical first responders and the policies of insurance companies who are afraid of lawsuits, many remain frozen in the impact trauma. For instance, if you are involved in a car crash, you will be immobilized and strapped down by an ambulance crew. There will be a collar put around your neck, and your head will be taped to a backboard. This action is a result of aggressive insurance company policies designed to prevent lawsuits if someone has a broken neck and is further injured by the medical response team.

You remain immobilized in a hospital bed for hours or days. You are reminded to be still. Constrictive devices are placed around your neck to prevent movement. All the while the memory of impact is becoming cemented into your nervous system and your musculature.

Every now and then when someone's neck is actually broken, this treatment is helpful. However, this is a rare occurrence and the vast number of people who experience this treatment will suffer further damage from this immobilization years later. Most people are further traumatized by the medical system because the energy of impact begins to settle in their body when they are immobilized. An animal found in nature would want to move the energy outward. We are taught to hold on to it.

Whenever you apply a cast to a body part, you attempt to immobilize that part so the area can heal. This is how a broken bone is set. While well intended, this approach often leads to the storage of the trauma memory, as well as a blockage in the flow of energy.

Sue was one of my clients who broke her femur in a car accident when she was ten years old. She had a cast placed on her leg from the bottom of her foot to the top of her hipbone. The cast was eventually removed, and Sue believed she was healed. Years later her back started to go out on her. When I began to work with her, I touched her leg and made a startling discovery. I told Sue that her previously broken right leg still felt like it had a cast on it.

The right leg was shorter than the left one. The muscles and the fascia on the right leg were much denser and harder, as there was less energy running through it. The physical cast may have been removed, but there was still an energetic cast on her leg. This helped to explain why she always felt so heavy and dead on her right side.

Muscles Hold On

When you are involved in a physical trauma, your muscles initially hold on. Whether it is a sudden fall or a collision with another car, your muscles grip in fear. These muscles then remain contracted around the areas of impact.

For instance, if you are driving and are hit from behind, your head is jerked forward and backward. The muscles in the back of your neck activate in a split second and try to catch your head. As a result, these muscles become "traumatized." They catch and hold on. This is commonly referred to as "whiplash."

Unfortunately, these muscles may not let go right away, or ever. There is a memory here of impact. The muscles still believe they are needed to protect your head from injury. They still believe that there is an accident occurring in this moment, although twenty years may have passed since the original trauma. Without the proper treatment, the memory of impact stays with you for a long time.

We engage the muscles around an injury as if we were creating a cast. Unfortunately, many years later the mind is still telling the muscles to hold on and our cast is still very much alive. If you follow nature's guidance and move the muscles of impact gently as soon as possible after a physical trauma, you will eliminate the memory in this area. Gentle movements are best at first. What this does is to teach the muscles that were impacted that it is safe to let go now.

Terry was involved in three car accidents over a five-year period. She was hospitalized for brief periods after each accident. Today, Terry suffers from a stiff neck and tight shoulders. In Terry's experience, her muscles and nervous system still believe that the accidents are currently happening. Nobody told the muscles that the accidents have passed and that it is safe to let go. Terry is frozen in a moment from the past. Her muscles activated to protect her from injury and have not let go since.

This does not always have to be the case. A stuntman can jump out of a moving car at forty miles per hour and not even suffer a minor scratch. When he hits the ground, he rolls and tumbles like a beach ball. Many of us slip and fall on the sidewalk and break our hip and have back problems for the rest of our lives. What is the difference?

The stuntman believes that the ground is his friend and does not tighten up as he falls. He just rolls with the movement and does not attempt to stop or impede the energy of his fall. He allows his body to be relaxed and flows with the movement. In this manner, the energy of his impact just flows right through him.

When you unexpectedly slip on the sidewalk, you tighten up every muscle in your body. You contract and hold on. The impact will store the energy within you. There is very little release of energy. Your mind fearfully causes you to go into contraction and you end up storing the energy of the fall. This energy then resides in you as if your body were a sponge soaking up water. The stuntman remains relaxed as he falls, rolling through the fall. He is much less likely to hold on to any residual physical trauma. He does not tighten up around the impact. This is quite different than how most of the rest of us experience a fall.

The same could be said if you were in an automobile accident with a drunken driver. You are much more likely to die or be seriously injured. This is because you are much more likely to tighten up and catch the energy of the impact that enters into your body. Within a very short time frame, seconds or fractions of seconds, you can absorb a tremendous amount of energy into your body as the car that you are riding in collides with another car. Your body becomes like a sponge and collects the energy of the impact. Your muscles activate to grab on to this energy. All of your bodily systems are threatened and your life may be in danger.

A drunk driver will not have time to tighten up and repress this energy. This is due to the fact that his nervous system is impaired and reacts very slowly. He is much more likely to walk away with far fewer injuries because he did not repress or store the energy of the impact. The energy just passes right through him as his muscles and nervous system are sluggish and cannot react quickly enough to grab on.

Muscles experiencing physical trauma, just like in repression and stress, grab on and prevent the energy of the body from flowing. A muscle that remains in contraction for an extended period of time will cause the fascia to harden and dry out. This results in a diminished flow of energy through the body.

A young boy who is hit in the groin by an elbow or a plastic baseball will contract the muscles of his genitals, perhaps for the rest of his life. The muscles learn to hold on to protect him from another blow of extreme pain. He subconsciously pulls his hips and genitals in to ensure safety. This initial physical trauma can have far reaching consequences many years later.

A good example of the similarity between repression and physical trauma is to look at the physical body. If you were to engage in a series of contact sports day in and day out, such as high school football, you would experience numerous blows to your body on a daily basis. Usually, one blow is not enough to do any serious damage. Over time, you might awaken with a sore back or a stiff neck (even years later) because of all the energy that you have stored. This is the result of repeated physical traumas.

This is the same as a child repressing his tears for many years. Energy is stored over time. The child might use his own muscles to repress the energy of emotion. This is very similar to how many use their own muscles to hold on when experiencing physical traumas.

Physical trauma does not have to be a careless or unexpected accident. Physical trauma can also be a well thought out surgery or medical procedure. The act of cutting into the body can cause just as much physical trauma as any car accident. A surgeon's scalpel or needle puncture can create trauma to the body just as easily as a car accident. Think of every time you have been jabbed and poked by medical needles when receiving shots or having blood drawn. The body does not distinguish between an accidental trauma and an intentional one.

Peter's Story

Peter was a young eight-year-old boy. He developed a tumor on his pancreas. The medical doctors decided to cut out the tumor as his treatment protocol. While certainly trying to help Peter, they ended up causing him many more problems throughout his lifetime.

Since Peter was still a young boy, he was continually growing. The surgery might have prevented the cancerous cells from spreading, but it also created a great amount of scar tissue. As Peter kept growing, the scar tissue was pulling on his spine. By the time Peter reached full maturity, he had a significant curvature of his spine. The scar tissue from the surgery had created enough physical trauma to Peter's body to prevent the spine from growing straight.

A pronounced scoliosis pattern had developed in Peter's spine over time. This was so significant that he was in physical danger. The medical doctors wanted to insert a metal rod into his spine. As an adult, Peter had to come to terms with a body that had been physically traumatized by a medical system.

Gerald's Story

Another example of how surgery can result in significant future consequences is Gerald's story. Gerald noticed one day that his leg was swelling. Twenty-two years prior, he had a several veins surgically removed from his leg and grafted to his heart as part of coronary bypass surgery.

The medical exam revealed that Gerald had a blood clot in his leg, which was causing the swelling. This was a major medical emergency.

Gerald spent seven days in the hospital and was given drugs to help dissolve the blood clot.

What Gerald and his doctors did not realize was that his surgery, more than twenty years earlier, had created a physical trauma and scarring to his body. Years later this physical assault showed up as a life-threatening predicament.

Emotions and Trauma

You are better able to let go of the energy of physical trauma if there is adequate comforting when you experience pain. When you are left to deal with the pain alone, you tend to hold on to the pain.

For instance, if you were to receive a cut on your foot and were left alone to be strong and not cry about the pain, you most likely would store that pain within your body. If you were comforted in your pain with hugs and kisses, you more than likely would release that pain.

Dan Kindlon and Michael Thompson describe this phenomenon in *Raising Cain,*

"In a very real way, this tactile sense not only protects us from pain-we withdraw our hand when we feel the heat of a flame-but it also allows us to be comforted, whether it is being cradled by a parent in infancy, caressed by a lover, or touched by a friendly hand on the shoulder when in grief. All kinds of touch result in the release of these natural painkilling opiates. When a child with a skinned knee runs to his mother, her touch not only brings psychological reassurances and the promise of safety, but it also literally helps relieve the pain."

A stubbed toe or a bumped elbow will more likely release the energy of impact if you can cry and scream it out. You are now using your muscles to express the energy of emotion. If you do not do this, you will use your own muscles in order to repress the experience.

Tears are like a faucet that release built-up pressure within the body. Not only are you releasing moisture when you cry, but you are also clearing out stagnant energy. When you cannot grieve, you are doing tremendous harm to yourself. John P. Conger writes in *The Body in Recovery,* "Many people do not know how to work through the losses life brings. Our body faithfully records the traumatic events in contracted musculature and energetically withdrawn tissue."

Learning to grieve is a key element in your healing. Sitting down and reading this book will not teach you how to feel your pain, nor will talking to a professional about your feelings. Taking a workshop will not get you beyond your pain. The only way that you will learn how to feel your feelings is to actually practice experiencing them until it becomes normal to feel everything.

Emotions are very much involved in the physical trauma to your body. If you can grieve your hurt and pain, you are much less likely to hold on to this energy. Grieving activates your surrender state of consciousness where you feel safe and your musculature is softened. The energy of trauma is better able to pass through you.

Candace Pert explains in *Molecules of Emotion,*

"It is this problem of unhealed feeling, the accumulation of bruised and broken emotions, that most people stagger under without ever saying a word, that the mainstream medical model is least effective in dealing with. When people do seek help, often what is offered through mainstream psychology and psychiatry is what I call "talk and dose" therapy of talking and even more pills, which are supposed to make the unacceptable feelings go away. A treatment, yes, but one that really only Band-Aids the symptoms and consigns people to a drug dependency rather than directing them toward an opportunity for really healing feeling."

Unfortunately, most are taught that control is a more important value than letting go of control. When someone dies or there is a family tragedy, it is often heard, "That family is so strong." We see this example played out all of the time, especially through the media. When there is a tragedy we so often hear how "strong" someone is when they hold their emotions inside and they are commended for "holding it all together." Someone who follows nature's guidelines and releases their emotions when a tragedy occurs is said to "break down."

A person committed to being strong when facing trauma more likely will hold on to this energy. He uses his own muscles to grab on to the energy from the physical trauma. When you maintain control you activate your muscles to store the energy of physical trauma.

After a while, the sensation of pain or discomfort is lessened. The area of physical trauma may actually feel better. This is because a numbing effect takes place due to impaired nerve signals. Candace Pert adds in *Molecules of Emotion,* "Repressed traumas caused by overwhelming emotion can be stored in a body part, thereafter affecting our ability to feel that part or even move it." By numbing out an area, we do not have to deal with it.

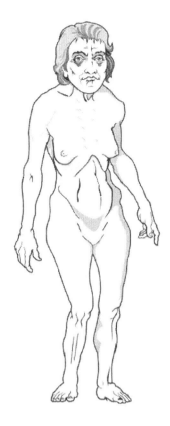

Your Myths Get Stuck in Your Body

Your body carries the story of your life. While your mind may be good at telling lies, your body continues to tell the truth. The mind may have its own unnatural agenda, but the body is like a lie detector. When you examine your body you begin to understand the myths that reside in your head.

What is the "truth"? The truth is not found in a book or religious tradition. The truth is found in nature, not in myths or stories. The farther you get from the intent of nature, the farther you get from the truth. When you forget the truth, you develop false beliefs that trigger your stress response, resulting in frozen energy that is stored in your body. When you deny or try to conquer nature, you take the path away from truth.

Two elderly women are shown side by side in the following picture. One is doing a yoga back bend while the other appears shrunken and compressed. Both are living the myths within their heads. The woman doing the back bend is telling herself the story that expansive movement leads to freedom in her body. Repression and holding on are expressed through the body of the other woman. This is exemplified by the shrunken and twisted woman on the right. Regardless of whether one is rich or poor, male or female, the myths within your head are reflected throughout your body. While the age of these two women might be the same the myths they tell themselves in their heads determines the outcome of their bodies.

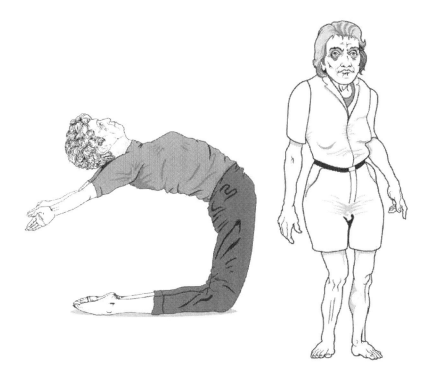

    Myths have become so much a part of every culture that it has become very difficult to distinguish them from the "natural truth." Sam Keen writes in *Your Mythic Journey,* "It is differing cultural myths that make cows sacred objects for Hindus and hamburger meals for Methodists, or turn dogs into pets for Americans and roasted delicacies for the Chinese." Your myths have become your "truths," and in essence, they are often false beliefs that you have come to honor as natural beliefs.

    Many myths begin within your own generation. For instance, there is a common myth that a "hard body" is a healthy body. From an energetic perspective, this is the farthest thing from the truth. A "hard body" usually is nothing more than someone who continues to build layers of "armor" around himself as a way to avoid feelings. Muscles are shortened and tightened while the connective tissue becomes hard and glued together. This type of person develops a suit of armor in the form of tight musculature and is usually frozen in the Fight Response.

The false beliefs that dictate your life may be as innocuous as, "Turn the other cheek and never get angry," or, "Don't let anyone see you lose control." These kinds of beliefs turn you into puppets. You lose your freedom to express who you are, as well as your relationship with the natural world. You become a false self, hiding behind a mask of false beliefs.

A good majority of your myths were created well before you were even born. To demonstrate how a false belief leads to pain in the body and subsequently to addictions, let's look at the religious belief that "the human body is evil." In the 12th Century, Saint Augustine wrote about the evils of the body, most likely because he was not comfortable with his own body or his own sexuality.

James B. Nelson writes in *Embodiment,*

"Of all the Church Fathers, Augustine deserves special comment. His imposing theology was to set the stage for many centuries of Christian thinking, including thought about sexuality (with which Augustine himself had a long and personal struggle).

"Augustine was deeply troubled about the problem of sexual lust and was almost exclusively concerned about genital aspects of human sexuality. Our subjection to the lust of 'concupiscence,' he believed, is a direct result of the Fall. One of the Fall's clear marks is that the genitals are no longer under our voluntary control, and our insatiable search for self-satisfaction (concupiscence) though evident in all spheres of life is particularly evidenced by the genitals' disobedience. Since Augustine sees a clear link between original sin and concupiscence, every sex act is not only directly connected to original sin (for which each of us is responsible) but also binds us more firmly to it."

This false belief was adopted by many different religions over the years and passed down for many generations. I can remember in my own Catholic upbringing that the Church extolled the belief that the body was dirty and that "pure" people never had sex. This is exemplified in the myth of the "Virgin Mary." Even today, some eight hundred years later, many people are still being taught that the body is evil. This is how a "myth" ends up becoming a cultural "truth."

When you experience your natural sexual desire, you may be confronted with the sexuality myths about your body. As a result of this conflict, you often end up repressing your sexual feelings by tightening your own muscles once again, specifically, the muscles around your genitals and inner thighs are held tightly. In this manner you can hold back the energy of sexual expression because you value the myth over nature's desire to release energy. As a result, you might often be plagued by physical manifestations of disease as the energy flow has been impeded.

Another source of Catholic mythology was the *Baltimore Catechism*. The *Baltimore Catechism* was a modern version of the centuries-old Catholic tradition of repressing feelings and bodily sensations. Here is just a brief example:

What are the chief sources of sin?

"The chief sources of actual sin are: pride, covetousness, lust, anger, gluttony, envy, and sloth, and these are commonly called the seven deadly sins."

Nature gave us feelings and sensations for a purpose, including lust and sexual attraction. Nature wants you to feel your sexual feelings. What happens if you are trained and controlled by a cultural myth to repress and deny all sexual feelings? When your sexual feelings arise (and they will), you contract your body in fear of feeling or expressing these feelings. You hold on tightly and falsely believe that your sexuality is the enemy. Instead of questioning the cultural myths you believe, you automatically assume you are wrong to have these feelings.

For instance, many women are taught to believe that they are "bad" because they bleed monthly. This false belief comes from a time-honored male way of thinking that a woman is unclean when she is menstruating. This brings much shame to a woman because she believes she is defective for what happens naturally to her body.

There are many myths surrounding the human body. According to Western cultural myth, a woman's breast should not sag. "The body is a source of corruption" is another one of those beliefs. "To self-pleasure yourself will cause blindness," "sex is dirty" or "all touch is sexual" are other false beliefs. Many young boys are shamed for having a nocturnal emission, or "wet dream." They are told that they are bad and have sinned against

God. They are ordered to repent their sin to a priest and to do penance, even though this is a very natural experience.

There are many false beliefs regarding the ideal body, especially the female body. In America, women are often taught to mold themselves after a Barbie doll, because this is the standard that American society rewards. Many men are taught to be rock solid with strong muscles and inflated chests. The human body continues to be shaped by many age-old myths.

There are many false beliefs about the position of the spine with regard to health and enlightenment. In the Sufi tradition, (considered the mystical branch of the Islamic religion), the way to harmony with the universe is to spin the erect spine in a counterclockwise direction a number of times. In the Catholic tradition, kneeling on one's knees with a straight spine is considered to be the gateway to heaven. One should never cross one's legs in the Catholic mythology. On the other hand, Eastern tradition claims that a crossed-legged position with an erect spine is the way to enlightenment. Being close to the ground is essential; a sagging spine is the equivalent of spiritual failure.

The body has become a journal for the beliefs and prejudices that we carry against it. Your attitudes about your genitals, skin and appearance are reflected in your body. When you cannot express your body's story, your body ultimately manifests that story.

Your muscles stay contracted when you try to mold yourself to honor this story in your mind. Fascia or connective tissue that surrounds your muscles shortens and hardens, which causes pain and stiffness. A man's lower back might become irritated or a woman's monthly period painful because they have learned to deny their sexual feelings and kept their muscles contracted.

Peter Levine says in *Waking the Tiger,* "When a young tree is injured it grows around that injury. As the tree continues to develop, the wound becomes relatively small in proportion to the size of the tree." You do the same thing with your body. You stay contracted around a physical or emotional wound, building layers of protection.

Traumatized muscles develop an imprint or memory of holding on. They still believe that the injury is occurring. When you are under stress or engaged in repression of sensory or emotional experiences, you tighten up areas that have already established a pattern of holding on. Some people refer to these areas as their "weak spots." Most likely these areas are places that have experienced a physical trauma. The memory or imprint of trauma still resides there. When you are experiencing the emotion of fear during the stress response, you might tighten up areas that are already accustomed to being tight.

Your myths become the false beliefs that trigger your stress response. Many times the myths you tell yourself teach you that your feelings and bodily sensations are the enemy. These myths get stored in your body as you try to protect yourself from feeling them. You stand on guard to defend your myths while attempting to destroy your own body.

One Christian myth states that, "It is better to give than to receive." Initiated many hundreds of years ago, this myth is still believed and makes it difficult for many people to receive. They give until they have nothing left to give and their bodies finally wear out. They may feel anger and resentment at not being able to receive. Many people may also be unable to directly express their needs, ending up in conflict due to another myth that anger is one of the seven deadly sins. Now they are stuck repressing their needs and feeling angry inside about it all, while not allowing themselves to express this internalized anger. The body ends up in Fight or Flight as this vicious circle continues.

Feeling anger is often interpreted as an imaginary life-threatening event based on the false belief that people who are angry are "bad." Muscles stay contracted when you are unable to say "No." You might search out addictions to numb your pain. This is the result of a myth created hundreds of years before that you have accepted as a "truth" in your life.

A common myth that gets stuck in the body is the myth that "good boys" and "good girls" are not supposed to say "No!" This false belief stems from religious-based traditions where you are supposed to obey your parents no matter what. Questioning a parent would be like telling the king of a country that he was wrong. Authoritarian systems are set up to keep the power at the level of kings, rulers and often parents.

Matthew was raised as a "good boy." He was not allowed to confront, argue, disagree, get angry, set boundaries or have his needs met. He believed that if he said "No," he would be a bad boy (shame). This false belief began in early childhood and continued throughout his adult years. This belief came to exemplify who he was. If Matthew were to say "No," he falsely believed he would be abandoned and not liked. He avoided all conflicts so as not to have to make a choice.

Matthew physiologically stored a tremendous amount of unexpressed rage in his eyes and neck. The Fight Response that he learned early on was to contract the muscles around his eyes and face, which eventually led to poor eyesight. He also suffered from frequent headaches. Matthew's body took on the anger that he could not express.

In order for Matthew to heal, it was necessary for him to reprogram the false belief that he had in his head regarding his inability to say "No." He had to constantly remind himself of the following messages:
• I'm not bad if I say "No."
• It is normal to say "No."
• I have the right to say "No."
• I will not die if I say "No."

Matthew had to continue to dialogue with his inner thoughts and create a new pattern. He had to learn to breathe deeply, receive bodywork to unblock his frozen musculature, and practice movement awareness work to keep his energy open. He had to go through many tiny deaths in order to heal from this myth that was stuck in his body.

Your myths about how to look and what to feel ultimately become lodged in your body if you are in direct contrast with what is natural. James Prescott, Ph.D., makes a very profound statement during an interview:

[Prescott] "We have to understand that moral, philosophical and theological religious systems become the gate keeper of our sensory experiences, particularly those that involve pleasure and pain."

[Interviewer] "Are you suggesting that our full development as human beings is being limited by the religious traditions of Western Civilization?"

[Prescott] "Yes."
James Prescott Ph.D., *Touch the Future Magazine,* Fall, 1995

Your myths or false beliefs come from many sources. Not only are you bombarded with Christian mythology, other religious traditions also pass their mythologies on.

James B. Nelson writes in *Embodiment,*

"The Christian culture is not the only one to have had problems with sexual alienation and dualisms. It is an unfair oversimplification to assume that only the Christian West has been thus afflicted while so-called primitive cultures and Eastern civilizations have escaped. For example, among the Manus of New Guinea sex was degraded and rigidly controlled. And the frank sexuality of Hindu art says little about the day-to-day sexual

life of the Hindus, which has been governed by strict caste-based rules and prohibitions. Further, in Buddhism, even more explicitly than in many strands of Christianity, the rejection of sex and bodily expressiveness is counted essential to the attainment of freedom. So, the problem is not unique to the Christian story."

Whether from the past or present, your myths often cause you to lose your own body. The myths behind the repression of feelings and sensations become more important than the expression of feelings and sensations. You then trap this energy within your body. It is a direct result of these myths that contribute to a repressive system, loss of self-trust, and many degenerative diseases. What you think about will ultimately change your body. Many times your thoughts are the source of your disease.

Energy wants to flow through you. Myths and false beliefs often cause you to live in a pattern of the stress response because these myths create so many imagined life-threatening events that operate in opposition to the ways of nature. Repression of energy becomes the norm when you allow your myths to guide your life. Only by dismantling your myths will you be able to free up your body. This is how the body-mind connection works.

Stress, repression and physical trauma are the main assaults to the body. They are also the greatest factors in aging. Learning how to bring yourself back into balance begins with creating the tools to remove these patterns from your body and the beliefs in your mind which initiated them. Recovery of the body is the next important step.

Pillar Number Two

Recovery of the Body

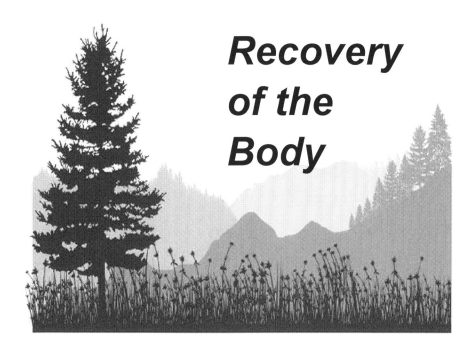

Recovery Through Bodywork

It is often said that your body is a temple. Many people though, wracked with pain and stiffness, feel as if their body is a prison. They feel trapped within a container that does not function to its full capacity. They might feel compressed and lack mobility. It is easy to become depressed because your body hurts. You feel as if you are the rusty old tin man in the movie *The Wizard of Oz*. You accept this decline in the vitality of your body as a natural progression of aging.

This does not have to be the case. You do not have to live life trapped within your own body. You do not have to accept age as the culprit for your decline. You do not have to accept another opinion from a medical professional who says there is nothing to do but accept your pain and live with it. You do need to take action though.

Your belief systems, not your age, are primarily responsible for the loss of your body. Years of reinforcing false beliefs, which helped to cause stiffness and immobility, led to the decay of your body. Much of the time you create your own prison. Many tend to escape into the world of the head, to that of intellectualization or an altered state of consciousness, because it is too painful to live in the body. Your body may continue to rebel against you daily as you become further alienated from it.

An essential part of healing is to recover your body. One of the most profound tools to recover the body is to receive *bodywork*. Your body is the only one that you will ever have. Maintaining its proper function is imperative to growth and well-being.

Mirka Knaster refers to the many bodywork styles as "bodyways" in *Discovering the Body's Wisdom*. She says, "Underlying all the reasons that lead us to bodyways is an instinctive drive toward wholeness. We all also yearn, consciously or unconsciously, to be at peace within the war zone of our own bodies."

What Is *Bodywork?*

Bodywork is a relatively recent term to describe many different techniques that help to remove pain and blockage from the body. Bodywork can be much more than just receiving a massage. Thomas Claire writes in *Bodywork,*

"The term bodywork, *which has only recently come to mean anything other than auto repair, is more encompassing: It includes both traditional massage as well as other approaches to working with the body. Nearly all bodywork practices are united in their common goals of relaxation, pain relief, improved physical functioning, heightened vitality and well-being, and increased awareness."*

Over centuries of attaining beliefs that have moved us away from nature, many people have become disembodied. We have forgotten what is like to have a body. We have left the body behind and moved off into our head. You might only change when you get a painful wakeup call from your body that something is amiss.

The purpose of bodywork is to bring you back into your body. Many people treat their body as if its only purpose is to carry their head around. Your head has become your only reference point for your world. Many have become split off from their body. These individuals have an energetic gap between their head and their body where their neck is. The body has become a foreign oddity. In fact, most people know more about the their cell phone "apps" and where the best sales are in town than about their own body. Most people have very little body intelligence.

When you become removed from your own body, you talk about your body as an "it" or "thing." Your body is no longer part of you but is some separate entity. Body parts are discussed and examined by the medical profession as if they were pieces of an automobile, split off and separate. Skin is referred to as "cutaneous flesh." A bruise is a "hematoma." Arms and legs are referred to as "appendages." When you are removed from nature, your body takes on the language of a cold and inanimate machine. This is the world of mechanized medicine.

Bodywork is an attempt to heal your confused and distorted views of your own body. Many were raised in families and cultures that scorned you for having any pleasurable bodily sensations. You might have been taught that to have a body and to use it consciously was akin to evil. Mirka Knaster writes in *Discovering the Body's Wisdom,*

"Somatics professor Don Johnson recalls growing up in a family in which sensual knowledge was associated with sin. As a small child, he went to sleep at night afraid that he would end up burning in hell for all eternity if he even let his guard down against following his own physical impulses. He remembers being warned, 'If you touch your penis with pleasure, or

enjoy looking at your naked body in a mirror, you're committing a mortal sin, worthy of eternal damnation.'"

Through bodywork you are better able to develop a healthy relationship with your own body. You begin to develop beliefs about your body that do not produce guilt and shame. You start to let go of the distorted beliefs that you were given about your body by experiencing it in a new way. You start to see and feel your body as nature intended.

When you experience bodywork sessions, you begin to receive more information about your body story. A practitioner will touch you in a certain way in a particular area. You become awakened to the sensations in this area. You might begin to learn where you are holding on tightly. The story held within the tissues begins to be released. A bodywork session is like watching a movie of your entire life. All of the events of your life that were never released have been stored within the body. As you lie down on the massage table, your story begins to unfold.

The body is like a sponge. Every car crash or physical assault to your body becomes stored in your tissues. Every emotion that has not been completely released is lodged inside you. All the fear that you have been holding tightly shows up in your muscles and fascia tissue. Just like a sponge soaking up water, your body does the same with the unreleased events in your life.

The human body is more like soft plastic than hardened stone. It is forever changing and molding to the forces that exert pressure on it. You begin to reshape your body when you continue to apply stimulation to it in a positive fashion.

Bodywork begins to heal the damage caused by the three main forces in life—stress, repression and physical trauma. These three forces are the primary reasons that the body rapidly degenerates in the first place. Let's examine them one at a time to see how the role of bodywork can help to reverse their damaging effects.

Stress

Stress is an emotional experience that sends you into a survival state. When you feel threatened by a real enemy, you react with the Fight or Flight Response and this could last for seconds or minutes. In a natural world with a real enemy or danger you enter into a state of relaxation shortly after the danger has passed.

If the danger is only imagined and in your own head, the Fight or Flight Response can last for a very long time, perhaps weeks or even years.

Your body then begins to act as if it is under constant siege, or in a state of war. Only now the enemy is within you. The stress response was designed by nature to be short-lived. Because of your ability to live in your head and remove yourself from nature's rhythms, the stress response often becomes a primary reference point in your daily life.

The long-term effects of stress on your body can be devastating. Not only are you plagued by an increase of stress hormones, you also suffer from other aspects of the Fight or Flight Response. In the Fight Response you hold on tightly. You tighten your muscles as if you were preparing to do battle with an enemy. If you remain frozen in this state of consciousness over time, your muscle tissue continues to shorten, harden, dry out and bond together. The fascia, or "connective tissue proper" as it is often called, forms layers around and between your muscles. When the muscles remain in a constant state of contraction, they bond together in a process called "hydrogen bonding."

Bodywork begins to reverse the hardening effects of the stress response on your muscles and fascia tissue. With hands-on bodywork, areas of holding begin to soften. Fresh blood begins to flow where hardened muscles had previously squeezed the blood flow out. Fascia tissue begins to separate from each other, similar to the separation of strands of string cheese. Bodywork calms your nervous systems and relaxes your warrior body.

Another aspect of the stress response is the Flight Response. This response occurs when you flee from your danger. You could do this in one of two ways: you either run as fast as you can with busy activity, or you leave your body. If you use this part of the stress response to run, you are almost always busy and occupied. Bodywork helps to bring you back into your body and also teaches you to slow down and stop running. You have to be still for a while to receive a treatment. This helps you come to terms with the source of your stress and to slow down long enough to let it go.

If you engage in Internal Flight, bodywork also helps you to come back into your body. When you feel threatened by either a real or imaginary enemy, you often leave your body as a survival strategy. With safe touch you are reminded to come back into your body. Bodywork uses tactile sensation to remind you that it is safe to live in your body.

Bodywork becomes an important tool to reverse the effects of the stress response. You are reminded to come back into your body when safe and skillful hands touch you. Your muscles and fascia tissue are encouraged to relax and repair any damage. As you slow down you no longer feel the need to stay constantly busy to run away from any enemy, either in reality or in your own head.

Repression

Your body is designed to be like a river in nature. Everything is meant to flow through you and be released, such as waste products, emotions and energy. Due to a force in your life called *repression*, this flow is often impeded. It is through the act of repression that you further alienate yourself from your own body. Bodywork becomes an essential tool to begin to dismantle the harmful effects of repression.

Muscles are used for many purposes. They are like tiny motors that provide the force to lift a load. Your muscles shiver uncontrollably on a cold day to keep you warm. Muscles are also used in the expression of emotion. If it were not for your very own muscles, you could not laugh, sing or cheer.

Muscles are also used for another purpose. This purpose is to withhold the expression of emotion through repression. You often use your own muscles to withhold or push down the energy of emotion. When you do this, the energy of emotion does not just go away or disappear but will lodge within the muscles that are used to hold it back. When this happens, you are now suffering from tightened and hardened muscles.

Imagine that you were going to sneeze. You have a belief that it not okay to sneeze. You might believe that it is rude to sneeze because someone told you not to pass your germs around. You might be afraid to make noise because people around you might notice you. You withhold the energy of the sneeze by contracting your own muscles to prevent the sneeze from being released. This is called repression.

Repression also occurs when you try to prevent yourself from vomiting. You can squeeze your esophagus and underlying muscles tightly to prevent the natural expulsion of the vomit. As a consequence, the muscles of repression hold on tightly, far longer than the action of wanting to throw up or sneeze. After a while these muscles will harden and shorten, and perhaps be unable to let go.

A muscle that remains frozen in place is not a healthy muscle. A healthy muscle needs to be able to relax and contract on a regular basis. A muscle frozen in a state of contraction is a muscle that loses its strength and vitality.

Imagine all of the emotions that you do not feel comfortable releasing. It is most likely that you have been practicing the art of repression for some time. Muscles remain hardened wherever you have learned to repress the emotion. This may be around your eyes, jaw or middle of the back.

Bodywork begins to soften the hardened muscles used in repression. Muscles that have been dammed up for years begin to let go. Many times this becomes a very emotional experience for the recipient of bodywork as the emotion that was stuck begins to flow once again. In return, the muscles and soft tissue begin to transform back to a healthy state.

Through skillful bodywork, the body begins to let go of what you have been holding on to. You may feel a sense of relief or a sense of freedom. You can finally take a deep breath as your spine becomes free. Bodywork encourages you to let go. With regular bodywork treatments, the long-term consequences of repression can be reduced and even eliminated.

Physical Trauma

When you experience an impact with another object, either stationary or moving, you experience physical trauma. This can be from a fall off a building, car accident or slip on the sidewalk. The body, acting like a sponge, will absorb the energy of the impact into the muscles and connective tissue. This energy does not necessarily go away by itself.

Bodywork begins to peel away the many layers of wounds in your body. You begin to have sensation in affected areas again. You might begin to live in your body again and not in your head. A body that is in severe agony due to a long history of physical trauma is not one that most people wish to occupy. Bodywork helps you to come back into your body.

I had the opportunity to work with a client who had just broken her neck in a horse riding accident. Shortly after the accident, we were able to release the trauma in her neck before it had a chance to settle into her body. Unfortunately, because of the fear of lawsuits and cautious hospital policies, most people are taped to a backboard and placed in cervical collars or casts soon after a traumatic accident. This just creates immobility and allows the energy to settle into the body even quicker.

As soon as it is safe to move or be touched, treatment should begin. After X-rays and other examination procedures prove negative for spinal fractures, broken bones or other serious injuries, bodywork or gentle movement can begin. When you are not allowed to move after an accident, the energy of the impact begins to settle into your body. While the practice of immobilizing a victim of an accident may help a few people from suffering further injury, most people are harmed in the long run. Years later, after the doctor is either dead or retired, you will continue to suffer from headaches and neck pain because you were instructed to keep still and you begin to imprint the memory of holding on.

Long after the ambulance crew has left, you then begin to suffer from the result of this immobilizing medical treatment. The paramedics, nurses and doctors might think of their job as heroic as they tape trauma victims to a backboard for immobilization, but they could be condemning a person to a lifetime of chronic neck and head pain. An animal that experiences a trauma will get up and shake itself a few times, as if it is shaking the traumatic energy right out of its body. There is less chance of holding on to the energy this way. We ought to learn from animals and nature.

When allowed to settle into the body, this energy will remain with you. This wayward energy makes muscles hard and weakens connective tissue. Because you are first and foremost energetic beings, the energy you receive from any impact is absorbed by your body if not released soon afterward. This energy then is converted into physical abnormalities, like hardened muscle tissue. The longer this energy stays within the body, the more problems that can occur.

Think back and recall every fall or unexpected stubbing of your toe. Recount every car accident or impact with an opponent on the football field. Each one of your traumas creates an exchange of energy. Sometimes you release the energy that comes in. Much of the time the energy of those traumas is stored in the body. Every time you stub your toe on the sofa and hold your breath afterwards, you may be holding onto the energy of the collision with the sofa. These traumas begin to add up, eventually leading to problems in the body.

Bodywork becomes a larger and larger tool to begin to release stored traumas in your body. These physical traumas, while frozen in time, need to begin to move. With varied and consistent bodywork, your body will begin to return to its dynamic and healthy state.

Memories Are Stored in the Body

Your body tells a story. The most truthful part of yourself is not your head, but your body. Your head often lies to protect your false beliefs and distorted view of your natural world. Your body is the greatest source of truth.

When receiving bodywork, it is very common for your stories to reveal themselves. Because a person's whole history is stored in his body, it is not uncommon for one or many different stories to reveal themselves during bodywork treatments. Many times when working with clients, I would touch a certain area and the client becomes startled at the sensations experienced.

The client is unaware of anything until the area is probed. Bodywork tends to wake up these hidden stories.

I have experienced numerous sessions with clients in which we were working on a particular area of their body and a traumatic memory would surface. Kristy was one such client. On one occasion, while receiving an *Intuitive Connective Tissue Bodywork* session, Kristy suddenly remembered the abuse of her ex-husband. As I relieved the tension in the fascia at the base of her neck, she recalled how her ex-husband would assault her by dragging her around by the hair. These memories had been pushed deep down inside. The bodywork provoked the memories to be released. As we worked through the session, we were able to release a long-held story that had settled into the base of Kristy's neck.

In another session, I was working to release the fascia in Kristy's lower back. She began to sense an enormous amount of anger toward her mother. Kristy had allowed her mother to control her life and had a difficult time saying "No" to her. This emotion was stored in her back. As I worked even further on Kristy, she was able to recognize the pattern lodged within her body and eventually release it. Kristy learned that memories, emotions and traumas do settle into the body. She also learned that bodywork could be very useful to help her release this story.

Penny was another client of mine. She was a breast cancer survivor. When we were doing a session of *Intuitive Connective Tissue Bodywork,* Penny began to have a strong reaction. I was working across her upper chest when she began to cry and shake. Her body was letting go of something.

As I began to dialogue with Penny, she revealed that she was reliving the moment in her life when her father had died. She was remembering when she was thirteen years old. Penny recalled having to be strong for her mother. Neither she nor her mother shed any tears at the loss of her father. Penny had kept it all inside. The energy of grief had settled into her chest, many believe leading to breast cancer years later. By working with the fascia tissue in this area, Penny was releasing this pent up emotion. The dam of emotions was finally being released. The long-held grief was finally coming out through the bodywork session.

Your life stories are revealed in your body. All of the memories and traumas that you do not completely release become stored within you. Bodywork begins to release your stories, even stories that have been hidden for a very long time. Bodywork becomes the instrument in which you can play your story out.

What Is a Healing Crisis?

There is a seldom-understood reaction to bodywork and other types of growth work called a "healing crisis." This reaction is indicated by a state of chaos or confusion as you change and release old information in your body. Many people experience this without even realizing it.

As you go through life, you create layers of protection around your body. You form habitual ways of moving to reinforce your stiff joints. You become accustomed to your way of experiencing the world. An old injury may be surrounded by built up muscle and hardened fascia tissue. When you begin to release some of this stiffness and tension in your body, you may enter into a phase where your body is "readjusting" itself. Bodywork can be one of the tools to help bring you to this place of readjustment. You enter into a healing crisis when the layers of physical and emotional armor begin to be swept away and you begin to feel what lies beneath. It is almost as if you are experiencing the old wound, either physical or emotional, for the very first time. It feels that real.

The body is like an onion. There are many layers. When you experience a wound, either a physical trauma or an emotional upheaval, this wound is stored in layers of your body tissues. When you begin to experience some types of bodywork, you may start to release many of those layers. As you do so, your normal way of experiencing your world becomes altered. This is almost as if you are peeling an onion in your kitchen and reach a layer that is not so appetizing. The layer of the onion looks and feels decayed and dried out. Bodywork can have a similar effect on your body.

This is what happened with Penny as I helped to release the grief held across her chest. Her body shook and trembled as a way to let the story out. The bodywork released a series of hardened layers of fascia tissue. As a result, an old and unresolved emotional wound was exposed. As Penny shook and cried for a few minutes, this layer of wounding was attempting to release itself.

The healing crisis can last for minutes or months. I have had clients who felt "off center" for weeks at a time. Others passed through the times of instability fairly quickly. Bodywork can be an instrumental tool to assist you in your growth and in letting go of the stories that plague you. The healing crisis may be a side effect to your work with your body that needs to be considered.

In another instance, Terry and I had just finished a very powerful bodywork session. I gave her what I call a *Kundalini Massage*. This massage is designed to release the blocked energy along her spine. A week later, Terry recanted her story of what happened to her after the session.

Terry had a normal pattern of not sleeping very well at night. She always had a difficult time falling asleep, and she woke up early in the morning to start her day. She did not feel safe when sleeping, so her body did not let go very easily.

Terry fell asleep that night after the *Kundalini Massage* and did not wake up for two straight days. She did not wake up to hear the telephone ring or to use the bathroom. She thought it was a joke when she finally did wake up and went to the front door to retrieve her newspaper. She found two newspapers waiting for her. Only after making several telephone calls did Terry finally realize that she had fallen into a very deep sleep for two straight days.

What happened to Terry is not uncommon. As you receive bodywork sessions and other growth oriented work, your body will often do strange things as it attempts to readjust. In Terry's case, she needed to go into a "semi-coma" for two straight days in order to integrate the bodywork that she had received. The *Kundalini Massage* was just the instrument to dissolve many layers of holding. I often find that people feel a sense of fatigue after different bodywork sessions, especially *Intuitive Connective Tissue Bodywork*. The side effects can be varied and diverse with each individual.

Some people experience sensations of freedom or release after bodywork. Others feel more pain in other areas as their body shifts about. Some people report a sense of giddiness or childlikeness. Still others feel confused and off balance for a few days.

It is common for some people to feel much worse before they begin to feel better. The body, being like an onion, releases several layers during bodywork sessions. Other layers may tighten up to compensate for these releases. I have known several clients who actually were hospitalized with different ailments as their body shifted and readjusted itself. The bodywork did not cause the ailment that sent the person to the hospital. The bodywork only released the layers that had held the issue in place.

One example of this comes from a bodywork session with Fred. Working with the *Intuitive Connective Tissue Bodywork* method, I released the fascia around Fred's kyphotic back (he had a very rounded back). He had an extreme curvature in his spine. The session was very successful as I helped to lengthen Fred's spine.

The next morning Fred could barely move. His pre-existing gout had flared up. The bodywork session had opened him up so much that a repressed disease process was surfacing. The bodywork did not create Fred's gout. The bodywork only released many layers that were holding the gout in place.

Bodywork of all sorts can be utilized as a powerful tool to repair damage to your body and release pre-existing trauma patterns. Bodywork can also send you into short-term chaos as you heal and repair. The healing crisis is not something to fear or avoid. The healing crisis is a way to let nature heal your body. Removing the blockages that hold you in place allows nature to bring deeper issues to the surface that might require healing. When you heal with nature bodywork becomes essential. A healing crisis may follow as you let nature take its course.

Fred's Bodywork Session

Single Session Only

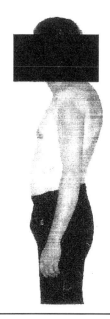

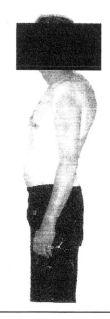

Before *Intuitive Connective Tissue* Session

After *Intuitive Connective Tissue* Session

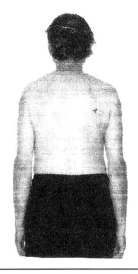

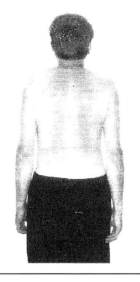

Before *Intuitive Connective Tissue* Session

After *Intuitive Connective Tissue* Session

Why Be Touched?

Touch is essential to your life. Touch is something that we all want and need but often take for granted. Bodywork not only employs specific hands-on techniques to begin your body transformation but also allows you to receive a safe form of human contact. Without touch you might feel starved.

The editors of *Prevention Magazine* write in *Hands-On Healing* about touch,

"It generally feels good to have another human being's skin come in contact with our own. Touching can reassure us, relax us, comfort us or arouse us like nothing else. In a way, the importance of touch is so basic that we tend to take it for granted, just as we do breathing. Or, if we're really forced to think about touch, we may blather something like, 'It generally feels good . . .'"

Your skin is the primary sense organ involved with touch and is the largest recognized organ in your body. The skin is your tactile playground. The skin is embedded with thousands of sense organs, from pleasure to pain, and hot to cold. One of the ways that you perceive whether or not your world is a safe place is through contact with your skin.

Deane Juhan writes in *Job's Body,*

"Skin and brain develop from exactly the same primitive cells. Depending upon how you look at it, the skin is the outer surface of the brain, or the brain is the deepest layer of the skin."

When you are touched, you receive information about your world. Without safe touch, you often tend to disassociate from your body, losing your sense of perception with your external world. When you are touched frequently in a safe fashion, this message is then transferred to your brain. You can relax and let your guard down. You feel safe in your world. Without this peripheral stimulation of your skin, your brain and belief systems are often caught up in the thought that the world is not a safe place. Being touched helps to make you feel safe.

Can you remember what unsafe touch feels like? When you share an armrest with a stranger on an airplane, notice how much muscle contraction is used to keep him away. Bumping into a stranger on a street corner often brings you into hyper-alert status. A physical or sexual assault most certainly causes your body to go into panic.

Now recall times when touch was safe. Can you recall what it felt like to pet a soft puppy in your lap? What does a lover's embrace feel like? A nurturing massage is most often a way to experience safe touch.

What were your first experiences with touch as you came into the world? Were you poked and pricked with sharp and cold medical instruments? Were you banished to an incubator or crib for long periods to fend off the world by yourself? These early memories of touch, or lack thereof, can still be instrumental in your attitude toward touch today.

Touch is food for us. In a natural world, following the laws of nature, touch is essential for survival. Thomas Claire writes about the benefits of touch in *Bodywork,*

"Ashley Montagu, anthropologist and author of the acclaimed text, Touching, *has shown that soothing, nurturing touch is essential to life. Newborn animals must be licked by their mothers if they are to survive; rats that are petted grow faster and develop greater immunity to disease than those that are not. Touch deprivation can be devastating. Victorian mothers, schooled in the emerging science of hygiene, maintained a respectful distance from their offspring with horrifying consequences: In the nineteenth century, more than half of all infants died within the first year of life from what was simply and tragically called "wasting away."*

The laws of nature are very clear. Touch is not an option; it is critical to your survival. Those working close to animals and the land already know this. Deane Juhan states it very clearly in *Job's Body,* "Animal breeders, farmers, veterinarians, and zoo-keepers all concur that the new animal must be licked if it is to live."

When you align yourself with the laws of nature, touch plays an instrumental role in your health and well-being. The editors of *Prevention Magazine* take it a step further. They quote Dr. Suomi, "Look at primitive cultures—they're all very touch-oriented," he says. "If you want to go further back and look at the higher primates (the closest biological relatives to humans), in every single species contact plays a very powerful role."

Animals of all sorts are constantly involved in touch. Dogs cuddle together for comfort. Chimpanzees hold and caress each other. Even wild and ferocious animals like lions and hyenas sleep in a pack with their bodies in contact with each other.

If this were not enough to convince one of the importance of touch, Deane Juhan writes in *Job's Body,*

"Margaret Mead made a study of two New Guinea tribes that throws some light on this influence of touch in such markedly different cultural circumstances. The members of the Arapesh tribe take great delight in children, and fondle them regularly; an infant is rarely out of someone's arms. The mother carries it in a sling around her body all day long, regardless of her activities, and if she is absent for any length of time she is careful to devote enough attention to the child upon her return to make up for the lost hours. Nursing continues three to four years, and mealtime is a happy affair to both mother and baby, with nuzzling, tickling, rocking, sucking, playful pats, and laughter being usual parts of the ritual."

According to Margaret Meade, the conclusion to all of this tactile stimulation is the following.

"The result is an easy, gentle, receptive unaggressive adult personality, and a society in which competitive or aggressive games are unknown, and in which warfare, in the sense of organized expeditions to plunder, conquer, kill, or attain glory, is absent."

In sharp contrast, Meade also explored a tribe to the south of the Arapesh called the Mundugamors. They did not have the same kind of joy with children. There is almost a harsh treatment of children and infants. As a result, Meade recants in *Job's Body,* "The Mundugamors are an aggressive, hostile people who live among themselves in a state of mutual distrust and uncomfortableness."

Safe touch is essential for your life. Bodywork can be an important tool in which to feed you with human contact. Your sensual self becomes fulfilled. Your contact with others is reinforced. You do not feel alone in the world when you are touched. Your ability to let your guard down when you are touched becomes a vital component in your life to help you feel safe. You feel connected and able to trust others more when you receive regular physical contact. Safe touch becomes just as important as proper nutrition when it comes to your development.

The best medicine that you can give someone is touch. Many who own animals already know this. Petting a dog or cat tends to help one relax. Sleeping with animals at night gives many the sense that they are not alone. In fact, most adults prefer to sleep with another person because it helps them feel safe at night when contact is made.

It has even been shown that touch can help an infant to grow faster. Thomas Claire writes in *Bodywork* about the research of Dr. Tiffany Field, Ph.D., at the University of Miami Medical School, " . . . premature infants who received massage treatments for fifteen-minute periods per day for ten days gained 47 percent more body weight than infants treated with standard therapy."

Touch brings reassurance. Your primal roots long for touch. Touch is natural. In a post-industrialized sterile society, many have forgotten about the importance of touch. Touch will bring you back to yourself and to your natural roots. Bodywork becomes an important element in your return to nature.

Myths of the Body

Nature holds the truth. Weather changes daily based on fluctuations in atmospheric pressure. Earthquakes make mountains rise up and floods bring loose soil back down to the sea. Seasons change at regular intervals as the earth's axis of rotation shifts. Nature continues to display its own fundamental truth.

When you follow the laws of nature, you find your own truth within your body. The mind may lie and create many convoluted stories to unravel, but the body always tells the truth. You cannot fool nature without adverse effects. The same holds true with the human body. You cannot continue to lie about what is happening in your body without severe consequences. When you listen to the story that your body is telling, you begin to recognize the truth about yourself. The body is constantly changing, as is the world around you.

Most people are in complete denial of their body issues. They seek painkillers to eliminate an issue the body is trying to release. They numb themselves out because they are too busy to listen to the messages that the body is attempting to tell them. Many deaden any adverse sensations because they believe it is more important to hold it all inside.

You live in a constant sea of change. Every day your cells are dying off and being replaced by new ones. You are not the same person you were just last week. Your body is constantly being reshaped and molded every day by the forces around you.

A popular myth is that you change for the worse as you age. Most people are taught to believe that you will contract, stiffen, shrink and lose your eyesight as you age. This is not true. This belief is a false belief stemming from a culture in denial about the body. Bodywork can help you change how your body ages and change your beliefs about your own body.

It is not the accumulation of years or your parents' genetic history that affects you most as you age. It is the effects of stress, repression and physical trauma that create the greatest assaults to your body every day. Denial of these three forces leads to a very old and degenerated body very quickly. *Age* is not the culprit; *how you age* determines who you are.

You may stiffen as you age because you have an old injury to a hip that was never released. The energy of this physical trauma has settled into your hip and made the fascia tissue glue together over time. This is not about age. This is about energy that was never released from your body and about the mind never letting the story go. Bodywork is a marvelous tool to begin to release this blockage from the body; freedom of movement can result.

Many people shorten as they age. This too has very little to do with age itself. What is really happening is that the effects of stress (I do not feel safe) tend to keep the muscles along the spine and front of the chest in contraction for long periods of time. Eventually, these muscles shorten and harden like a vice being cranked tighter each day. Over time, the skeleton has to curl forward as the compression continues.

Bodywork can prevent this from happening as well. Many types of bodywork attempt to reverse the effects of a lifetime of holding on to muscles. I have worked on many people as they lengthened and regained their youthful posture. Age is no barrier. I have worked with several clients in their mid-seventies who gained significant amounts of length and flexibility while working with bodywork techniques.

Many have accepted the loss of their body as a normal aspect of aging. You are told to slow down to prevent injury and that old people are supposed to be frail. Bodywork begins to change all of this. After receiving many bodywork sessions you will begin to reverse much of the effects of stress, repression and physical trauma. This is true no matter how old you might be.

Changing your beliefs about your body is the first step. Letting go of your body myths helps bring you back in balance with nature. The body is not a machine to be conquered, just as nature is not a force to be denied. When you heal with nature, you use bodywork techniques to help you return to the rhythm of nature.

Specific Bodywork Techniques

People often ask, "What is the best bodywork technique for my particular condition occurring in my body right now?" There are hundreds of different bodywork techniques. There are many variations of each technique because each practitioner interprets the work differently. There are some important questions to ask before beginning bodywork treatments. Here are a few of these important questions:

- What are my expectations?
- What have other people's experiences been like?
- How much time am I willing to devote to a series of bodywork treatments?
- How much money am I willing to spend for treatments?
- Do I feel comfortable with a certain practitioner?
- What are my issues with my body?
- How comfortable am I being touched?
- Do I work with a man or a woman?

There are many different types of bodywork—deep, intermediate, light, off the body, and integrative (using more than one technique). Every bodywork technique works on a different level. Some techniques address the client by attempting to free up the lymphatic system. Other styles palpate the muscles to bring circulation to an area for healing. Still others attempt to move energy through a brittle and dried out layer of fascia.

There are many styles, techniques and approaches. One particular style or technique may not solve all of your body issues. The body systems are interrelated in an elaborate way. Perhaps several styles over a period of time might be more beneficial to address the complexity and inter-connectedness of your body.

The following pages give a brief synopsis of a few different bodywork styles. These represent only a small sampling of the many various techniques available.

Swedish Massage

Swedish massage is probably the most well known of all massage styles. This type of massage attempts to increase circulation, nourish muscles and stimulate nerves through a series of long and short strokes. Oil or lotion is used to help create a lubricating effect. Joints become more mobile, and the Fight or Flight Response (your reaction to stress) is reduced. The hopes are that by relaxing the person and bringing nourishment to the cells, the body and mind will be renewed.

Reflexology

Another example is the practice of Reflexology. This technique stimulates the feet, hands and ears for the purpose of releasing energy in particular organs, glands or other body parts. For instance, by pressing on the center of the underside of the big toe, it is thought that one is able to create a reaction in the pituitary gland of the brain. It is not yet known how or why this works, whether nerves are linked or meridian channels follow the same pathways. From my own experience, I have been able to relieve the symptoms of severe migraine headaches on clients simply by pressing on a client's toes.

Reiki

Reiki is an ancient technique thought to originate in Tibet more than ten thousand years ago. This is a technique of "laying on of hands" that helps to open up the energy flow of the recipient. Thomas Claire writes in *Bodywork,*

"Practitioners draw on two techniques: They can place their hands over key areas of a receiver's body, where the principal organs and glands are located (these areas correspond to the chakras, or subtle energy center, of esoteric tradition), or they can visualize special symbols, enabling them to send healing energy, even at a distance. Hands-on touch can be combined with visualization in a bodywork session for a particularly powerful effect."

Craniosacral Therapy

Unbeknownst to most people, the body has a fluid pulse that expands and contracts every six to twelve seconds. This pulse affects the bones, nerves and organs within the body. Based on the movement of cranial fluid leaving the brain, the blockage of this rhythmic flow of fluid often leads to many complications in the body. Craniosacral therapy is designed to help in correcting these imbalances.

This is a very gentle yet profound bodywork technique. There is very little pressure applied to the specific body area (only about five grams of pressure). When the balance of fluid flow returns, patients report phenomenal results. Practitioners of craniosacral therapy are extremely sensitive with their touch and have a tremendous amount of patience. Those who suffer from an assortment of complaints, including headaches or jaw pain, seem to find this technique extremely helpful. This is also a very useful technique to use on young children. Any remaining childbirth traumas can be released before they lead to further complications.

Intuitive Connective Tissue Bodywork

One bodywork technique that I have created myself is called *Intuitive Connective Tissue Bodywork*. This technique melts and molds the fascia in the body. I have seen some dramatic results with this work. Skin returns to normal from years of aging and sagging. Dark spots are removed as the energy is returned to a long stagnant area. Scars and burns melt away over time. Chronic stiffness and pain are gone as the dried out fascia returns to its fully functioning vitality. The results are remarkable.

I have worked with many clients utilizing the *Intuitive Connective Tissue Bodywork* style. I have witnessed a severely crooked spine straighten after several sessions. Necks have lengthened, frozen shoulders have loosened, and headaches have been relieved.

Working with fascia becomes an important aspect of conducting bodywork sessions. This bodywork style is very different than working with muscles in a Swedish massage. It is through the fascia, or sometimes called *connective tissue proper*, that energy is thought to travel in the body. When the energy channels through the body are opened up, increased vitality to the muscles and cells result.

Lengthening of fascia with *Intuitive Connective Tissue Bodywork* is almost the direct opposite result of what most practitioners of physical therapy attempt to achieve. In many physical therapy treatments, the therapist most often tries to strengthen the area around an injury with weights or machines. Why would you want to tighten up an area that is already tight? For instance, most people who suffer from back pain are told by their therapist to tighten up their stomach muscles. Now they not only are tight in the back of their body, but they are tight in the front of their body as well. In *Intuitive Connective Tissue Bodywork*, the emphasis is on lengthening and loosening rather than tightening and contracting.

Intuitive Connective Tissue Bodywork

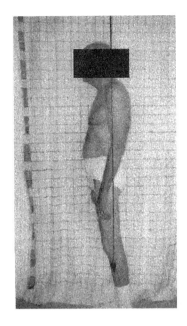

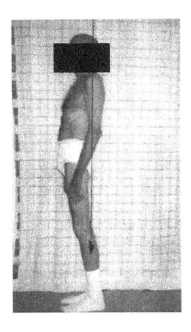

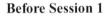

Before Session 1   **After 24 sessions**

Intuitive Connective Tissue Technique

Only 1 session

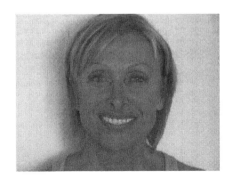

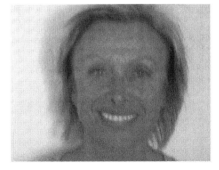

Intuitive Connective Tissue Bodywork is more like art than science. There is a keen sense of listening to the fascia tissue as you work with it.

The way I describe the work is like walking a dog. In essence, you are not walking a dog while the dog remains tethered to a leash. The dog is walking you. This is the same for *Intuitive Connective Tissue Bodywork.* By dialoguing with the tissue, it tells the practitioner how much pressure to apply throughout each stroke. It is about listening to the fascia and asking it what it wants to do. The results can be profound.

How to Begin

Recovering your body requires releasing past physical traumas and allowing the natural flow of energy to continue to flow. Many people are familiar with bodywork, while others are treading onto new ground. Many people want to know where to begin. Here are a few suggestions.

1. Learn How to be Comfortable with Touch.

Many people grew up with a belief that it was not okay to be touched by others, especially strangers. Because of family practices or religious belief systems, they might not have a healthy attitude about their own body. Some might have experienced touch in a negative way while growing up, perhaps through sexual abuse or assault. Others might regard all touch as sexual or erotic.

Learning to be comfortable with touch is an important first step. This means finding a bodywork practitioner whom you can trust and let go with. This might not happen immediately with the first person that you try. Often, trust is built over time. Word of mouth or a referral from a health care provider or health spa might be a good place to start.

A professional will keep you fully draped and respect your fears and desires. Many times I encourage a first time client to wear as many articles of clothing as desired. What I find is that over subsequent sessions, a client is able to feel more comfortable trusting. At this point, he or she may be completely unclothed when lying under the sheet used for draping. Learning to trust is an important first step in the recovery of your body.

2. Learning to Let Go

Stress keeps you wound up. You feel as if you need to always be on guard. Something as simple as receiving a Swedish massage can shut off your Fight or Flight Response for a short while and allow you to enter into your Relaxation Response. When this happens, you feel dreamy and are able to surrender and let go. Learning to lie still and receive bodywork is an important step. Many were trained to focus on others and to place their own needs last. Massage time is your time to have someone take care of you. This should be a time for quiet and learning to receive nurturing from someone else.

Surrendering not only means being willing to receive safe touch but also allowing yourself to participate fully in the letting go process. This can be by verbally informing the practitioner during your session as to your level of comfort or distress. Communicating your areas of pain to those working on you will greatly enhance the massage session. Try not to just lie back and let someone treat you like a piece of meat. Instead, be active in receiving a massage by providing important feedback.

Breathing complete and full breaths is another important aspect of participating fully in a massage. As the practitioner works from the outside to release tight areas, you can breathe fully to help let go from the inside. Surrendering with the breath means a complete letting go, especially with the exhale. Stress is a time when we tend to hold on to our breath. Let your massage be a time when you can practice letting that breath go again.

Being an active participant in your massage or bodywork treatment also means allowing any and all emotions to rise up and be released. Many people will release strong emotions; others will not. Your body will let go more deeply if you can allow your emotions to come out. These are many of the same emotions that were frozen in your muscle and fascia tissue from the effects of repression. Bodywork often brings these emotions back to the surface. The massage session is a wonderful way to free yourself from this trapped energy.

3. Ten Massages in 30 Days

Many people are so wound up all the time that it is irrational to expect one massage every so often or even once a week to solve 30 years of stress or 150 hours a week of repression. This is not possible. One radical treatment I often suggest for those who have a difficult time getting out of their Fight or Flight Response to stress is to receive ten massages in 30 days. Through this radical treatment, your body has more time to remember what it feels like to be relaxed. The more time you stay wound up in stress, the harder it is for the body to unwind.

Each massage activates the Parasympathetic Nervous System (the Relaxation Response) and reminds your body what it feels like to be relaxed. A significant amount of bodywork stimulation in a relatively short period of time will help to remind the body how to relax.

4. Three Massages in One Day

Another radical approach to relaxation that I teach clients is to receive three one-and-a-half hour massages in a single day. When we feel overwhelmed in our stress response, sometimes you have to input a significant amount of release work to turn off the fear response. Clients looking for a new way to relax or "reboot" their overwhelmed nervous system spend a whole day receiving bodywork. They arrive for a one-and-a half hour massage where we peel away the first layer of stress. After the session they go away for two hours to be alone. They return for their second session where we unwrap the next layer of tension. Once again, they leave for two hours after this session is over. They return for their third session where we imprint the memory of what relaxation feels like. It is truly a remarkable program for those who desire to relax.

4. Paradoxes of Bodywork

There is no right or wrong way to receive bodywork. There are many techniques and many styles. Each therapist has his own interpretation of the skills that he has studied. There are some treatments that are very painful, yet you often feel much better afterward. Others are so subtle that you can hardly imagine that anything can be happening at all. Each type of work affects you on a different level of healing—some superficially, others on a very deep level. Each client requires different types of work dependent on the levels of armor and resistance in his body.

There are many contradictions in bodywork. There are some techniques that teach to massage the belly in a clockwise direction. Other styles promote massaging the belly in a counter-clockwise direction. There are good reasons for each style. Some styles teach to never take your hands off the body while others claim that the body needs time to integrate the work, and moving away from the client for short periods of time is totally acceptable. Some techniques teach to only push toward the heart while other styles reverse this direction.

What is right? Unless causing obvious harm, most techniques are entirely acceptable. The rule of thumb is to educate yourself about what kind of treatment you want and what it is supposed to do for you. Always ask questions if you are concerned about a practitioner's intent and techniques.

Bodywork is the second pillar used when learning to return to nature. Recovering through bodywork is an essential step. There are various styles and techniques to be explored. One technique may have significant results, but it may not be enough for you. Just as there are many parts of your car that you need to keep in working order, the same is true with your body. Receiving bodywork treatments is not just for pampering. The long-standing affects of stress, repression and physical trauma begin to be released. In order to return to vitality and heal with nature, regular bodywork is a necessity.

Pillar Number Three

Expansive Movement

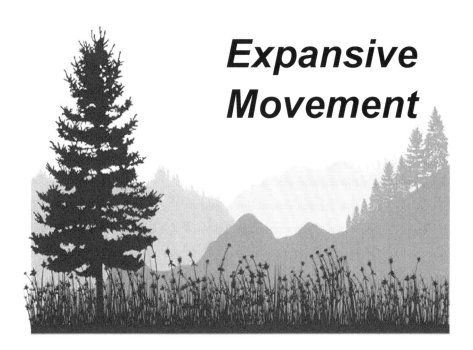

Movement Is Life

Nature is all about movement. Rivers will flow from the mountains to the sea. Storms will blow in and just as quickly disappear. Birds migrate with the annual seasons. Canyons are slowly eroded away by the forces of nature. Nowhere in nature do you see absolute stillness all of the time. Some movement is faster than other types of movement. A cheetah chasing after a prey at sixty miles per hour is certainly much quicker than a glacier crawling down a valley floor at sixty inches per year.

We are just as much a part of nature as the glaciers and the migrating birds. A young child learning to walk is demonstrating his ability to follow natural movements. A man climbing a tree to gather coconuts is using his natural body movements to seek out food. Movement is who you are as well. With natural movement, you continue to enjoy vitality and radiant health.

Movement is occurring within you at all times. Your heart continues to pound at a rhythmical beat for the duration of your life. Red and white blood cells travel through your vascular system like clockwork. Waste products are continually being transported and released from your body. The muscles of respiration provide you with oxygen through your lungs twenty-four hours a day. You are a vast sea of movement. When you sit down to release the waste in your bowels, you even call this a "bowel movement."

The body was meant to move. From the constant beat of the heart to the flow of cerebral spinal fluid around your brain, movement is who you are. Your entire body will move with every breath. A sneeze will shake and rattle you from the inside out. Even the act of vomiting will move your insides violently. Without movement, you will die.

The distancing ourselves from natural beliefs has often led to adopting movements that are contractive movements. It is through contractive movements that you begin to limit your growth and range of motion. Movements that originate from unnatural beliefs only lead you into decay and the breakdown of your body. Contractive movement begins to deaden your tissues and prevents you from moving efficiently.

The more you honor your relationship with nature, the more you honor your own movement. With natural movements, you expand and grow. Through expansive movements you will regain your lost body. When you honor nature's rhythm to move, you achieve optimal health. The third pillar of healing is learning how to honor nature's guidance through expansive movement.

The Loss of Our Movement

Movement begins in your head. The beliefs that you carry with you will help to dictate the movement patterns that propel you down the street. As you become farther and farther removed from nature, an interesting change begins to happen. As your beliefs change, so too does your movement. Often you no longer move in the same way as your natural ancestors. Many times you seem to have become a victim of your own body and of your movement. When you acquire false beliefs, you begin to move your body in a very unnatural manner. If you wish to change your movement, you must first change your beliefs.

There are several forces at work that undermine your movement. In order to recover your movement, these forces need to be addressed. These forces are once again, stress, physical trauma, and repression. Added to this is the fact that many people are now more sedentary in their movements because of high-tech ways to create movement for them. Along with this lack of movement comes contractive movement that many times is more damaging than lack of regular movement. When you put it all together, the denial of nature has led to the loss of your body and the loss of your movement.

The History of Movement

Throughout the course of human history, movement has been a large part of our survival. In generations past, we went on hunts to bring home food for the tribe and family. We built homes with our own hands. We carried water from nearby streams to cook and clean with. We traveled with all of our possessions on our backs to follow migrating food supplies and the seasons of the year. We chopped wood to keep us warm at night. Movement has been essential to the story of our survival.

For most of history, we did not have to think about movement. We celebrated with a dance around a fire at night. A wedding ceremony often included some form of ritualistic movement. We moved our bodies in a natural way, often mimicking the animals around us. We were connected with nature. Movement came naturally. These natural movements went on for thousands of years.

Between five to ten thousand years ago, a dramatic shift occurred. This was the shift in our brain. We gradually became more interested in left-brain stimulation. Languages were created. Numbers began to emerge. We were slowly beginning to move away from our natural roots. Movement begins in the brain; as the brain began to change, our movement was quick to follow.

Before the shift in our brain to cognitive brain dominance, we used our own movement as a way to survive. We did not have a lot of free time to move unnecessarily. Women usually stayed close to the camp and foraged for roots and berries while watching the children. Men were normally out hunting when demands for food necessitated it. Our bodies were kept strong by these natural movements. A hunt for the food supply not only brought home nourishment but also helped to maintain the strength in our legs. Chopping wood for a fire to keep us warm at night kept the muscles in our upper body strong and toned.

It was during this hunting cycle that men would use their bodies to chase down and kill prey to be brought back to the tribe or clan to eat. As the brain began to shift into more cognitive brain dominance, men began to expand the hunt. The hunt for food soon became a hunt against other tribes. Men were now hunting each other over land rights and hunting territory. Men were killing other men over the beliefs in their heads. "My god is better than your god" and "my skin color is better than yours" became the instigators of these fights. This shift came to be known as war.

The concept of the warrior was developed. In order to be the best warrior possible, men would train for war. A strong body was desired to be an efficient warrior. In order to be prepared for the battlefield, men soon forgot about their natural ways of moving and began to move in ways to train for battle. Men began preparing their bodies to be strong warriors by running faster and becoming stronger. They developed their hunting skills even more. But they were no longer hunting animals in the forest; men were now hunting other human beings.

Around two thousand years ago, the Olympics in Greece began. Contrary to popular belief, this was not a friendly display of camaraderie. The Olympics were started as training for war. Ancient Greek city-states would cease their actual battles for a period and come together to engage in "mock" war. The discus throw was a way to perfect one's throwing skills with a large stone. Running races prepared one to be faster at combat. Wrestling was just another way to train for hand-to-hand combat. These mock battles came to be known as "sport."

In other words, competition was developed as a way to move the body. Competition is movement that originates from the cognitive brain and is synonymous with stress. When you move competitively, your mind still believes that you are at war or are being hunted. This reaction is then translated to the body. My definition of competition is the following: "The need to dominate another or self because of the fear of being dominated."

Out of the first competitive movements, other types of competitions followed over time. From basketball to hockey, bowling to badminton, boxing to tennis, we have created a culture of movements based on competition. We have slowly lost our relationship with natural movements and replaced them with warrior movement. A boxer is still a warrior fighting for his life. This time it is his fear of losing that kills him more than a knife to the abdomen. A fencer is still dueling with competitive movements. Even a professional bowler is practicing stressful cognitive brain movement when he rolls the ball down the alley. A warrior is a warrior is a warrior. No matter what the sport or event, competitive movements are equivalent to being a warrior. Competitive movements are movements that are based in fear and war. Even though the enemy might be an imaginary game-like scenario such as an opponent across the tennis court, the body still remains at war and fighting for its life.

Artificial Movement

The more we have come "out of the woods and into the city," the more we have lost the natural movement of the body. We are no longer using our body to survive. Our survival requires more skill with our head and our logic. Our body just seems to be going along for the ride.

In the last few generations, technology began to creep in. Horses replaced foot travel. Cars took over for horses. Soon the airplane took us wherever we needed to go in a hurry. Little by little, technology has created labor-saving devices, from the food processor to indoor plumbing. We are no longer as dependent on our own movement for our survival. We have become more passive. We have become less of a movement-oriented species and more of a thinking-based species. This seems to be another aspect of our evolution.

As we have become more used to living in cities, we have had to create artificial movements to replace the natural movements we once enjoyed. This artificial movement has come to be known as "exercise." When you are using your body to survive, every daily activity helps to keep your body strong. Relying on your head for survival means you must learn to replace these once natural movements.

A sedentary lifestyle does not favor the body. Regular movement is important in order to maintain optimal health and vitality. Unfortunately, in a valiant effort to create artificial movement to replace our natural ways, we have created something that has ultimately removed us from our natural ways. In many instances, our modern movement has created more problems than even a sedentary lifestyle. The movement experiment has gone astray. Our original intentions of creating movement to duplicate what was lost when we became sedentary by moving to cities has turned against us. Movement that was once natural has been replaced by war-like movements.

In the latter half of the nineteenth century, cities began to flourish. More and more people found themselves moving from the rural farm into large-scale metropolises. No longer burdened by the physical tasks on the farm, these new city dwellers had to be more conscious of their movement. It was at this time that a notion developed uniting the puritanical religious institutions with movement. From here started the belief in what was called "muscular Christianity."

Alan M. Klein writes in *Little Big Men,*

"The first successful gymnasiums in North America were built during this period. The YMCA dates to this time-period in which physical conditioning and religion grew compatible. Muscular Christianity was most popular in just those Northern cities with the largest populations and, presumably, the most congestion and urban-defined problems.

"The aesthetics of the muscular body also grew popular during this time. Although Eugene Sandow is often thought of as bodybuilding's pioneer, the groundwork was first laid in the fusion of the look of robust muscularity with ideological religious purity."

Health clubs, gyms and regular exercise routines are a very recent addition to our evolutionary history. With the advent of the Industrial Revolution came the progression toward more and more labor-saving devices. We now had more free time and we still needed to place some physical stress on our body to make it function efficiently. In the last couple of decades, more emphasis has been placed on getting exercise—something that used to happen naturally before our many labor-saving devices came into existence.

The source of our learning about movement has not been very natural. Physical education teachers, aerobics instructors and fitness trainers have helped to shape our beliefs about movement. Unfortunately, these new beliefs may have helped to do more harm than any good they could ever have done. Our new ways of moving have taught us how to be contractive and to move in an unnatural way. Most of us learned to move our bodies the same way we learned about our mind. We were graded on our movement in P. E. classes like we were graded on our ability to remember cognitive and rational information. Push-ups, sit-ups, and other "war-like" movements were how we learned to move. Our movement was based on performance and achievement.

Contractive movements have arisen out of a cognitive brain myth that we can dominate our body as well as other aspects of nature. The concept of bodybuilding derived from attempting to conquer the body. Building big muscles and "rock solid" physiques originated from a belief that the body was something that could be conquered by the mind. Unfortunately, this is the same mindset that has attempted to conquer almost every other aspect of nature.

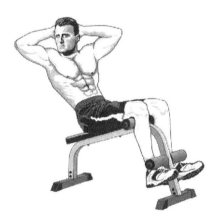

Out of the Industrial Revolution arose a callous, machine-like attitude toward the body. New bodybuilding machines were developed that could mimic the way machinery acted in a factory. Back and forth movements became standard exercise routines. The actions of a piston in a factory became a model for developers of bodybuilding equipment. Counting the number of repetitions became a universal format. Contractive movements began to become institutionalized in our culture.

New myths about movement began to spring up all over. From the laboratory to the fitness studio, we had one hero after another who began to emerge to show us what movement was all about. A flood of celebrity exercise videos burst onto the scene to teach us how to move. Unfortunately, most of these new ideas were contractive in nature. These new ideas were very much in line with this emerging philosophy—the body is something to be conquered.

In the middle of our developing trends toward unnatural movements began to emerge the leaders of "exercise science." These men and women in laboratory coats began to design the philosophy about what health was and was not. Unfortunately, they created movements based on machines and not on nature. Most of these myths created by laboratory scientists have survived to this day.

One of the pioneers of the exercise science revolution was a NASA scientist named Dr. Kenneth Cooper. It was Kenneth Cooper who would monitor astronauts in training on treadmills to test the "fitness" of their heart. Dr. Cooper invented the historic philosophy of strengthening the heart by "cardiovascular conditioning." This came to be known as "aerobics." It was believed that if you could elevate your heart rate up for at least twenty minutes several times a week you would be healthier and live longer. This was the famous "220 minus your age" formula. You would subtract your age from the number 220. This would give you your maximum heart rate. The concept taught one to elevate your heart rate from anywhere from 50 to 80 percent of this number. According to Cooper, you were now healthy.

This philosophy spread like wildfire. In fact, this belief is one of the founding principles of almost every gymnasium. This is called "aerobic fitness." There is only one problem; it doesn't work. It is a myth. You are not guaranteed to live any longer nor be any healthier if you practice "aerobic fitness." In fact, the practice of aerobic fitness may even shorten your life quite a bit.

Peg Jordan elaborates in *The Fitness Instinct* about the training manuals many of us were taught to follow. Besides limiting fat to no more than 30 percent of total daily calories, not smoking, stress management and maintaining ideal weight, she also mentions "perform consistent aerobic exercise." As a nurse, Peg Jordan recalls a man who did all of this.

"When I was a cardiac care nurse, for example, I knew a 40-year-old runner who surpassed every one of those guidelines. He followed a heart-healthy diet, even sprinkling lecithin (a fat emulsifier) on his breakfast cereal. He had the blood pressure of a teenager. He had no family history of heart disease or any other identifiable risk factor. Thus, when he dropped dead from a sudden heart attack, it made me question the value of the numbers game."

This man was not alone. The famous author of *"The Complete Book of Running,"* Jim Fixx, also died of a heart attack. Fixx was in his early forties and died while he was running. Over and over the stories keep coming in. Accounts of men and women dropping dead of heart attacks during or after aerobic activity have become commonplace. Aerobic activity performed over long durations is not a natural behavior. How many animals do you see exerting themselves like this, except for short durations?

Even more startling is the admission by Dr. Kenneth Cooper himself. Dr. Cooper states in an interview in the April 2000 edition of *Fit Magazine,* " . . . it should be noted that the 'godfather of aerobics,' Dr. Kenneth Cooper, has changed his mind about running: *'What made me change my mind was telephone calls from distraught widows whose husbands had followed my guidelines and had died of heart attacks,'* says Dr. Cooper. *'I now recommend walking at any speed for 30 minutes, three times a week. I used to think that to be exercising aerobically you had to be in your target heart rate or you were wasting your time.'"*

After hearing from the man who started the aerobics myth recant his theory, do you see any gymnasiums shutting their doors? Unfortunately, the aerobics myth has become institutionalized in our culture. Unnatural and often "unhealthy" movements have become normal. Adding more fuel to the fire was celebrity exercise queen Jane Fonda who would help popularize the aerobics myth. We learned how to move our body from an actress who was struggling with an eating disorder.

Peg Jordan writes in *The Fitness Instinct,*

"Jane Fonda told me that she believed she was on a mission to help women discover the hidden athlete within themselves. Her disclosures of bulimia and body self-loathing were applauded by sympathetic fans. She was credited with having transformed a sick obsession into a healthy pastime. And the tapes kept coming. She made 15 videos in 15 years, creating the largest-selling video library in history. Every year, she seemed to look younger, and the public believed that the queen of aerobics was energetically and metabolically superior. Only the editors of the national magazines watched closely as a tuck here and there, a breast lift, or a face lift became evident."

The heroes and creators of our body myth-making were all around us. Charles Atlas demonstrated what a body should look like if you were a man. Dynamic tension had chiseled his body into a statuesque spectacle of "rock solid" hardness. Jack La Lanne, considered the "godfather of physical fitness," pushed us through routines of push-ups and sit-ups on his morning exercise hour. Arnold Schwarzenegger drove bodybuilding to the limit with bulging biceps and "washboard abs." Arnold became our hero to try to emulate. (We did not realize at the time that much of Arnold's success was due to his admitted steroid use). Soon Joe Weider entered into the fray with *Muscle and Fitness Magazine*. We now had a recognized training program by an "authority" on how to "bulk up" your body using weights and supplements. We were being programmed on how to move our bodies even more like warriors and machines.

It is often said that knowledge is power. With this in mind, whoever establishes our beliefs for us holds the power. Unfortunately, a consortium of celebrities and laboratory scientists have created the myths that we believe about our bodies. Misinformation can be just as powerful as natural truth. Add to this the commoners' way of experiencing this knowledge, (the fitness trainer), and now you have real trouble. Fitness trainers were a new branch of service industry professionals designed to capitalize on the myths passed down by the laboratory scientists and the overzealous celebrities. Fitness trainers helped bring unnatural movements to the masses, believing that they alone had access to the knowledge designed to better a person's life.

Our heroes who taught us about how to move and be in our bodies laid down a foundation for the rest of us to follow. Unfortunately, their model is anything but natural and, in most cases, goes completely against our own health practice. Just as we have learned how to brush our teeth and to go to the bathroom, we have also learned how to move our body. This learning came predominantly from warriors. The result is a culture that has learned to move while in a state of war.

Fitness Is Not Health

By and large, this new model of how to move our bodies that was created for us was met with eager acceptance. Scientists in laboratory coats, actresses, models and unknown bodybuilders became the heroes of the time. We emulated them. We attempted to be like them. Gymnasiums became our social clubs where we would hang out for long hours. We wanted so badly to be like our heroes that we forgot about our natural ways.

What came out of this period was a concept called "fitness." We all jumped on board to become "fit." Terms like "workout," "conditioning" and "fitness level" became household words. Being "in shape" or "out of shape" became our way of measuring up to the new standards set by society. We were measuring our body fat regularly. This number told us if we were a good person or had something to feel ashamed about. Contrary to popular belief, fitness is not necessarily health. In fact, most of the fitness world is contrary to a health practice.

Peg Jordan writes in *The Fitness Instinct,*

"Fitness is a concept, a word, an image in the mind, shaped by decades of advances in exercise science along with corporate-sponsored images and publicly broadcast messages. Fitness as a cultural phenomenon is controlled by a cartel that includes several industries, among them beauty, fashion, sports, sporting goods, and media."

The phrase "health and fitness" is thrown around like we all know what we are talking about. There are even some magazines that incorporate this phrase into their title. Despite the fanfare, fitness is not necessarily health. The fitness industry is more closely associated with the beauty and cosmetic industry than it is with the health and wellness industry. Fitness is primarily interested in shaping the body to appear according to socially acceptable standards. This might include a flat abdomen, inflated chest and firm buttocks. Health is associated with feeling "good" and the complete and full functioning of all the bodily systems. Only on a rare occasion will fitness be associated with health.

For instance, if you are severely overweight, your heart might be forced to pump more blood throughout your body. In this instance, a fitness program designed to lose weight might actually be helping your health. However, in most instances fitness is attempting to look good and sacrificing your health in return.

Most of the exercise in this culture is contractive, meaning it attempts to keep you tightened down. You might perform stomach exercises not for the benefit of healthy organs but so you can "look" good in a swimming suit. You might lift weights not to make your body healthier but to create a body that is tighter with less ability to feel. We are still trying to be soldiers, even in our exercise. You might jog five miles a day because you are afraid of dying of a heart attack. You get on the stair climber each morning because you are afraid of getting fat. Much of our exercise is fear-based movement.

In fact, most people who work out or are exercising in a gym are doing so from fear, creating further contractions in their body. Fear of being fat, having a heart attack, being ridiculed, being beaten up, (the bully concept) and fear of aging are the primary motivations of most people attending gyms and health clubs. This is not health but war for your body. While heavily promoted by most medical doctors, personal trainers and celebrity talk show hosts, this philosophy adds little to your natural ways.

The language of fitness is based on the warrior body. When practicing fitness, most attempt to tighten their bodies and get a "hard body." This is exactly what a warrior needs in order to go into battle. People might lift weights and call this "pumping iron." They seek "buns of steel" and" "rock-solid abs." When practicing fitness, most often people attempt to turn their bodies into a machine in order to go to war. Exercise science has created a new myth called "fitness." While these contractive movements have been promoted as adding to one's health, in most cases the very opposite is the case.

Fitness practice attempts to keep you in your Cognitive Brain. You are taught to move your body by the numbers. You count the number of repetitions when you lift a weight. You measure the number of calories burned when running on a treadmill. You constantly check your heart rate (another number) when performing an aerobic activity. You count the laps when you swim rather than just enjoying being in the water. You have forgotten what natural movement is like and are now practicing movement by the numbers. You find yourself reading a magazine while sitting on an exercise bicycle. Reading is another cognitive brain pursuit.

While fitness was an attempt to counter the effects of obesity, there have been some significant miscalculations. The adverse effects of fitness, (a tight and hard body), far out-weigh anything a few extra pounds might incur. Science has declared war on fat and has tried to conquer the effects of obesity and a sedentary life with contractive movements and hardened bodies. A person with a low percentage of body fat is the equivalent of having reached sainthood. Trying to fit into an image that gossip magazines and celebrity talk shows have created, we have all fallen victim to unnatural beliefs about what it is like to have a body.

Human beings are the only species that has created movement to improve the way we look and bolster our appearance. Centipedes are not doing push ups to look better. Squirrels are not out running around all day long to lose a few pounds. It is only human beings that move to change our looks.

Over time the idealized body has changed. At this juncture, the media has created an image of the idealized male body to be one of a bulging chest and large biceps. Women are expected to have large breasts, tiny waists and slim hips. Fitness has attempted to box us all into this model. In the end, we have forgotten about nature and about our own health. While fitness may be found in a gym, health is usually not. In fact, calling a workout facility a "health club" is another oxymoron. Health clubs do very little to serve up health.

Sport and Competition

Out of our primal roots we have developed sport and competition. These were war games designed around the principles of hunting animals. Conquering nature meant hunting animals for sport, not necessarily for food. Animals were called "game" and killing an animal became known as "dropping game." Eventually these rules of hunting carried over to hunting other human beings. This was called war. Out of war emerged training for war. This became known as "sport."

When you are engaged in a sport, you are still engaged in hunting or war; only this time you are hunting a human opponent. The rules of the battlefield have become symbolically transferred to the playing field. Opponents are now considered the enemy. Those "others" from various schools, teams, cities or countries are now yours to defeat. Through sport you have learned how to symbolically kill your opponent. Coaches, sending their troops into battle, have replaced generals. Soldiers have become players. Time-outs are now symbolic of battlefield truces.

In the same manner, rocks and clubs have been replaced with balls and bats. Swords have given way to racquets. Chain mail and iron helmets now show up as shoulder pads and knee braces. Instead of throwing a stone at your enemy, you are now hurling a baseball 90 miles per hour at him. The war strategy meeting between commanders in now replaced with a huddle where a play is called to try to deceive the opponent. There is still a battlefield to play out the skirmish. Only this time, it might be on a clay tennis court or a 50-meter swimming pool.

Killing the enemy remains the goal even to this day. The language of sport resembles the verbiage of war. "Kill them," rings out on the field. "Knock his head off" comes from an enthusiastic parent. "Kick someone's butt" is the coach's rallying cry. A boxer is knocked to the canvas by a menacing pugilist standing over him. The masses in the stands jump up with glee when a member of the opposing team is "annihilated." Does this sound any different than the Gladiators massacring the Christians in front of thousands of exuberant fans within Rome's ancient Coliseum?

The field may have changed, but the impact on your body remains the same. A warrior in battle is no different than a warrior in sport. The body still moves from a place of fear and combat. Instead of conquering someone's kingdom in war, you now earn a hefty paycheck or the rights to own another's ego. This is akin to the owning of slaves. If I can defeat you in a sport, whether it is in fencing or in the sport of ice hockey, then I symbolically own you and your team, city or country until the next time that we meet in competition. To defeat an opponent means that they are yours to own. To defeat an opponent is symbolic of taking them prisoner. You have imprisoned their ego. There is an attitude of "to the victor belong the spoils" when it comes to sport. The enemy is dehumanized and is prey to be conquered. A victor has bragging rights until the next battle ensues. This is how we train our bodies.

Sport soon developed a new way to engage in battle. This became the cognitive brain numbers game. Instead of "playing" a "game," now the most important aspect became to count statistics or to keep score. Points and goals began to be the equivalent of conquering territory. Batting averages served as reminders of who the superior warriors were or who had the most kills to their names. Yards rushed and the most points scored became the statistical numbers game. The team that had the most victories in the season was rewarded for winning the most battles and conquering the most territory. Movement continued to be about playing war in our heads. The cognitive brain, with its statistics and analysis, now ruled our movement.

A new category of person developed. This became the athlete, who is the modern day version of the warrior. Athletes come in many shapes and sizes. From petite ballet dancers to monstrous rugby players, athletes share one unique characteristic: they are primarily concerned with training their body like a warrior and moving from a place of fear in battle.

Muscles have been used to conquer nations and armies. The man with the biggest muscles many times was the best warrior and won the most battles throughout the ages. Things have not changed that much. The higher one jumps or the faster one runs usually helps to make him or her a better warrior. People still win more battles with better training. This time they win championship trophies rather than another's kingdom or city. The scorecard still lists the warrior's physical dimensions, like height and weight.

Now this may seem easier to notice from a boxer's perspective, mimicking a very ancient sport that has not changed that much. How could a tiny ballerina be considered a warrior? To derive that answer, we must look at the nature of competition and stress.

Stress and Movement

Competition is movement based on fear. Much of the fear is not real, like in a real battlefield scenario where you could actually die. However, there are some sports that do involve a sense of danger where physical harm could result. This is not necessarily the result of a battlefield experience; this is just the effect of natural forces at work.

Competition begins with the beliefs that you are given. You learn competitive movements as children in your childhood games. Your parents, teachers and older playmates pass down the beliefs of competitive movements. Kickball, dodge ball, tag and relay races are all based on winners and losers. These games are all based on performance and fear. You learn how to be a warrior from the very moment you begin to socialize with other children.

Training boys and girls how to be men and women often begins with your movements. Movements have come to be rites of passage. For young boys, hunting, killing animals and joining the military are rites of passage. Competitive sports and aggressive movements are akin to these hunting rituals. A young boy, in order to be a man, is often expected to go out and kill. Sometimes the kill is a real animal; other times the kill is defeating a symbolic enemy on the battlefield. This could be soccer, baseball or basketball. As men and women have gained more equality in our culture, women have learned how to harden their bodies and become warriors as well. Whether a military or a sports warrior, women have begun to lose their relationship with nature as well as men and now practice movement from a place of fear.

Most competition is based on internalized fears. We believe we will die if we lose a match. We believe will be destroyed if we fail. It is common for people to believe if they are not perfect at their particular sport they will have no worth or value. Failure at a given sport will lead to loss of love and alienation from others. These are some of the many beliefs that run through your head as you engage in sport. You have created an artificial enemy so that you can continue to conquer. You are rewarded with accolades for conquering others. You fear failure more than anything.

When a professional golfer misses a shot, it is symbolic of a hunter who misses his mark. The hunter fears coming home to his family without something to eat. The professional golfer is still hunting. This time the meal comes in the form of a paycheck. An amateur golfer still suffers from this fear. His competitive mind believes that if he loses the round of golf, he loses status in his social circle. This is equivalent of the runt of the pack having to eat last or not at all. The golfer fears ridicule. Losing the match means losing social status.

Competition derives from fear. Whether in business, war, sports or any individual competition, you are still measuring your worth against another when you are competitive. You might be measuring yourself against a clock time or against your previous best score. You are still moving from fear and moving as a performance. Competition almost always equals moving from a place of stress.

When you watch a finely tuned athlete running down the track during the 100-meter race, the surroundings of the stadium might seem safe, but within the athlete's mind his stress response is most surely activated. He is hyper-alert. His mind believes there is a wild tiger chasing after him. His brain, in its competitive state, believes that losing or failure is the equivalent of death.

A ballerina dancing across a large stage floor in front of an expectant crowd is almost surely in her Fight or Flight Response. She too is hyper-alert. She is competing against herself to perform at her best. Whenever you are measuring your performance in your movement, you are now creating fear-based movement. Moving from a competitive mind still brings on war mentality.

When movement stops becoming playful, it starts becoming stressful. If you are moving your body while concerned about your performance, you are most likely activating your Fight or Flight Stress Response. Competition, either from outside or from within, is almost always about measuring your performance as you move your body. This means stress.

Stress is a reaction in your body that is produced when you do not feel safe. This reaction occurs when you experience any situation, either real or imaginary, that creates a sense of fear. Competition, whether in a group or self-competition, is almost always stressful. Competition draws you away from nature and turns you into a warrior. Warriors almost always move from fear.

There are essentially two nervous system reference points from which you move. These are the Sympathetic branch and the Parasympathetic branch of the Autonomic Nervous System. The Sympathetic branch is the part of your nervous system that speeds you up and tells you that there is danger ahead. This is your stress response. The Parasympathetic branch is the part of your nervous system that slows you down when you are feeling safe. This is the relaxation response. There is no middle ground. There is no compromise. You either feel safe or you don't. Your nervous system does not lie.

Moving from a place of competition is most likely to create a Fight or Flight Reaction in the body. You are afraid of losing a tennis match. Your shoulder tightens up. As a sprinter running down the track, your hamstring might go into spasm. What is happening in your mind is that you are terrified. Instead of a grizzly bear chasing after you, you are now afraid of losing or of not being perfect. The Fight or Flight Response is no different, even if the event is only imagined. Your body still reacts with tightness as if the danger were real.

Whether you are competing on the basketball court or at a track meet, it does not matter. Your "killer instincts" are still alive. Your movement is still based on fear and contraction. You are still moving as if a lion is chasing after you.

Most people approach exercise already stressed. Imagine a twisted rubber band. Now try to stretch this rubber band. The rubber band will not stretch as far as if it were straight and free of the tangles. Your body is the same. When already contracted by the forces of stress, you become even stiffer when you move. Why would you want to create more movement that makes you even tighter?

There is a common myth that exercise will relieve stress. It generally does not. Exercise only helps to repress the feelings associated with stress. If stress is a feeling that makes one "feel unsafe," then it is rare that contractive exercise will make you feel safer. It is hard to feel anything while exercising in a contractive manner. Emotions are usually pushed down even farther.

The Fight or Flight Response to a life-threatening event will do one of three things. You will contract your muscles, keep incessantly moving or leave your body. Just because you are moving does not necessarily mean that you are out of Fight or Flight. For instance, a dancer might leave her body as she performs. Her movements might be expressive and flowing, but her sense of self is gone. She is still reacting in fear. A runner might be compressing his neck and shoulders as he runs because he is afraid of getting fat and wants to make sure that he gets his run in unimpeded. An exercise addict might go from one aerobic activity to another, unable to slow down. If she stopped, she would have to feel some kind of pain. She is still in her Fight or Flight Response.

A branch of sports science has emerged called "sports psychology." This area of interest includes training in teaching athletes to perform at their peek while they are relaxed. This is what is referred to as the "zone." It is while performing in the zone that your body is free of fear and remains in its Relaxation Response, maximizing performance. While an honorable pursuit to try to achieve, this is seldom accomplished in training or in performance. Most athletes' movement will generally come from the place of fear. To be truly relaxed, both the mind and the muscles of the body need to be relaxed. If the body is not also in a state of relaxation, then the Relaxation Response has not been activated.

Competition is fear-based movement that will contract and shorten the body. Over time, with continuous competition, the body will continue to shorten and harden. The body is hardened in its armor.

Stress and repression are forces in our lives that tend to tighten and harden the body. As you endure the Fight or Flight Response of stress, your body is pulled tight to protect you from danger. Repression causes muscles to tighten to hold back the waves of emotions from being released. Participating in regular contractive and competitive movements only pulls your body tighter. Practicing contractive movements magnifies the effects of stress. In other words, the types of movements that most of us are accustomed to performing only make the effects of stress and repression even worse.

When you go to the gym, you might notice people of all ages who are already well versed in the effects of stress and repression. Their movements may be restricted. Their posture is hunched over. Their chest muscles are already overly tightened, causing their shoulders to roll forward.

What do you notice most of these people doing? In most cases, they are creating movements to contract their bodies even more. They are tightening up already tight muscles. Already constricted abdominal muscles and chests burdened with layers of tightness will get their daily dose of more tightness through strength-training workouts. An old injury to a leg or arm will get worked out with a weight machine to build up muscles around an already stiff joint. Acting against nature, people are only magnifying the effects of stress and repression when they move their bodies as warriors.

Two of the common practices of warrior training are cardiovascular endurance and weight training. Both are contractive behaviors designed to prepare the body for war. Both help to undermine the health of the body.

According to the weight-lifting philosophy, a "hard body is a healthy body." This is a classic myth developed by the fitness world. A hard body is usually a hyper-tonic body devoid of healthy muscle tissue. For a muscle to be healthy, it needs to be able to relax and contract. A hard body usually has only one option—to stay hard and contracted. When this happens, the connective tissue surrounding the muscles will harden and fuse together. The result is a process called—*Hydrogen Bonding*. Muscles are fused together and the normal energy that travels through the tissue is diminished. A hard body is a body filled with muscles that are dried out and sensitivity deadened. Muscle tissue that resembles beef jerky is the result.

The cardio myth is another precursor to stress. When exercising at high levels for significant periods of time, the body almost always enters into the Fight or Flight Response. Breathing through the mouth as a way to gasp for air is a big part of this. Peg Jordan recalls the work of Ayurvedic physical therapist Allan Douillard in *The Fitness Instinct:*

"Douillard knew that breathing through the mouth tends to inflate only the upper lobes of the lungs, which are connected to sympathetic nerve fibers, the branch of the nervous system that activates the fight-or-flight fear response. Breathing through your mouth prepares your body with adrenaline for an emergency response. Your pupils dilate, blood is shunted to your extremities, peripheral blood vessels expand, and so on. The problem with exercising at this level all of the time is that you are consistently dipping into a full-alarm state with every workout."

Exercising aerobically is a sure way to activate your stress response. When you are out of breath, the body triggers a danger signal. The body attempts to defend itself by activating the stress response. This certainly kicks you into high gear, but now you are operating from the place of stress. Not being able to breathe creates stressful movement.

Add to this the endorphin myth. Endorphins are real. Laboratory scientists discovered these bio-chemicals during the times of the jogging craze in the 1980s. Endorphins are chemicals released in the brain that produce a euphoric feeling. This experience was dubbed the "runners' high." After a period of twenty minutes or so of heavy breathing and moderate to intense aerobic activity, the brain releases these "feel-good chemicals." Needless to say, they are much sought after by most exercise enthusiasts.

Endorphins are the body's natural painkillers. These bio-chemicals were intended by nature to help one numb out pain during battle with a wild animal or other natural threats in order to help you continue to fight to stay alive. During a natural disaster (like a tornado), endorphins numb your pain to ensure your survival.

The fitness world discovered these natural painkillers and began to teach people how to create more of them to increase their performance. In essence, the competitive mind created an artificial high. By stressing your body for a certain amount of time, the brain would release endorphins. This would numb you out from the neck down. You could now continue to battle, only the battle was not against a wild animal. The battle was against yourself. Most people have grown accustomed to stressful movements so that they can keep numb in their head as everything from the neck down continues to perform. Stress and contractive movements continue, but most have discovered an artificial way to not feel them.

How Do Warriors Age?

A good test of movement will determine how this movement stands up over time. How does a person who is involved with competition and contractive-based movements age? What are the effects on his or her body years down the road? The results are staggering.

In my clinical experience, I have noticed some disturbing trends. Those people who are engaged in the traditional types of movement and exercise as outlined by the fitness world are not necessarily the healthiest people as they age. In fact, those who have practiced years of stress-based and competitive movement may very well be less healthy than some people who were never that athletic to begin with.

Athletes in general do not age very well. Athletes practicing competitive and contractive movement have spent many years, perhaps a lifetime, learning how to harden and tighten their bodies. These effects will show up as they age. All of the contraction, physical assaults and armoring of the body will still be there. Many people want to blame this on age itself, yet this is not so. Those practicing expansive movements will have a different relationship with the aging process.

An aging aerobics instructor or a fitness trainer will not necessarily be the healthiest of specimens. A body builder will feel the effects of a warrior's body for years to come. A long-term committed jogger is not necessarily going to have the healthiest hips and knees. The many miles of pounding that his body has endured will begin to show up years later.

An athlete, whether a "weekend warrior" or a professional, is not necessarily going to have the healthiest of bodies years later. Look at the problems that many former professional football players experience with their knees and backs. Many of them limp their way through life after they are forced into retirement. In fact, a retired professional football player will have a life expectancy of 55 years, 52 if he was a lineman.

How often do we hear stories of professional athletes needing to retire well before their career ought to be over with? Early retirement is commonly blamed on back pain or another nagging injury. Charles Barkley and Larry Bird are two such basketball players who come to mind. Even martial arts master Bruce Lee suffered from excruciating back pain that nearly ended his career.

Imagine yourself as a youth playing soccer. Every time a soccer ball bounces off your head, it is the equivalent of a sword coming down on your metal helmet. The impact trauma will remain for a long time afterward. A crash on the ski slope while racing down the giant slalom course will create a tremendous amount of energy impacted into the body. Broken bones and bruises may or may not be the initial result. Years down the road, the impact will certainly make itself known to you.

As a jogger pounds his way down the pavement, all of the impact energy of his feet hitting the ground will be stored in his ankles, knees and hips. It is rare to find a runner who glides through his stride and stores very little of the energy of impact.

Bicycle riding creates an enormous amount of impact trauma for cyclists. All of the bouncing around will result in small amounts of energy collecting in the body. Over the course of many years, the results could be staggering. The perineum and lower abdominal cavity receive significant jarring over time. Long-time cyclists have been known to have inflammations in their prostate glands. The constant jarring of the bicycle seat into the pelvic floor might also lead to other health issues including testicular cancer and inflamed prostates.

Athletes move their bodies like warriors. As a result, the body will hold the remnants of war. Joints will continue to stiffen as muscles harden. Posture continues to decline as the effects of contractive movements take hold. Movement begins in the mind. A warrior is still practicing war even though the battle might have ended years before and it was only "make-believe" war as in sports. Many ex-athletes continue to move their bodies in the same manner as they did while preparing for their earlier battles. If the mind does not change, neither will the body. Most former athletes are still practicing war mentality.

Competition and sport is a way to continue to practice war. Whether playing team sports or individual competition, it does not matter. If you are more interested in the score, a particular time or your performance, you are most certainly practicing stress-based movement. Movement based on competition is movement that denies the body its life and vitality. Warriors will show the effects of war for a very long time to come.

Myths of Movement

The myths that you live your life by go very deep and seem so normal to you. You might rarely stop to question their purpose or their origins. Movement is no exception. Take the case of martial arts as an example of movement myths gone astray.

We all have the right to defend ourselves. Practicing movements that satisfy our fears of being attacked are quite legitimate. However, the practice of martial arts still keeps one training for war. The word "martial" means military. When practicing movements of martial arts, you are practicing military or warrior movements. You are operating from a position of fear, or Fight or Flight, hence contracting the body. You are using your body to push away another human being.

The ancient practice of tai chi was one of the first martial arts systems developed in China. "Tai Chi" means "peaceful energy." First developed as a means to protect travelers from roadside thieves, tai chi continued to gain popularity over the centuries. Other martial art systems soon developed.

Today you might notice someone practicing tai chi in a quiet park or on a serene beach somewhere. While the movements appear to be graceful and flowing, even tai chi can be a fear-based movement system. Arm circles are symbolic of a warrior blocking an opponent's punch thrown at him. A leg kick is symbolic of attempting to push away a sword thrust. Even tai chi, one of the tamest of all the martial arts, is still based on warrior mentality. Other martial art systems are even more contractive in nature. A warrior's body will contract with movement, even while performing in a serene park. The mind is still engaged in a defensive and fear-based posture.

The myths of movement are diverse and varied. Most have accepted them as nature's reality when in fact the majority of them are just myths.

The following are some of the other myths of movement that have been perpetuated throughout our culture.

Myth #1: If Your Back Hurts, Tighten Your Abdominal Muscles

It is often heard how someone's back "just went out." The irony is that backs do not just go out. The muscles of the back and spine do not simply fail one day by chance and it is your unlucky day. Despite your denial, a whole series of events have led up to this day. Perhaps a lifetime of stress and repression has been stored in the back muscles. Along with this holding, there is the possibility of physical trauma being collected in the muscles and connective tissue of the spine. Your spine has been a tightly wound spring for some time and you have chosen to ignore it.

Your medical doctor or fitness trainer advises you to do more "sit-ups" to strengthen the abdominal muscles; you are told that this is the cure. Wrong! Imagine adding gasoline to a fast moving house fire. This is exactly what you are doing if you continue to tighten your abdominal muscles. The back and surrounding tissues are already locked into a contractive pattern. The muscles have hardened and shortened, compressing the vertebral disks and often putting pressure on a nerve.

Tightening your abdominal muscles might stabilize the lower back area. Now you have a tight back, a tight stomach and everything beneath the abdomen is locked in a contractive pattern. Your diaphragm, the primary muscle of respiration, is unable to move efficiently. The intestines, designed to digest food, become compacted within the abdominal cavity, hampering their effectiveness. Overall, you have created many more problems for yourself now and in the future.

Again, the myths of sports medicine and athletic trainers have misled you. Hard, compacted abdominal muscles are not normal or natural. Cultures that are not ruled by fashion magazines and celebrity gossip television shows allow the belly to hang out and chest to sag. These cultures do not necessarily suffer from the same ill effects that a hardened abdomen or a frozen chest will create. No, if your back hurts, it is ill advised to tighten up the back or the stomach muscles. Wouldn't you think it natural to lengthen these muscles instead? Backs do not just go out one day. Back pain is a well-orchestrated series of events based on your mythologies of movement.

Myth #2: A Hard Body Is a Healthy Body

A hard body is anything but a healthy body. The parameters that establish health are not relegated to strength alone. Just because someone is strong does not necessarily mean that he is healthy. Having a tight and hard body usually is the furthest thing from health.

Muscles kept rigid by constant training lack the ability to relax. When a muscle cannot relax and be at rest, it actually weakens. The connective tissue of hardened muscles will also bind together like cement, lose its liquid nature and dry out like beef jerky.

Health is not about hardness. When your body is hard, you are stiff. Shortened muscles and tendons pull your joints together. Mobility is restricted. Organs and glands are compressed which causes improper functioning of these organs and glands. Your body becomes shortened, as a tight body will cause your skeleton to be incased in hardened and compacted tissue. This shortening leads to a hunched over posture.

Hardened body tissues lack sensation and sensitivity. Muscles and connective tissue frozen in place will lose their ability to distinguish sensation. Hardness will help to create reduced sensation and lack of mobility. Movement is life; stagnation equals death. A body that remains frozen behind walls of hardened tissue is a body that is slowly dying. A popular myth is that lifting weights will add years to your life. Lifting weights does get people of all age ranges to move their bodies; however, there are better ways to move your body. The act of tightening muscles by itself only adds to the effects of stress and repression.

Weight training derives from the myth that the body can be used to dominate others. A skinny kid who feels threatened by the neighborhood bully will lift weights to make himself feel safe. Often, bulky muscles help one to feel safe. These hardened and armored bodies created by weight training have been used to dominate others who are weaker. Women, children, animals and other elements in nature have been the recipients of the muscled body used to attain and keep power.

Many people were taught that they could isolate a muscle and make it strong when they lifted weights and performed strength training. This is another myth. Muscles rarely move individually. Muscles will move in groups. Peg Jordan writes in *The Fitness Instinct*, "Rarely in life do you have to use one muscle to do something. The act of reaching for a heavy dictionary and lifting it across a table involves numerous muscles in your shoulders, chest, and arms—more muscles and tendons that you can imagine."

Muscles move as a team. In fact, muscles at the other end of the body where the weight is being lifted might be engaged. Notice how a person who is performing a shoulder press is tightening up his neck. A hamstring strengthening exercise usually will cause one to engage the lower back and psoas muscle as well. Even arms curls cause the back of the neck to tighten and the eyeballs to bulge. Hardening a part of the body usually means hardening most of the body. I have witnessed people throwing out their backs as they were performing something as simple as an isolated bicep curl.

Performing a bench press lying down may create more strength in the chest muscles. However, organs and glands beneath the chest muscles are tightening as well. This includes the heart and the muscles of respiration, including the intercostal muscles between the ribs. A hardened chest usually means hardness all the way through the thorax. While a degree of tone is important, a hard body is the antithesis of health.

Myth #3: Cardiovascular Fitness Improves Health

The average diet has continued to change as we have developed more high-tech foods and labor-saving devices. It is true that since most of us do not grow any or all of our own food these days, we are reliant on commercial companies for our food supply. These new food products often contain more fats than we once ate. But fat is not the enemy.

Some years back, science declared war on fat as the primary instigator of heart disease and many other ailments. Scientists pointed their fingers at the amount of fats that we consumed as the reason for illness. This myth has endured for quiet some time. It may be time for a new idea.

Classically, we were told to exercise and move our bodies as a remedy for prevention of heart disease and obesity. The classic medical finger pointing told us that in order to reduce the risk of heart disease, we must keep our blood pressure lowered and avoid a high cholesterol diet. Most of the emphasis had been placed on focusing on what we were putting into our body. It may be true that our diet may add to our risk factors, but diet is only a minor factor. The primary factors are stress and repression. The interesting fact is that many cultures eat a very high fat diet, much higher than Americans, and suffer far fewer heart problems.

Dr. Dean Ornish has done some amazing and groundbreaking work in the area of heart disease and fats. Dr. Ornish uses a low calorie diet, yoga, meditation and group support to achieve phenomenal results with his patients. Dr. Ornish writes in *Dr. Dean Ornish's Program For Reversing Heart Disease,*

"The use of cholesterol-lowering drugs is based on the presumption that cholesterol is the primary determinant of atherosclerosis, whereas I am

becoming increasingly convinced that other factors, including emotional stress, perceived isolation, lack of social support, hostility, cynicism, and low self-esteem, also play important roles."

In my experience, stress and repression are the primary factors in heart disease. Diet is only a minor influence. It is our emotions that we cannot release that lead to heart disease. Having too much fat in our diet is only a minor problem.

Dr. Ornish writes about the effects of stress on the heart.

"When our stress mechanisms are chronically *activated, the same responses that are designed to protect us can become harmful—even lethal. Arteries constrict not just in our arms and legs but also inside our hearts. Blood clots are more likely to form inside our coronary arteries.*

"Thus, most of our muscles constrict during times of chronic, intense emotional stress, ranging from the large muscles (causing tension and pain in the neck, back, shoulders, etc.) to the smooth muscles that line the coronary arteries (leading to spasm), to the fibers of the heart muscle itself (leading to contraction band necrosis . . .)."

Stress and emotional repression are the primary factors involved in heart disease. Whenever you are in fear, whether from a real or imagined threat, your body responds with the stress response. This includes your movement as well. When you are running, performing aerobic activity, panting for breath and pushing yourself to the limit, you are most often moving your body from a place of fear. This will actually put more stress on the heart as the muscle of the heart and the arteries contract.

Arteries are primarily made of connective tissue and smooth muscle. Under stress, the arteries will narrow and over time the connective tissue will harden. Moving your body from a place of fear is no different. As the arteries continue to narrow, tiny cracks are formed. Dr. Ornish writes,

"In the late 1970s studies in Italy by Dr. Attilio Maseri and others demonstrated that the cause of heart disease was more dynamic and complex than had previously been thought, and that other mechanisms besides blockages played important roles in reducing blood flow to the heart. He demonstrated that the coronary arteries are not rigid, like lead pipes; the arteries are flexible and are lined with smooth muscle that can constrict,

thus reducing coronary blood flow. This constriction of the artery is known as coronary artery spasm, or just spasm.

"When a coronary artery goes into spasm, it can injure the lining of the artery, leading to cholesterol deposition and plaque buildup as described earlier."

When you move your body from a place of fear, you often cause your own coronary arteries to constrict with the stress response, damaging the lining of the artery. The body's wisdom sends cholesterol to the damaged lining of the artery in an attempt to plug up a crack or hole. Dr. Ornish adds:

"Blockages form when the lining of a coronary artery is damaged. The body attempts to repair this insult by putting the physiological equivalent of a Band-Aid over the damaged area. This band-aid is made of cholesterol, collagen, and other materials."

So much emphasis has been placed on the heart being a pump and the need to strengthen the heart in order to be healthier. Making the heart stronger does very little to improve the tight muscles and frozen fascia that surround the arteries and veins that cause the heart to have to work so hard in the first place. Many times striving for a strong heart rate is a very stressful behavior. If cardiovascular fitness actually helped the heart, one would think that those who were the most fit would have the healthiest hearts. Unfortunately, this is not the case.

Many would consider firefighters as a group to be at the top of the fitness profile. With the physical rigors of their job, they must stay in top shape in order to perform at the highest level. Their lives and that of others depend on it. However, according to the U.S. Fire Administration, 44 percent of active on-duty firefighters die of heart attacks. One of the most fit professional groups has one of the highest incidences of heart disease death. You see, fitness is not necessarily a measurement of health, and in most cases will be a detriment to health.

Moving the body from a place of fear can actually lead to deterioration of the heart and surrounding blood vessels. Limiting the amount of fats that one consumes is only a minor influence.

Dr. Ornish explains that most of the cholesterol in your body does not come from a fast food restaurant or your refrigerator. Your own body produces most of the cholesterol in your body. "Your body makes all the cholesterol it needs, even if you don't eat any cholesterol in your diet and even if you reduce your saturated fat intake. In fact, three-fourths of the cholesterol in your blood is made by your own body."

A lifetime of practicing stressful movements leads to a heart under duress. Dr. Ornish furthers his reasoning this way. "In people with coronary artery blockage, exercise actually *increases* the tendency of blood to clot and arteries to constrict during the time of activity—one reason why even athletic people sometimes die while jogging (like Jim Fixx), or playing basketball (like Pete Maravich)."

While it is true that adding muscle allows the body to burn fat more efficiently, it is also true that we are obsessed with fat in our culture. Building muscle for esthetic looks and trying to conquer our obsession with fat can have an important impact on how we move. Building muscle can be another way to reduce our movement.

The body will store fat for a reason; it believes it is in survival mode and will need the fat later. This is what the stress response does for you—it places you in survival mode. Often this reaction continues for months and years on end. Colleen A. Sundermeyer, Ph.D., writes in *Emotional Weight,* "Your body sees fat as survival, even though you see it as gross and ugly." It is our inability to relax and release our stress response that is the problem, not fat itself.

We need to stop blaming fat for our problems. Fat is necessary for our survival.

Myth #4: It Hurts to Move so Why Move

When there is pain in our body, we learn to protect that pain by limiting our movement. When we do this, we tend to lock the pain in even more. Movement is vital to working pain out of our body. Much of the time, our fascia is frozen and needs to be loosened. Sitting still will only make matters worse. The body needs to be stimulated in order to grow. Stopping movement because it hurts to move will only make matters worse in the long run. When we learn to have kinesthetic intelligence of our own body, we know when to rest our body from further injury and when to apply gentle movements to keep it loosening up.

An animal in nature will move through most injuries. It will shake itself out after a fall. A frantic moment will be followed by a complete head to toe shake to dissipate the trauma from its body. When we move slowly through a trauma, we do not lock the trauma into the body.

Myth #5: We Need to Slow Down as We Age

Many believe that we need to stop moving as we age, so we do. We limit our activity and then we can't move anymore. I have witnessed many people in their fifties, sixties, and seventies who have made a commitment to begin a regular yoga practice. Within weeks their movement is much more expansive and fluid. I have noticed changes in their breathing and their posture as well.

Most people believe that to age is to slow down, shrink in size and retire to an easy chair to wait out the rest of their lives. The belief for many people is to work hard while you are young, save your money, and then when your body is no longer able to move, you can retire and sit back and do nothing. This is a myth. It does not have to be this way. But if you reduce your movement as you age based on the assumption that you need to slow down, then you will be doing yourself a disservice.

Summary

Most of what we have learned about movement is just a myth. These myths have added to the loss of our body and the restrictions of our movement. Leaning to recover our movement means learning to change our beliefs about movement.

Expansive Movement

A sedentary life will lead the body to obesity and decay. A life filled with contractive and fear-based movement is not much better. Movement based in nature is expansive and life giving. Learning to heal your body and maintain your vitality means learning to move in an expansive way.

Movement begins in the mind. Where did your beliefs come from about movement? When did you first begin to lose your relationship with natural movement and become committed to artificial movements? Who were your role models who taught you how to harden and stiffen your body?

Expansive movement begins with your beliefs. When you are moving your body in this manner, you are moving without fear. You are not counting calories or measuring your heart rate. You are not concerned with your performance. You are not timing yourself and racing against another individual, group or yourself. When you participate in expansive movement, you are opening up rather than contracting. Moving with nature means not being a warrior in your movement.

When you watch young children and animals, you can learn how to change your beliefs about movement, hence changing your movement itself. Your role models might come from nature rather than from a publisher of a glamour magazine or a promoter of a body building competition.

Movement Is Learned

When you were first born, your movement was limited. You could move your eyes but not focus too well in the distance. You could move your hands and feet yet still had difficulty in grasping things. A cry would move your rib cage up and down. Your movement was limited to the development of your brain. You had not yet learned how to coordinate your movement nor did you have the strength to move even if you tried.

That quickly changed. With every day you began to experiment by using different muscles. You learned how to roll over and to lift your head. You began to grasp objects. You started to crawl. The crawl led to a walk and then you learned how to run. Pretty soon you learned to run from place to place. You had a difficult time slowing down. You would climb on furniture and swing from everything in your path. Movement was fun as you explored your world. Your development was dependent on your carefully orchestrated use of your movement. As your brain developed, you soon learned how to coordinate muscles more efficiently. You gained strength as you used your limbs. From infant to child to adolescent, you continually learned new ways to move. This was just a normal aspect of your personal evolution.

For most people, expansive and playful movement was left behind when they began to grasp language and the rules in their culture. Most were introduced to competitive games early on where they were measured on their performance and not on their curiosity. Fun was replaced with winners and losers. Entry into the school system continued to reinforce these beliefs about movement.

You were most likely forced to sit in a chair for most of the day and memorize information that you were told would be useful for the rest of your life. You learned that rational knowledge was more useful than anything your body might tell you. Body knowledge, the type that you were learning the first few years of your life, was now being replaced by intellectual knowledge. You were only allowed to get up out of your chair and move your body during pre-arranged times throughout the day. This was called "physical education."

Unfortunately, your teachers attempted to educate you about your body in a manner similar to what was going on in the classroom. You became more cognitive brained and competitive in your movements because this is what you were learning in the classroom. You were now being graded on your movement. The students with the most competitive and athletic bodies received the best grades. This was just like the student who was the best at spelling or math. Movement that showed up on a report card now replaced your natural beliefs about movement.

Nature created movement. Science came along and attempted to recreate it to fit into the emerging model of the cognitive brain. Movement now came from head knowledge rather than from body knowledge.

Expansive movement is your natural birthright. As movement is learned, you can either continue to develop this natural approach to movement or you can repress these beliefs and replace them with beliefs that run counter to nature.

Each culture teaches movement differently. A culture that values natural movement will teach this to its children. Notice cultures that do not place such great emphasis on intellectual knowledge. Here you will find people who live much more of their lives in their body. Their awareness of their body is very profound. They tell stories with their body. Their movement and facial expressions are more vivid and alive. They celebrate with a dance or a song.

This is unlike a culture that spends so much time in its head, favoring intellectual knowledge. Here you will find people who live in their heads and have numbed out their body. They find it startling when there is a problem in their body, almost as if they were a victim of their own body. They tell stories with words from their head transferred to paper or a computer screen. They celebrate with a written card from a popular greeting card company.

It is amazing to watch a culture of people who live in their body. They come alive with movement. Watching a hula dancer in Hawaii always amazes me. The movements are flowing and expressive. The story of their history comes alive in the dance. A belly dancer from a Persian culture will communicate the seduction story of her dance. Words are seldom used to convey this message. It is her hips that speak the language of the story. A Brazilian speaks of the passion in the Samba with costume and dance. Each muscle is used to express the rhythm and the passion of the culture. The body is used as a tool for expression rather than a tool for war. In fact, it has been a very long time since Brazil has had a war. Warrior mentality is almost non-existent.

Expansive and playful movement comes to us naturally but is quickly replaced with contractive movements. For many cultures, warrior movement becomes the norm. Cultures that spend more time in their heads, reinforcing the cognitive brain, are more apt to develop war-based movements. Cultures that practice war develop citizens that move like warriors. A head-based culture will be very different than a body-based culture. This can be seen in the movement of the people who live there.

Movement to Unite or to Repel

Expansive movement is aimed at uniting bodies rather than at repelling an enemy. If you watch very young children at play, their movements will draw them together. Children will roll around together with their bodies intertwined. Their movements are designed to merge them all together. Look at the childhood game of "Twister." Bodies are interwoven amongst each other on a giant fold out mat. Laughing and playfully mixed together, these young children are using their movements to make contact.

When you engage in expansive movements, you merge rather than push away. Movement to soften rather than to harden is used. Notice two lovers embracing. Their bodies are intertwined. They are enjoying each other. They are soft and relaxed. They are merging with their movements. When you engage in movement that is expressive, you are more likely to be in a state of relaxation and not moving from fear. You do not fear contact with another. You are not hardening in defense.

In contrast is the warrior's body. This contractive and fear-based movement is designed to repel and keep people away. A warrior practicing martial arts will use his movements to keep an opponent or attacker away from his body. A football player will use his arms and body to avoid being tackled to the ground by the opposing team members. A soldier will use hand-to-hand combat to keep an enemy from getting to his body.

Expansive movement brings us closer together. Competitive and fear-based movement will keep others away. Healing is very difficult in isolation. Learning to merge with others, either as lovers, as friends or in playful situations, only adds to your health. Using your movements to push others away only keeps you defended from the world. When learning to reclaim your body and your movement, it is important to begin to incorporate expansive movements designed to merge you with others.

The Body Is Like Soft Plastic

The body is constantly changing and evolving. It is not a piece of concrete that is stuck in place but can be equated to a piece of soft plastic. The types of movements that you are engaged in will mold and shape your body. These forces could be internal as well as external.

Notice the variety of different bodies in a crowd. They are all unique and different, indicating that there are many external forces at work. Take for example the body of someone who surfs quite a bit. His upper body will usually be larger than his lower body. The effect of the repetitive paddling on a surfboard to catch a wave will develop a very large upper body and a less developed lower body. The surfer's movements over time have shaped his body.

A person who rides a horse often is more prone to developing bowed legs. The position of straddling a horse will cause the legs to be shaped according to the midsection of a horse. This is usually in a bowed pattern. The constant stimulation of the plastic-like quality of the tissues of the body will conform to the forces applied to them.

Wearing high heels frequently might look socially appealing to women, but the strain to the legs and back is real. Wearing high heels causes the calf muscles, hamstrings and lower back muscles to shorten. Over time these add up to real and significant changes.

A professional tennis player will usually have one arm larger than the other. This is the arm with which he normally carries his racquet. A frequent backpacker may have shoulders that roll forward from the heavy weight of the backpack. The human body is constantly changing and being shaped by the forces applied to it. Ask any woman who has ever been pregnant if the body is capable of change as a baby grows inside of her.

Many times you will see an elderly person hunched over a walker as he pushes himself around. The act of hunching over for a long time will accentuate any hunched-over posture already occurring. Hunching over while using a walker to move around will only create more hunching over.

When you move around from place to place, you are moving with pre-established patterns. When you add artificial movements to your already unbalanced body, you only accentuate these imbalances. If your left hip is stiff due to an old bicycle injury, you may walk with an uneven gait. What happens when you try your hand at jogging? When you do this, you not only perpetuate the unbalanced gait, you actually begin to make it worse.

Your movement patterns will shape your body. An exercise program designed to create contractive movements will only contract the body even more, as the forces at work designed to harden and stiffen the body will do just that. An exercise program based on expansive movements will also change the soft plastic quality of the body. Instead of tightening and compacting around and old injury or pattern, an expansive movement system will lengthen and open up the body.

There is a notion that you are supposed to shrink with age. This is just a myth. You only shrink because of the contractive forces that you keep applying to yourself. While it may seem strange in your mindset, expansive movements can actually make you taller. The body is constantly changing based on the forces applied to it. If you apply movement that allows your body to lengthen and expand, this pattern becomes the predominant shape.

The only reason that you might shrink is because you have stopped moving and have chosen to contract instead. The fear that you have stored within your body is still pulling you downward, causing your muscles to contract, the fascia to harden and the spine to compress. Bones do not move by themselves. Bones are being pulled out of balance by the soft tissue (muscles and fascia). A person who continues to move and practice expansion will show very little signs of shrinkage as he ages. He might even be taller than he was when he was a young adult.

A good example of this is demonstrated in how some women in Balinese and other cultures wear necklaces around their necks. These necklaces are a status symbol in their culture. The woman with the most necklaces usually has the highest standing in the tribe.

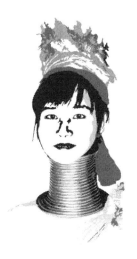

These necklaces also stretch the neck. Every so often a new necklace is applied. One woman was even measured to have a 17-inch neck. If you are to shrink with age, then how is it that these women's necks continue to grow longer each day as they age? The consistent lengthening forces that they apply in the form of necklaces are the answer.

Movement is also shaped by physical trauma affecting your body. A blow or an impact will settle into your body. When this happens, the tissue that is affected will contract and harden as the muscles remain frozen and the connective tissue hardens. Unfortunately, most rehabilitation programs will reinforce an impact injury. By utilizing strength training to build muscle around an injury, you are just surrounding the injury with layers of armoring, not necessarily healing the damage.

The problem with many rehabilitation programs is that they are based on science and not on nature. Science generally attempts to conquer nature. When following many rehabilitation programs, you are still hardening your body like a warrior, not necessarily healing the damage created by the impact trauma. Most traditional rehabilitation programs are based on warrior mentality where hardness is equated with health. The key mistake being made is that fitness is being used as a health treatment. As we have already seen, fitness and health are usually two entirely different concepts.

This hardening around an injury seldom gets to the heart of an injury but only builds walls of muscle so you won't feel the energy that is stored deep inside. A better approach would be to loosen the area around an injury with bodywork and gentle movement. This would be more natural.

Expansive movements are designed to re-educate an injury sight. If the muscles already were frozen in place, why would you want to tighten them up even more? Expansive movements attempt to teach the muscles and the nervous system that it is safe to move now. The fear and the energy that were once locked into place during the initial trauma begin to dissipate when you practice expansive movements.

Just as the external forces in your life will shape your body, so too will the internal forces at work. Stress and repression will continue to pull your body tighter. Expansive movements start to move the body in the opposite direction of stress and repression. Expansive movements are an antidote to many of the effects of stress and repression.

If you keep moving your body in the same way, you will continue to get the same results. Stressed-based movements will give you the same results—more contraction and stiffness. The results are predictable. Only when you begin to move in a way that is unfamiliar will you begin to get different results.

Emotional Weight

While working for a well known health spa for years, I would often notice how some people could lose 20 pounds or more in a week of intense physical exercise while others would scarcely let go of half a pound. Both would consume the same amount of calories and experience the same level of physical activity. I started to ask some deeper questions. What I came to realize was that those who did not lose any weight during this rigorous week of activity seemed emotionally repressed. They just would not let go. Their bodies were holding on tightly. Their muscles were stiff. They breathed shallowly. Their body would not let go of anything, including weight.

What I discovered after working on a number of people like this was that much of the time was that their energy was slow to move through their body. They were literally holding on tightly in their emotional world and their body was just a physical reminder. They were so fearful about getting fat and not being loved that their body was in a constant state of contraction. The fat cells could not be released because there was no energy getting to those areas.

Alexander Lowen writes in *Pleasure: A Creative Approach to Life,*

"Tense muscles can only be released by expressive movements, that is, movements in which the activity expresses the repressed feeling. As long as a movement is mechanically performed, the repressed impulses are held back and no release of the tension is affected."

Lowen goes on to add, "Suppression of feeling is produced by chronic muscular tensions which restrict and limit the motility of the body, thereby reducing sensation. In the absence of movement, there is nothing to sense or feel."

A better choice for exercise with an expansive quality is to choose something like yoga or dance therapy. Depending on the type of yoga and your internal goal, this could be a very effective tool to use in helping the body to free itself from its contractive state. Yoga tends to lengthen muscles and connective tissue. Dance therapy can also be another good choice. Just playing some music to move to when you are feeling contracted could be a way of using exercise to expand out of your contracted nature.

Another movement tool that I have found important to help expand through contraction is Reichian therapy. Reichian work attempts to unlock the temper tantrum stuck deep within us. Once this happens, your energy flows more freely. For many people, cathartic releasing can be a way to heal. Candace Pert believes this to be an effective method for some people. She writes in *Molecules of Emotion:*

"Based on the drama and rapidity of some therapeutic transformations, I believe that repressed emotions are stored in the body—the unconscious mind—via the release of neuropeptide ligands, and that memories are held in their receptors. Sometimes transformations occur through the emotional catharsis common to the many bodymind therapies that focus on freeing up emotions that have gotten lodged in the psychosomatic network, but not always."

I notice people of all ages who start an exercise routine and get even stiffer and contracted rather quickly. Whether it is a walking, running or a weight routine, if you are not breathing fully and using movement to expand, the movement might be keeping you even tighter.

Your medical doctor telling you to go out and exercise or you will die is not enough. If you do not breathe deeply and use expansive movements, the exercise could be doing you more harm than good. Just because someone in an authoritarian position (many times your medical doctor) advises you to get out and run on a treadmill three times per week, does not necessarily mean that this type of movement is best for you. If you are angry, repressed and stressed out, with every step you will be holding on to more tension rather than letting go of it.

People of all ages can begin to practice movement therapy rather easily. Choosing the right type of movement with the right attitude will make all the difference though. Just because you are walking three miles per day does not necessarily mean that this movement is the most beneficial for you. The attitude and manner in which you move your body is extremely important as to how your body responds to it. For instance, if someone goes out regularly for her "power walk" with her rigid attitude and shortened movements, she may be stiffing up with each outing.

Recovery of your movement means practicing expressive and expansive movement on a regular schedule. Movement needs to be playful rather than stressful. To stop moving is to freeze up and die; practicing fear-based movement can be just as fatal. Fear-based movement will lead the body into contraction, build armor and will shut off more feeling and sensation. Recovery of the body must include expressive and expansive movements.

Examples of Expansive Movement

Learning to change your movement begins by learning to change your beliefs about movement. Your goals have to change. Your approach has to change. You often must learn to let go of many years of reinforced conditioning. Changing your movement means being willing to try something new.

Just as there are many ways to tighten and harden your body, there are also many ways to practice expansive movement. Three examples of an expansive movement practice are yoga, Feldenkrais and Continuum. Some of these approaches have been around for thousands of years while others are relatively new. They all share one thing in common—they are all expansive in nature.

Yoga

Yoga is an ancient system of beliefs and movement that originated in India. It is through the yoga practice that expansive movements are used to create a healthier body. Yoga allows you to capitalize on natural movements and use them for your advantage while being a wonderful tool for wellness.

Yoga works by creating heat in the muscles. Every time you engage in a pose (asana), you heat up your muscles. You take the heat and stretch the warm muscles. This is like pulling warm taffy. The muscles and surrounding connective tissue will lengthen and develop into an even more open pattern. You can actually get taller by practicing yoga regularly.

Yoga attempts to create space. This space is created between spinal vertebrae, or in knee and hip joints which become more open as the muscles and connective tissue warm and lengthen. As flexibility increases, so does health. Yoga will be in sharp contrast to Western exercise principles that attempt to harden and tighten the body.

Yoga also employs a nasal breath. When breathing through the nose, the air passes through the First Cranial Nerve, massaging it and calming the mind. When you breathe through the nose, you are more likely to stay out of your Fight or Flight Response. This is unlike Western exercise where the mouth is primarily used to breathe and the breath is often a panting and shallow breath.

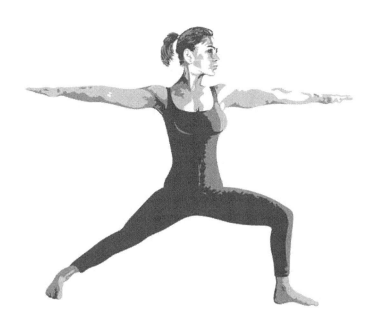

Another fascinating aspect of yoga is that as the body warms and is stretched, the connective tissue will change shape. This tissue, primarily a water-based, gelatin-like material, will lengthen along with the muscles. As the connective tissue lengthens, the energy in the body changes. The connective tissue is responsible for the transfer of "chi" or energy through the body. The lengthening of the connective tissue helps it to maintain its liquid nature, transferring energy more efficiently. In contractive movements (like weight training), the connective tissue will tend to dry out and harden as the muscles bond together. Energy does not travel very efficiently through dried-out connective tissue.

In this respect, yoga is much more than just an exercise practice—it is a wellness practice. Yet the yoga system is not without fault either. Yoga is many things to many people. Just because you claim to be practicing yoga does not necessarily mean that you have this magical bubble around you to protect you from all illnesses and keep you out of harm's way. When practicing yoga with a rigid or competitive mind, the practice will help to create more rigidity and more competition. Some of the tightest bodies I have ever worked on belonged to long-time yoga practitioners and teachers who practiced yoga in a competitive and rigid manner.

Some styles of yoga are more analytical than others. These particular styles of yoga, which emphasize the precision in the pose, help to activate the Fight or Flight Response. This will tighten up your muscles in the long-term. When you emphasize the "right" and the" "wrong" way to move, you set yourself up for a stress response because judgment of movement can lead to stress. When you critique your movement, you are now performing. In order to use yoga as a healing tool, the emphasis needs to be on relaxation and feeling sensation while being in the pose. Any form of perfectionism or competition with yourself or others will only lead to stress. This applies to yoga as well.

Incorporating a non-competitive and relaxation-based yoga practice into your life is much more in line with natural and healing movements. The body will lengthen every day. The body will become more dynamically alive with regard to organs, muscles and glands. Lung volume will increase and your energy level will rise. Yoga is an expansive type of movement system. When practicing yoga, it is easier to follow nature's guidelines of moving the body.

Feldenkrais

Moshe Feldenkrais, an Israeli physicist, designed the Feldenkrais Method. It is through the work of Feldenkrais that you may learn to re-educate your body's movement rather than reinforcing a pattern that does not suit you well. With this type of movement, you begin to move your body without fear or competition. The emphasis is on exploration rather than on goal-setting. Feldenkrais labeled his system "Awareness through Movement."

In *Alternative Medicine: The Definitive Guide,* the editors describe the Feldenkrais Method as follows,

"Participants of Awareness through Movement are guided through a slow and gentle sequence designed to replace old patterns of movement with new ones. As the client learns how to listen to these 'lessons,' he or she develops an awareness of subtle changes in habit and movement. Feldenkrais wrote that the lessons are designed to improve mobility, 'to turn the impossible into the possible, the possible into the easy, and the easy into elegant.'"

It is through this type of movement that you expand and let go. Rigid holding patterns are reduced or eliminated. Your range of motion is increased. You are learning how to move your body not as a warrior, but as a curiosity seeker. This is similar to how you first learned how to move when you were young. You explored range of motion as a form of self-discovery.

With the Feldenkrais work, you begin to heal the damage done by stress, repression and physical trauma. In a serious traumatic accident, many times the muscles will remain frozen in place, often for many years after the accident. Through *Awareness through Movement*, you might begin to teach your muscles to let go. You are finally coming free from a trauma that was locked into your physical and energetic body for quite some time. Leaning to move your body while relaxed becomes a key component of the Feldenkrais Method.

Continuum

In the Feldenkrais model, you are taught to move in a way to explore and re-educate your own body. In the Continuum model, you learn how to be playful with your movement. It is this playful and silly method that teaches you how to let your body story go, to be free of your past held tightly in your body.

When was the last time you went for a walk and were not concerned about how fast you were going or how many calories you were burning? Playful movement is something that many have forgotten how to do. You have become so accustomed to performance-oriented movement that you have lost your ability to play.

Emilie Conrad Da'oud says that movement is something that we "are" rather than something that we "do." She is the originator of Continuum. With Continuum, one is taught to move as if you were water, feeling the fluid-like nature of the body. There is an emphasis on moving in a wave-like pattern, just like the flow of water. This is another type of movement therapy that is expansive and liberating rather than the traditional types of contractive movements to which many people have become accustomed.

Suggestive "micro-movements" are used to allow the body to re-create a new sense of itself. There is an attempt to bring you back to your primal nature with these micro-movements and the underlying breath patterns that accompany the work. The movements are unpredictable and draw you deeper into your reptilian origins.

With Continuum, one begins to sense the freedom that movement can bring. When practicing these expansive movements, you begin to release the memories stored within your tissues. Emotions and old injuries have a chance to release themselves as the body moves in a way that provides safety and freedom instead of moving from fear. Continuum, as an expansive movement lesson, allows you to begin to heal.

Four Corners of Movement

As you get up and move your body each morning, have you ever asked yourself what your intentions are with your movement? Are you on "auto-pilot" and just do what you have always done? What motivates you to move? Are you exercising because you are afraid of getting fat or dying of a heart attack? Are you moving because you are obligated to move, as in a professional sport?

If you keep moving in the same manner all of the time, you will continue to get the same results. Most people continue to move their body in the same way as they have always moved. They continue to get the same results. In order to get different results, you may have to begin to change how you move. Your goals may have to be different. Your intentions and your method of movement may have to be updated. Are you still moving your body with pre-historic beliefs in mind? If the answer is "Yes," maybe it is time to update your belief systems.

In order to bring balance to your life, it may be necessary to begin to use your intuition rather than your habits to guide your movement. Health is much more than just strength and a lowered resting heart rate. The following are some guidelines that can be important as you begin to bring balanced movement into your life. I call this the *Four Corners of Movement.*

1. Disciplined Movement

Disciplined movement involves a pattern or routine. Emphasis would be on flowing and lengthening. This is an organized set of movements that is either interconnected or practiced separately. There is a structure, a formula and a method for practice. Examples of this type of movement might be: tai chi, yoga or Pilates.

2. Cardio-Strength Movement

Cardio-strength movement focuses on strength and endurance. A special emphasis might be placed on fat burning and increasing the heart rate. Examples of this type of movement could include the following: hiking, swimming, walking, jogging, aerobics, weight training. It is important when practicing cardio-strength movements to emphasize full range of movement and not be so concerned with numbers (i.e., calories burned, heart rate, etc.).

3. Integrative Movement

Integrative movement is important for healing from injuries or trauma. This may include a series of unifying lessons aimed at re-patterning the nervous system. There is a keen emphasis on moving without fear. An attempt is made to make the movements slow and repetitive so the body remembers. Examples of this type of movement are the following: Alexander work, Feldenkrais, and Continuum.

4. Playful Movement

Many of us have forgotten how to play. Playful movement is freeing and has little or no structure. There are few rules, discipline or prizes attached. There is no "right" or "wrong" way to move your body. You are not graded on how you move. There is no failure or shame. Examples of this kind of movement might be the following: playing Frisbee on the beach, kayaking, dancing to music or swimming in the ocean.

Summary

A balanced life begins with balanced movement. Incorporating many aspects of movement into your life will begin to stimulate you to grow and change in many ways. Changing your beliefs about movement begins with examining how you learned to move and the beliefs that you have taken on about movement.

Moving with health in mind means to let your arms swing when you walk and your hips to swivel as you jog. You won't be concerned about any numbers, calories or repetitions. You will move without fear.

"In shape" does not necessarily mean "in health." The guidelines that you once thought of as health may have to change. Many people may not be practicing much health at all when it comes to their movement.

Movement is natural; exercise is not. When you stop using your body to push others away, you begin your healing. When you end the long reign of teaching your children how to be warriors, you take the courageous step in changing your world. Movement begins in the mind. When you are willing to change your mind about your movement, you will begin to change your body as well.

Pillar Number Four

Recovery of the Breath

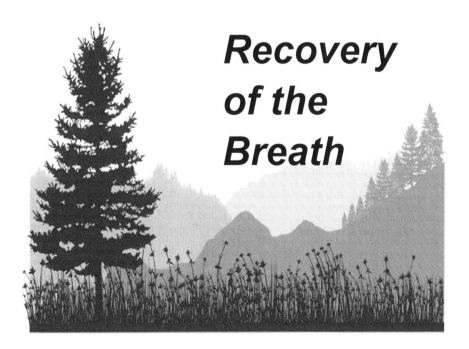

The Physiology of Breathing

Most people believe that breathing is as natural and easy as waking up in the morning. They assume the way they breathe is adequate to get them through life. They do not take much notice of their breath. They just know that if they are still alive, they must be breathing sufficiently.

The truth is that most people have lost their breath. They have lost their ability to breathe in and out fully and completely. They do not realize that deep breathing is missing from their lives until they attempt to take a deep breath and find it difficult. From the very first to the very last breath that people take, many pay little attention to how oxygen enters into their body. They assume that breathing comes naturally and is something one does not have to think about.

This is not necessarily so. Many Eastern cultures recognize the importance of the breath. There are several yoga practices that encourage the stimulation of breath. In fact, the traditional hatha yoga practice that many Westerners have become familiar with does not exist without the breath. The breath is just as important, if not more so, than the individual postures themselves.

How can you hope to recover something when you do not even realize that you have lost it? When you are aligned with nature, you breathe efficiently and fully. The breath is not labored or shallow. Rather, the breath flows deeply and fully. Returning to nature means learning how to dismantle the rigid breathing patterns that you have acquired. When you can allow nature to guide you, you establish a full breath that supports your wellness rather than adding to your body's decay. When you can attune with your natural breath, you help to recover your body.

The act of breathing is a very vital and necessary function in your life. Breathing is both very simple and very elaborate at the same time. Accessing the breath in a conscious fashion can enhance your health. When the breath is left to unconsciousness, you may suffer adverse health conditions. Recovery of your body includes the recovery of your breath.

The breath is primarily controlled by the Autonomic Nervous System. This means that you do not have to think about breathing. The process of breathing is automatic. While sleeping, eating or exercising, your body automatically breathes.

There are many variables to this automatic process. You can change the rate, rhythm and depth of your breath by learning to breathe, or learning to *not* breathe. You have the ability to alter this automatic process one way or another.

When you breathe, you are doing a number of things. The diaphragm pulls downward. The intercostal muscles between your ribs draw the ribs outward. The posterior scalene muscles in the neck help to lift the top portion of your rib cage upward. All of this muscle activity creates a vacuum within your lungs so that air will rush in to be absorbed by the body and travel to your cells. Many muscles are involved in the process of breathing.

The lungs themselves cannot move. The surrounding muscles affect the lung tissue. These muscles are like motors that create movement. Without these muscles of respiration, the only way you would be able to breathe would be with the help of assisted respiration.

The lungs are suspended between groups of muscles and connective tissue. As these muscles contract, they stretch the pleural cavity (the membrane compartment where the lungs reside). As this cavity is stretched, air is forced in on the inhale and waste products (carbon dioxide) are forced out on the exhale.

Imagine a round barrel. The lungs would be in the center. The diaphragm would be below and the scalene muscles above. The outer edges of the barrel would be the rib muscles (intercostals). As you inhale, the whole barrel would expand. On the exhale, the barrel would become slightly smaller and more compact in shape. The chest cavity acts like an accordion to change the volume of the lungs. This is how the body receives oxygen and removes carbon dioxide—by the chest cavity changing shape, due to muscle activity.

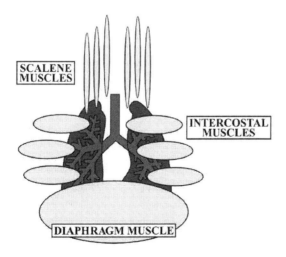

SCALENE MUSCLES

INTERCOSTAL MUSCLES

DIAPHRAGM MUSCLE

Why Is Breathing Important?

Besides the obvious "We need to breathe in order to stay alive," why is breathing important? There are many reasons that the conscious use of your breath is important. These reasons are stated below.

1. Conscious Breathing Helps to Focus Your Mind

Oxygen is critical to the survival of all living things. This includes human beings as well. The brain and eyes require more oxygen than any other part of the body. When insufficient amounts of oxygen reach the brain, the result is a mental sluggishness. Vision and hearing can begin to decline. As the oxygen levels to the brain are increased, so is mental activity. The brain requires up to three times more oxygen than the rest of the body.

2. One Feels More Energized as Breathing Increases

Oxygen is food for the body. An increase in oxygen gives the cells of the body more energy to provide mechanical action. Reduced breathing often leads one into a state of depression or sluggishness. Oxygen drawn into the lungs with the breath combines with nutrients from food at a cellular level to fuel your body. Without oxygen, this biochemical reaction cannot take place.

3. Digestion Is Increased

When the stomach and intestines receive adequate amounts of oxygen, the digestion and assimilation of food is greatly increased. Digestion can be sluggish when oxygen levels are reduced.

4. Improvement in the Quality of Blood

Oxygen acts as a means to help purify the blood and destroy toxins that travel throughout the blood stream. As increased amounts of oxygen reach the blood stream, more toxins are removed and the immune system is enhanced. Carbon dioxide, the bi-product of cellular metabolism, is removed from the blood stream when you breathe. Seventy percent of the body's waste products are removed through the lungs by way of exhalation.

5. Glands Are Rejuvenated

The functioning of the glandular system is increased by an adequate supply of blood to them. Glands consist of connective tissue and smooth muscle that require steady and consistent blood flow. As glands function at their most optimal level, all other parts of the body that depend on these secretions are improved as well.

6. Breathing Massages the Organs

As the diaphragm and other muscles of respiration are engaged, the internal organs are massaged. This assists these organs in their capacity to function. The heart, liver, kidneys, intestines and pancreas are some of the organs affected by the breathing process.

In The Beginning

Learning to breathe was one of your very first tasks when you first came into this world. Failure at this first lesson often meant that you would not survive to meet the next challenges that lay ahead.

Your pattern of breathing goes back to your birth. You spent nine months in a watery world. Your lungs were useless as you relied on your direct linkup with your mother's blood stream and the amniotic fluid in which you floated for your nourishment and oxygen supply. You never had to think about taking a breath nor worried about what it would feel like if you could not breathe. Your lungs were still very useless.

The lungs are one of the last vital functions to develop fully before you are born. A premature birth is especially traumatic because most of your organs can already function on their own, but your lungs may not be able to keep you alive unless fully developed.

The act of being born quickly changes all of that. When the water sac that you are floating in breaks and signals the mother that birth is on the way, what happens to you inside the womb? Your environment quickly changes. As the water rushes out, air rushes inside the womb. You go from the world of the fish to the world of the air breathers in a very short time. It is as if you need to exchange your gills for lungs very quickly in order to survive in this new world. Air begins to fill your lungs, even while you are still within your mother's body. You have no choice. You must begin to start breathing during your transition into the world.

If you have an easy birth that goes smoothly and quickly, you suffer fewer traumas to your body. Imagine a difficult birth that is delayed by many circumstances. You are within the womb trying to gasp for breath. You are learning to breathe while experiencing quite a bit of stress. Breathing then becomes associated with stress.

You finally emerge into this new world. Learning to breathe sometimes is not an easy process. You take your first few breaths on your own outside of your mother's body. For some, these first few breaths were very traumatic. The air stings your lungs. It hurts to breathe. Think of what it is like to be born outside of an air-conditioned hospital. Imagine what 35 degrees Fahrenheit feel like in a newborn's lungs if he happens to be born in a teepee on a cold wintry day out in a snowy pasture.

Joseph Heller and William A. Henkin write in *Bodywise,* "Breathing is the very first act we must all perform on our own. It is our proclamation, the single event that signifies we are alive."

Stuart Ira Fox writes in *Human Physiology,* "Even under normal conditions, the first breath of life is a difficult one because the newborn must overcome great surface tension forces in order to inflate its partially collapsed alveoli."

A doctor might have slapped your bottom to stimulate you to breathe. You now learn to associate breathing with pain. A strange world of lights and noise awaits most newcomers to this new world. Breathing may be associated with a feeling of panic or sense of unease. You may not feel safe when removed from your warm and watery world. A shortened breath may become imprinted as your normal way to take in air.

If you perceive the world as a scary place or experience a great deal of trauma as you are being born, you might have a difficult time learning how to breathe. A happy baby is one who breathes at ease. A frightened child will have difficulty taking breath in fully. Your first breath and subsequent breaths after that may become very important in how you breathe later on in life.

Dennis Lewis writes about his birthing process in *The Tao of Natural Breathing,*

> *"It is obvious to me today, however, that my 30-hour struggle to reach light and take my first breath left deep impressions in my body and nervous system, and laid the foundation for some of the fundamental fears and insecurities that have motivated my behavior as an adult."*

The way you first learned how to breathe often becomes the pattern that you continue to use the rest of your life. A traumatic early experience with breathing often continues to be replicated. Farther down the road you are confronted with other experiences and beliefs that further compromise your breath. These later conflicts with your natural breath combined with your early experiences with learning how to breathe often spell disaster for your breathing process.

Frederick Leboyer, M.D., writes about the early imprinting your first breath has on the rest of your life in *Birth Without Violence.*

"But is birth really so important, one might ask. It doesn't last long, you could say, compared with what comes before and after it. Maybe it's just a nasty moment to get through. But that is perhaps somewhat glib. After all, there is another 'nasty moment' which, although equally brief, nonetheless casts a long shadow, and that is death. Yes, birth and the moments that follow, however few, will leave a mark for the rest of life. It is as if we are heading off in the wrong direction, starting on the wrong foot. It's like a boat leaving the harbor, with the poor captain not knowing he has a faulty compass. This compass, one might say, is breathing."

Losing Our Relationship
with Our Breath

Stress

The relationship that you have with your breathing is founded on your experiences throughout your life. When you lose your relationship with nature, you also lose your breath. The three major forces that affect you are stress, repression and physical trauma. As already noted with other ways you lose your body, the breath is no different.

Once again, stress is an emotional experience that translates to your body as a fear response. Essentially, when experiencing the stress response, you do not feel safe. This can happen during your birth, being placed in an incubator in a hospital or any other experience. Any experience in your life can trigger the stress response. The common result is that you breathe in a shallow manner when you do not feel safe.

A child who grows up in a family that has a high degree of conflict, out of control parents, substance abuse, sexual abuse or uncertainty may grow up with a shallow breath. Because it is never safe to relax in her household, she is not able to let her guard down. She is constantly frozen in terror, not knowing when the next outburst or assault will occur. She keeps her breath shallow so as not to attract too much attention. This pattern becomes imprinted in her as an adult. A deep, full breath is a rarity in her life. She has made an unconscious commitment to hold on to her breath. Even as an adult, breathing deeply means that someone might find her and hurt her.

Rebecca was one such child. Her childhood home was never safe. Her father was a raging alcoholic who was both emotionally and physically abusive. She cowered in terror, not knowing when the next outburst would occur. Rebecca held her breath as her stress response was nearly always activated. She was living with the enemy and had nowhere to run and hide.

As an adult, Rebecca still suffered from a shortened breath. She still believed that she was unsafe; this belief had been imprinted in her. Only with much guided process awareness and breathing exercises was Rebecca able to take a deep breath again. She had to change her beliefs to remind herself that she was safe now and out of harm's way.

A child who grows up in the perfect model family might have the same stress response and subsequent shallow breathing. This response is due to her fear that she is not perfect all of the time. She pressures herself to perform. Failure is equivalent with death or denial of love. The stress response constantly keeps her on guard, and she continues to strive toward heroic goals. Relaxation is difficult because it means wasting time when she could be producing. The end result is that she often loses her natural breath. The child who is encouraged to always be good or in control to meet her parents' expectations might have a difficult time of breathing in fully. Even as an adult, she is still staying in control of everything, including her breath.

Joe came from a model family. His biggest fear was making mistakes because his family emphasized performance and perfection. He seldom let down his guard. He rarely stopped achieving. He lost his ability to take a deep breath and relax. His anxiety continued, and breathing became a chore by the time he was an adult. Joe had lost his relationship with his natural breath.

The pressures that ensue through elementary school, high school and college continue to add to your loss of your natural breath. Family traumas, deaths, relationship conflicts and world events only assault your breath even more. Sleeping alone at night can be enough to trigger your stress response and alter your natural breath. A day stuck in freeway traffic might create a shallow breath. Weddings, business transactions and even a "bad hair day" can be enough to drive your natural breath into hiding.

Steve was a client who suffered from shallow breathing. On closer examination, it was revealed that the source of Steve's stress was an old pattern he had developed while he was a child. He knew that his parents loved him and cared about him, but his father had irregular work hours and would often come home late at night. Steve recalls how he would lie in bed at night, frozen and alone. His stress response was triggered. His breath remained shallow. He could not completely relax and take a deep breath until he heard his father returning home. It was only then that Steve finally fell asleep. He felt safe now.

Stress is an interpretive experience. We all have different triggers that initiate our stress response and shorten our breath. Over time, stress shortens the breath to next to nothing. The average lung capacity for an adult is about three and a half pints of air per breath, yet most people only take in about one pint of air with each breath. This is how the stress response minimizes our oxygen intake.

Taking a deep breath is equated with relaxation. A shallow breath comes with the stress response. When you have a difficult time learning how to relax, you also have a difficult time breathing fully and deeply.

What do we know about stress and muscles? Stress tends to shorten muscles. The longer the stress is occurring, the shorter the muscles become and the more difficult it is to free them to their full length. Muscles of respiration are no different.

From the very first stress of your birth to every subsequent episode of stress in your life, your muscles of respiration will contract. This contracting of respiratory muscles prevents the complete expansion of your rib cage resulting in a reduced flow of oxygen to your cells. In essence, due to stress many people have lost their ability to breathe fully. The only problem is that most do not even realize what they have lost.

Repression

You practice repression when you hold back your emotions. The behavior of repression affects many areas of your body; the breath is no exception. When you withhold the energy of emotion you begin to alter your breath. Over time, just like with stress, repression destroys your natural breath and limits your ability to breathe.

Emotions are meant to flow. This includes joy, sadness, grief and anger. When you believe that a certain emotion is not acceptable to feel and express, you use your own muscles to push the emotion down. The end result is a series of muscles that feel like tight belts across your chest and belly. After these muscles habitually hold on over time, it is almost impossible to take a deep breath even if you wanted to.

Repression of emotions can often lead to disease and illness. Where there is stagnation and lack of movement, there is a breeding ground for illness. The muscles of respiration are no different. Jeanne Elizabeth Blum, author of *Woman Heal Thyself*, says that the lungs are the part of the body that process grief. The repression of grief is much more likely to lead to the development of lung conditions like asthma, chest colds and even lung cancer.

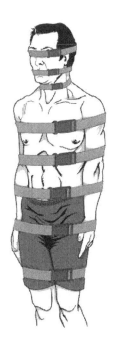

The act of repression across your chest and belly will feel like you are bound with straps and are unable to breathe.

Any expression of emotion, either intense or mild, will utilize the breath in a different way. When you are angry, you may hold your breath or breathe very quickly through your nostrils. When you are anxious, you may have a difficult time catching your breath. When you laugh, you use the muscles of respiration to help you express your pleasure.

When you hold on to or repress your emotions, you are also repressing or holding on to the muscles of respiration. You tend to store energy in these muscles when you repress your natural emotions. For instance, if a sneeze is about to emerge and you were raised with the belief that sneezing is rude or unacceptable, you might hold back that sneeze. In essence, the energy that needs to be released with the sneeze gets stored in the respiratory muscles and throughout the body. Most often, what you learn in childhood is carried with you into adulthood. This includes the repression of your breath as well.

Joseph Heller and William A. Henkin write in *Bodywise,*

"As with other physical holding, one occasion or two or a dozen is unlikely to damage the body. But if repression becomes a repetitive pattern, the muscles accumulate a little more tension and then a little more in addition to that, until the rib cage, chest, and diaphragm become set, and the child's torso becomes chronically tight. Then he breathes less and eventually develops a physical inability to express sadness—or even to be aware of feeling the emotion—by crying."

You often lose the ability to even know what emotions you are experiencing, as your physical body remains hardened and numb while your emotional wisdom is curtailed. The more you get cut off from your natural breath, the harder it becomes to find it once again.

A child who has not yet learned how to repress her emotions cries with her entire body. Not only do her tears flow steadily, but her rib cage heaves up and down as her entire body becomes engaged in releasing the sadness. When you learn to repress your sadness, your cries are reduced to a whimper, or they become non-existent. A child who remains free of repression laughs with his entire body until it hurts to continue. He rolls on the ground with laughter. There is a tremendous amount of air exchanged as the diaphragm and rib cage work overtime to help release the energy of the emotion of laughter. When he learns to repress his laughter, his torso becomes frozen as he moves into adulthood. He might show a mild sign of laughter on his face, but it is hardly the full body experience that he felt as a child.

Your experiences of repression teach you how to breathe inefficiently. The vicious cycle of repression of feelings is further complicated by the hardness in the respiratory muscles. Once this cycle is engaged, it requires a concerted effort to change this practice. Shallow breathing prevents you from taking in much less than the maximum capacity of air. As this pattern continues, you lose more and more of your body. Repression is another force that takes you away from your natural roots.

Physical Trauma

The third major force that affects your breath is physical trauma. When you experience an impact injury, your body takes on the energy of the impact. The muscles and connective tissue that absorb the impact often hold on tightly, even long after the initial impact. When the physical trauma affects your torso and the muscles of respiration, you often lose your ability to breathe fully.

When your muscles remain shortened for a significant amount of time, the fascia that surrounds those muscles dries out, loses its elasticity, and becomes glued together. The fascia connected to the muscles of respiration is no different. When the fascia loses its elasticity, it feels as if your rib cage is frozen in place. It hurts to breathe. This happens because the muscles of respiration are no longer able to expand and contract due to fascia that has lost its vitality. This feels as if you are wearing a corset around your torso.

Trauma that affects you comes in two varieties: sudden impact trauma and repetitive trauma. Both forms contribute to the loss of your breath.

Sudden impact trauma occurs in many automobile accidents. As a driver impacts with another car or stationary object, his torso might be thrown into the steering wheel. His chest might be crushed or bruised. The energy of impact causes the muscles of respiration to freeze up. When he lies in the hospital bed recovering from his injuries, it may hurt when he tries to take a deep breath, so instead he breathes shallowly. He then unconsciously trains the muscles of respiration to be still. Over time this pattern imprints itself and he is unable to take a deep breath. The memory of the crash gets stored in his chest. Long after the memory of the accident has faded, the shortened pattern of breathing often remains. Nobody reminds him that the accident has long sine passed, his body has recovered and it is safe to breathe fully again.

Tabitha was a client of mine who came to me for a variety of reasons. One issue was that she had great difficulty taking a deep breath. On closer examination of her trauma history, it was revealed that Tabitha had been in several automobile accidents. I observed a line of tension across her chest in the same pattern that a seat belt would align itself. It turns out that the seatbelt might have saved Tabitha's life, but it created a holding pattern along the same line across her chest. Only with several sessions of *Intuitive Connective Bodywork* and some breathing exercises was Tabitha able to finally take a deep breath.

Any accident can cause trauma throughout the respiratory muscles and affect the breath. A sudden and unexpected fall across a bicycle handlebar can create chest trauma which impacts the breath. Getting hit with a baseball in the rib cage might seem like a minor incident at age nine, but years later it may still be very difficult to breathe in fully. The fear of experiencing any more pain remains as the energy of impact has affected the surrounding muscles.

Being punched in the stomach during a street fight can impair a child's diaphragm with long-lasting consequences. The diaphragm might still be holding on. The child may believe that the pain will return if he lets go and takes a deep breath. The memory of the trauma has been imprinted. Even long into adulthood, this pattern has been repeated often enough to become normal.

Sudden impact trauma is only half the story; repetitive traumas are the other half. Repetitive traumas occur on a much smaller scale but add up over time. The result is often a shortened breath. Playing competitive sports is one way the breath might be affected over time by repetitive traumas. The collisions and impacts of competition can remain for years to come and can influence the ability to breathe fully.

A football player might have many small impact traumas to his rib cage. These impact traumas cause the intercostal muscles used in breathing to hold on tightly. Lifting weights to prepare for athletic competitions only adds tightness across an athlete's chest. He has to overcome this bulkiness made up of muscle mass if he wants to take a deep breath. A tightened and hardened abdomen locks the diaphragm in place. Now the primary muscle of respiration is clamped down by hardened muscle tissue.

The clothes that we wear are another way to hamper the breath. For women, wearing a corset or girdle might help to improve her appearance by narrowing her waist, but the breath is sacrificed in return. While not as popular as in days past, the girdle means death to the breath. A bra is not much different. A bra is worn to keep breasts from sagging even though sagging breasts are a natural occurrence.

As a bra tightens across the chest, it also prevents a woman from taking a deep breath. The muscles across a woman's chest now learn how to hold on. Stagnation and hardness in the connective tissue across the chest are likely to occur as lack of mobility is encouraged. As this pattern continues, a woman is teaching her nervous system that it is not safe to breathe deeply.

Another compromise to a woman's breath occurs in the form of breast implants. A silicone or saline implant in a woman's chest alters her breathing in a disastrous way. The muscles and connective tissue are stretched to accommodate these new bulges beneath the surface of the skin. The muscles across the chest are already stretched to their limit, but they have to struggle to stretch even further for normal breathing. Efficient breathing becomes almost impossible.

Men who wear tight belts and neckties are no different. A tightened belt and waistband might ensure a professional look but certainly does nothing to enhance the breath. Over time, the belt becomes a training tool to teach the diaphragm not to move, just as the bra has trained women not to move their chest as they breathe. A necktie gives a man a certain look but continues to restrict his breathing pattern. Many people have sacrificed their ability to breathe deeply because they are more interested in their appearance.

The breath is compromised by both sudden impact trauma and repetitive trauma. The ability to breathe naturally has vanished for most people. As these patterns continue, many people are forced to suffer the consequences of a reduced breath.

Learned Patterns

Along with the aforementioned forces that shape your breath, there are also several learned patterns of breathing. These patterns are reinforced over time to become habitual ways to breathe. These three patterns are the *military breath,* the *breath of depression,* and the *looking good breath.* I will explore these patterns in this next section.

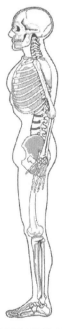

THE MILITARY BREATH

The Military Breath

The military breath occurs in the upper chest with a lifting of the shoulders. The diaphragm's action is sluggish or non-existent. There is very little movement while the breath is shallow and rapid. The primary focus is to maintain stillness and attention.

A military breath is often taught in the military but is also a common training pattern in controlled environments, such as in rigid families, businesses and academic environments. The military breath is associated with "type A" behavior, which is akin to extreme focus, intellectualization and pressure to succeed. A person who breathes primarily with a military breath seldom knows how to slow down and relax.

Stand at attention. Stick your chest out, tuck your belly in and lock your knees. Look straight ahead and be at attention. This is the classic military breath that many people are taught. Very little oxygen is exchanged with this kind of breath. As a result of long-term adaptation to this style of breathing, one develops a weakened diaphragm muscle and a tightened neck. The muscles of the neck, most notably the scalene muscles, have to perform most of the work to exchange air. This is an extremely inefficient way to breathe. The muscles and connective tissue across the chest remain frozen and immobile. The connective tissue has hardened into something resembling hard rubber or plastic.

The consequences of the military breath over time are dire. Not only does one suffer from hardened muscles and connective tissue, but a tightened neck may lead to complications down the road. Reduced blood flow to the head may help to contribute to conditions like Alzheimers disease or strokes.

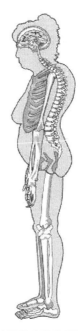

THE BREATH OF DEPRESSION

The Breath of Depression

The second learned breathing pattern is associated with depression. Depression has been classically misdiagnosed in our culture. Depression is essentially an emotional condition where the energy of emotion has not been released. Rather, the emotions have been repressed. Depression is a symptom of repression. When you do not allow your anger, grief, sadness and other emotions to be released fully, you trap these emotions within the body. This pattern shapes the breath.

A person who is practicing repression and suffering from depression can visibly appear hunched over with a caved-in chest, rounded spine, collapsed torso and shallow breath. It is almost as if he does not dare take a deep breath. He fears that he will feel something painful if he does. As a result, he protects himself from feeling by not breathing very deeply at all. His posture is just a protection mechanism from feeling.

The breath of depression may be associated with hopelessness or a sense of giving up. There is a lack of motivation and energy. It is too much work to struggle to get out of the situation, so one just collapses in despair.

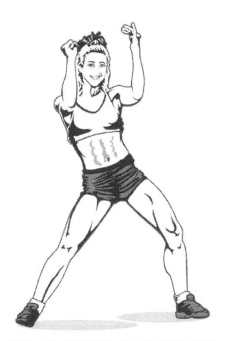

THE LOOKING-GOOD BREATH

The Looking-Good Breath

The third learned pattern of breathing is the *looking-good breath*, which many people have been taught to emulate. This is similar to the military breath, but a special emphasis is placed on pulling in of the abdomen. While the military breath focuses on absolute control, the looking-good breath emphasizes appearance. When you learn to breathe this way, you lift your shoulders and pull the belly in. Made famous by models and bodybuilders, you now redefine your societal worth by the hardness of your abdominal muscles.

Over time, this type of breathing is very detrimental to the body. Rock solid abdominal muscles keep the diaphragm locked in place. The diaphragm, the primary muscle of respiration, has no chance of moving to help create a decent air exchange. You impose a cast to prevent the diaphragm from moving. This cast consists of unnatural beliefs and rigid abdominal muscles. The abdominal cavity remains hardened and compacted, affecting digestion and the functioning of other nearby organs and glands.

The looking-good belly is a phenomenon developed by Western culture. Encouraged by fashion magazines and fitness trainers, the looking-good belly has become an accepted goal in Western culture. Most other cultures of the world do not share this flat stomach concept. In fact, many cultures pride themselves on the roundness of the belly. The looking-good stomach is another unnatural belief system that many have adopted as their own. Striving for a rock solid belly only takes you further away from nature and limits your ability to breathe efficiently.

When you pull your belly in with your exercise and your garments you hinder the function of the internal organs that lie beneath. Poor breathing habits become instrumental in helping to create disease. Dennis Lewis explains in *The Tao of Natural Breathing,*

"In short, such breathing weakens and disharmonizes the functioning of almost every major system in the body and makes us more susceptible to chronic and acute illnesses and 'dis-eases' of all kinds: infections, constipation, respiratory illnesses, digestive problems, ulcers, depression, sexual disorders, sleep disorders, fatigue, headaches, poor blood circulation, premature aging, and so on. Many researchers even believe that our bad breathing habits also contribute to life-threatening diseases such as cancer and heart disease."

The looking-good breath is just another unnatural pattern that has become common in our culture. Along with the *military breath* and the *breath of depression*, the *looking-good breath* leads you away from your natural breath.

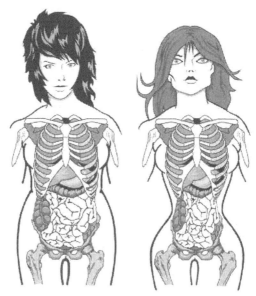

Normal   Constricted

**The abdominal cavity and many of the internal organs
become negatively affected when you chronically pull your belly in tight.**

There are many learned patterns of breathing. These are just a few. When you develop false beliefs about yourself, you alter your form and physical body. Your breath is no different. The beliefs that you have about yourself determine how you breathe. You learn about yourself from the role models in your life. Unfortunately, most have had very poor role models for the development of their natural breathing. When you step away from natural beliefs, you are shortchanged by inadequate breath. Disease is often just one short breath away.

The Natural Breath

Coming back to your natural roots means learning to breathe as nature intended. This kind of breath is free and easy. A natural breath is not restricted by tight articles of clothing nor altered by societal standards of control. A natural breath is like bringing the body a feast of energy to absorb.

While it may seem odd, for some people a natural breath was their first contact in the world by entering into the world with a conscious and supported birth. This happens in many of the natural birthing practices. This natural breath is defined as the entire body involved in the exchange of air, not just an isolated small area of the upper torso. For most people though, the natural breath was shunted by a traumatic and artificial birth process that included drugs given to the mother (affecting the infant's breathing), delayed labor by placing a woman on her back and forcing her to push up against gravity, and the overall trauma of the hospital setting. While this might have been traumatic, it is not something that one is condemned to live with his entire life. The natural breath can be learned and can come to replace many unnatural breathing patterns.

There are several parts to the breath. There is the inhale; next comes a pause. Then there is the exhale when the carbon dioxide is released from your body. Finally, there is another pause before the cycle continues. Each part contributes to the entire process of bringing oxygen to your cells and removing waste products. When your breath is lost due to shortened muscles and stress induced patterns, you lose a very important aspect of our life.

Nancy Zi writes in *The Art of Breathing* about the exhale being just as important as the inhale.

"We are used to thinking of breathing as a process of inhalation-exhalation, in that order of importance. We seldom give any thought to how we exhale. Most advice on breathing emphasizes inhalation, as in 'take a deep breath.' The truth is that exhalation is just as important. Exhalations are cultivated and refined inner energy being selectively channeled the reaping of what we sow when we inhale."

When you begin to learn a new way to breathe, it is important to identify where your breath remains held hostage to your old pattern. Do you falter on the inhale, or do you rush through the exhale? Does each of your breaths run together with hardly a thought to your breathing at all? Are you afraid to pause between breaths for fear of running out of air or of having to experience a quiet moment in your life?

The breath acts as a symbol for underlying beliefs. Beliefs reflect past experiences. For instance, someone might learn to breathe short and quick breaths. He might have had a suffocating experience during his birth. He could have learned that the world is not a safe place so he is continually on guard. By breathing short, quick breaths, he continues to relive his repression of feeling.

Another person might inhale very deeply but have a weak exhale. This might indicate that he is unable to let go. In this case, he fears letting go of the oxygen in his lungs. He does not trust that there is another breath coming next. This is a learned pattern that developed as part of a traumatic experience while young. Letting go meant death in some way to this person. As an adult, he continues to have difficulty letting go, even of his breath.

There are many ways to breathe. Eastern authors have written scores of texts on the diverse ways to alter the breath. However, most of these contrived means of breathing are not natural and do not achieve the goal of the natural breath.

Donna Farhi says in *The Breathing Book,*

"For now know that the deep level at which this process is taking place is the level we must enter to return the breath to its original flexibility. This is why attempting to alter the breath through mechanical exercises has a limited effectiveness, since we are not changing the underlying structures that support healthy breathing. On a deeper level, highly controlled breathing practices such as those employed in yogic pranayama *can backfire because*

they can act to repress the underlying psychological fears and issues that are driving poor breathing habits in the first place."

The science of the breath has been a large part of the Eastern world for some time. Included in this study also is the control of the breath. Unfortunately, the East has set out to control everything, including the body, mind and breath. The result is a person who is caged behind a rigid set of rules and a plethora of control. With most Eastern traditions, the natural breath has been lost.

Dennis Lewis reaffirms this idea in *The Tao of Natural Breathing.*

"Unfortunately, few people who experiment with their breath understand the importance of 'natural breathing.' This is the kind of spontaneous, whole-body breathing that one can observe in an infant or a young child. Instead of trying to learn to breathe naturally, many people impose complicated breathing techniques on top of their already bad breathing habits."

A classic example of the controlled breath comes to us from the yogic tradition. A popular breathing technique practiced by many is called the "ujaii" breath. It is through the ujaii breath that the yoga practitioner is taught to constrict the back of his throat, (the glottis), to create a slight hissing sound while inhaling and exhaling. The tight and constricted throat that the practitioner is left with could not possibly offset whatever benefits this kind of breathing could create. The yoga student is now encouraged to tighten and hold on to the muscles of his throat long after a yoga class has ended.

Dennis Lewis adds in *The Tao of Natural Breathing,*

"Breathing exercises involving complicated counting schemes, alternate nostril breathing, reverse breathing, breath retention, hyperventilation, and so on make sense only for people who already breathe naturally, making use of their entire body in the breathing process."

Much of Eastern culture places great emphasis on the breath, but the natural breath has been hijacked as a tool to induce a trance state. Learning to breathe is <u>not</u> learning how to focus on the breath. When you learn to recover your breath, it is important to learn how to be present with your feelings and not let your breath take you into a trance state. Unfortunately, many people have been taught to use the breath to alter their consciousness, as practiced by many Eastern traditions.

The breath is very powerful. Thousands of years ago, it was discovered that by focusing on the breath one could change his mood and enter into a trance state. He hoped to achieve higher levels of consciousness by continually focusing on his breath. Actually, trance state can be very misunderstood. Frequently these "other" internal states are not higher levels of consciousness but "altered" levels of consciousness. Altering of consciousness just becomes another way to mood alter.

One addictive thought is traded for another. Instead of thinking about that glass of wine that might minimize your pain, you now think about the air passing through your nostrils. Not much has changed. Instead of getting high on the alcohol in your blood stream, now you are getting high on the endorphin rush in your brain created by the focus on your breath.

Returning to nature is learning to be present and willing to accept all of your thoughts, feelings and sensations. Creating trance states with your breath is not learning how to reach a state of relaxation. Focusing on your breath throughout the day to change your moods is not recovery. Learning to breathe is critical to learning how to recover your true self. Getting high from focusing on your breath will do nothing to help you in recovery. Focused and controlled breathing might be a tool that you learn along the way in order to minimize your pain. Only when you are ready to face your pain will you be ready to let go of all of the trance states that mask feeling. These trance states include the age-old practice of focusing on the breath as a way to alter consciousness.

Learning to breathe naturally is *not* learning how to hold your breath. Another age-old yogic practice is the competitive practice of holding the breath for long durations. Once again, this does not lead you back to the natural breath but keeps you in a state of control. Control and relaxation are not the same.

Recovery of the breath is critical in the recovery of your body. Without full and complete breath, your movements, thoughts and body will stay contracted. Without the breath, emotions and sensations will be minimized and repressed. The breath is vital in your complete expression of your self. Learning to recover the breath is one of the necessary pillars of recovering your entire self.

A natural breath is a breath that is free of restrictions. This type of breathing is easy and effortless. When you breathe your natural breath, you take in life and let go of your holding patterns. Natural breathing means you are relaxed. The natural breath sends waves of aliveness through the body; these ripples touch you to your very core. The natural breath is neither an unconscious breath, nor is it an over-controlled breath found in the yogic tradition. Someplace in between is where you find the natural breath.

There is another fascinating aspect to the natural breath. When the diaphragm is free to move up and down as nature intended, the internal organs, lungs and heart are all massaged. This movement helps to stimulate your glands and organs. The diaphragm also helps to relax the lower back when it moves freely.

The heart is massaged by the back and forth movement of the diaphragm. There is a "seesaw" effect that happens when the heart and diaphragm move in unison, which helps to bolster the health of the heart muscle. When the diaphragm remains frozen, the heart tends to become more rigid and locked into place. The heart is connected to the diaphragm by fascia. These two muscles were designed by nature to move together. A hardened set of abdominal muscles will not allow this to happen.

Donna Farhi writes about studies conducted with heart attack patients. She writes in *The Breathing Book,*

"There have been a number of significant studies showing a correlation between upper chest breathing and heart disease. In one stunning report, patients who had already experienced a heart attack were taught how to breathe diaphragmatically and to generalize this behavior into everyday activities. In doing so they significantly reduced their chances of having a second heart attack. Another study showed that all 153 patients of a coronary unit breathed predominantly in their chests. Similarly, essential hypertension (high blood pressure of unknown cause) has been shown to respond favorably to a regimen of diaphragmatic breathing."

As indicated by Donna Farhi, heart attacks may have much less to do with your diet and more to do with the lack of movement in the diaphragm and heart.

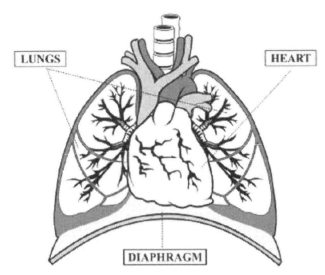

When the diaphragm is allowed to move naturally and completely, the heart is massaged with every breath. This allows for a more relaxed and healthy heart muscle.

The Breath and Energy

The breath cycle has another very important dynamic. Breathing operates like a pump that generates *chi*, or *life force energy*, throughout the body. *Chi* is the current of electrical energy that travels to every cell. It is through the complete and full breath that *chi* is generated and transported throughout the body.

Lack of adequate breathing tends to reduce the flow of *chi*. A person with a lung condition such as emphysema has a reduced flow of *chi* in his body. This is due to the fact that he cannot exchange oxygen and carbon dioxide efficiently. Someone who feels depressed might also suffer from a reduced flow of *chi*, because her emotions are bottled up. Subtle energy is very real and dynamic. Unfortunately, most Westerners rely on a very limited scientific viewpoint of anatomy which cannot measure or explain *chi*.

Speaking more about *chi* energy, Nancy Zi explains in *The Art of Breathing*,

"Modern science has done wonders to elevate the standard of human existence, with the expectation that new inventions and medical discoveries will raise our physical and mental well-being to ever-higher states. Advanced education systems sharpen our minds, while vitamins and nutritional supplements insure that our bodies are well nourished. Great

efforts are devoted to developing innumerable variations of exercises that promise to enhance our physical shape and condition. All these avenues for generating and maintaining a high level of energy are pursued with the intention of producing a better, more exciting person.

"Ironically, in our search for energy resources to maintain this modern lifestyle, we have overlooked the potential of the greatest energy source available to everyone: the current of vital energy that can be generated within our bodies, using the air we breathe. The Chinese call that energy chi.*"*

One way to begin to defrost the emotional energy that is stuck in your muscles is to participate in Bioenergetic exercises, which is part of Reichian work. In these exercises, the breath is used along with movement to energize the body. Alexander Lowen writes in *Pleasure: A Creative Approach to Life,*

"A contracted muscle cannot move until it is recharged with energy. This energy is brought to the muscle in the form of oxygen and sugar. Without a supply of additional energy, it is impossible to release contracted muscles. The important factor in this process is oxygen, since without sufficient oxygen the metabolic process in the muscle comes to a halt. This fact points up the importance of breathing for relaxation and for the lifting of repression. When a patient's breathing is deepened, his tense muscles will go into spontaneous vibration as they become charged with energy."

Shallow breathing tends to slow down the energy in the body and keeps you contracted. Your chest and diaphragm stay contracted as if squeezed by a tight belt. Over time, shallow breathing causes long-standing contraction in the musculature of the chest so that it becomes very difficult to voluntarily breathe fully. You might not be able to take a deep breath even if you should want to. Your muscles will not allow it. Your chest does not move, your muscles remain frozen, and the energy that travels through the body is weakened.

In *The Body in Recovery*, John P. Conger writes,

"Over time, our full breath has been reduced, our ribs grown inflexible, the pulse dimmed, our sea of energy thrown into an enforced and chilling calm. With diaphragm tightened, our breath no longer reaches down to our genitals, no longer connects the upper and lower body. How have we suppressed our life energy?"

In response to stress, what you normally do is stop breathing and stop moving. The natural antidote to this problem is to learn how to breathe fully, so you are prepared when your body goes into Fight or Flight in response to a stressful situation. When you breathe fully, you send oxygen to your cells where it is needed. Your body becomes "energized" by full, deep breaths. When you breathe fully, you send *chi* (life-force energy) through your body. This is what keeps you alive.

Bill's Story

Bill came to me as a last resort. He was seventy-seven years old and had been diagnosed by the medical community as having a disease called idiopathic pulmonary fibrosis. His doctors told him they did not know the cause of the disease or how to cure it. There was no known cure. Seventy percent of people who have this disease die within the first three years of diagnosis. The prognosis is almost always fatal.

Idiopathic pulmonary fibrosis is a condition in which the connective tissue of the lungs hardens and the ability to exchange gases is significantly diminished. The tiny air sacs (alveoli) that collect oxygen and release carbon dioxide remain hardened and are unable to stretch efficiently. Over time, those who are afflicted with this disease die of suffocation or drowning by way of pneumonia.

Without hope or knowledge about where else to go for help, Bill came to me. I first noticed his posture. He was hunched over and shuffled his feet. It took him a while to climb a flight of stairs as he was out of breath. Bill's neck was rigid and hardened as well.

As I got Bill on my treatment table and had him take off his shirt, I ask him to breathe. His chest barely moved. I touched his upper torso with my hands and felt a significant hardness across his chest. His belly and diaphragm were hardened as well. "Of course this man has a breathing disorder," I said to myself, "There is no movement here."

During further conversations, Bill revealed his engineering and military background. He remembered learning how to breathe by sticking his chest straight out, sucking his belly in, and locking his knees—classic military man. He also revealed his "type A" personality traits. Bill had a difficult time slowing down and was constantly on the go. "Type A" personalities tend to take shallow, short breaths, using only their neck muscles. I concluded that among other reasons, Bill's inability to use his lungs efficiently caused them to harden; they would not be able to stretch to take a deep breath. He had trained himself not to breathe and now was suffering the consequences.

I do not believe that a genetic anomaly or a virus he picked up while traveling in some remote region caused this. Bill had created beliefs which restricted his lungs and prevented them from moving. Bill's lungs had hardened over time because of lack of movement. In my opinion, this was the root of his pulmonary fibrosis.

In our first few sessions, I softened Bill's chest by using the *Intuitive Connective Tissue* technique. I began to see movement. We then progressed to teaching Bill how to breathe, incorporating several breathing techniques for him to practice and take home with him. Eventually he had a full assortment of breathing techniques that he could practice on his own.

Part of the challenge was to eliminate all that the medical world was doing to worsen Bill's disease. First, I had to give Bill hope. I had to assure Bill that his condition would change if he kept up the healing work on a regular basis. He was in a major medical crisis. There was no time to sit back and wait for a medical cure. We had to be proactive and work at Bill's breathing problems. The medical community had convinced Bill that there was no hope and no cure. He did not believe he could conquer the disease. Bill was forced to hear fatalistic testimony from the medical experts and read what seemed like an obituary in medical texts and informational web sites.

Here is an example of one such pessimistic outlook by Dr. Francis V. Adams, a "breathing expert," in *The Breathing Disorders Sourcebook*. "In pulmonary fibrosis, the air sacs of the lung are permanently destroyed and replaced by scar tissue." When someone says "permanently," that gives very little hope.

Seeing improvement in his ability to expand his chest started to give Bill the hope he needed to continue. Bill's posture also improved greatly as he was no longer hunched over as in the beginning.

Another obstacle was the hospital's rehabilitation program, which hardened and tightened Bill's body. He was placed on a program of weight lifting and abdominal exercises. This is the worst kind of exercise for deepening the breath. Tightening the chest with weights only shortens the breath. Abdominal exercises constrict the diaphragm, the primary muscle of respiration. Bill's hospital program was adding to his disease, not helping it. The hospital program was actually contributing to the death of patients with lung conditions. Through his work with me, Bill learned how to take a full and deep natural breath—perhaps for the very first time in his life. Bill's healing meant not just recovering his breath, but acquiring new beliefs that were more truly aligned with nature. He was better able to take a deep breath and let go of his belief in the military-type breathing that kept everything in control. While the medical establishment had grasped onto the belief that his genetics were to blame for his lung disease, this was hardly the case. At the root was nothing more than a belief that it was not safe to take a deep and full breath.

Learning to regain the natural breath is an integral part of healing and returning to nature's own way of healing. Breath becomes medicine for you. When you reclaim your lost breath, you also reclaim part of your body that was held in place by unnatural beliefs. Reclaiming your breath means making a commitment to live more fully in this world.

Exercises to Regain Your Natural Breath

When you were very young, every laugh and cry shook through your whole body. Learning to recover your breath might mean to learn how to allow the entire body to become involved in your breath once again. Let every cry, laugh or expression of anger be full and complete. Use your whole body and let your breath be as encompassing as possible. Try not to minimize your expressions of emotions but allow your body to release the energy entirely. Do not be stoic with your breath.

When learning how to breathe, it may be important to have reminders around that reinforce your new intention. We easily forget and these reminders are a good training aid. I like to provide for my breathing patients small stick-on dots that can be placed in key locations. Each dot will have a predetermined message that one attaches to it. For instance, a person learning how to expand his breath might place a small orange dot on the door of his refrigerator. Each time he opens the door, he is reminded to take a deep breath.

 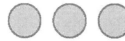

A set of three green dots placed on the steering wheel of your car reminds you to take three deep breaths every time you see the dots. This helps during times of traffic and this is a good time to practice your breathing. A single blue dot placed on the inside of your check book or the corner of your medicine cabinet is a simple reminder to exhale out completely. The dot carries a message that only you know. As a result, the natural breath is encouraged and fostered throughout the day.

When most people are in either physical or emotional pain, they tend to hold their breath and remain contracted. Recovering the breath means learning to breathe fully into your pain. A good way to begin to learn to breathe more fully is to practice regularly the following exercises.

Breathing Exercise # 1 The Five Count Breath

- *Sit quietly for a few minutes with your eyes gently closed*
- *Begin to count slowly from one to five*
- *As you do this take a slow, deep breath, feeling your chest expand as if you were blowing up a balloon*
- *Pause for a moment with your chest fully expanded*
- *Begin to exhale very slowly, counting from five to one, slowly releasing the air from your chest*
- *Pause briefly at the end of the exhale*
- *Repeat this sequence, paying careful attention to the expansion of the ribcage, letting the numbers be less important than the breath*

Breathing Exercise # 2 Three Part Breath

The diaphragm is the largest muscle used in respiration. Up to seventy percent of your breath comes from the diaphragm. Learning to activate the diaphragm becomes an integral part of finding the natural breath. Abdominal breathing creates a feeling of calmness as the parasympathetic nervous system is affected.

- *As you inhale, allow the lower belly to expand outward*
- *Continue to inhale and let the rib cage and torso expand*
- *Allow the shoulders to raise up gently as the inhale continues*
- *Pause*
- *Begin to exhale by first lowering the shoulders*
- *Allow the rib cage to compress as the exhale continues*
- *Complete the exhale by allowing the lower belly to pull in*
- *Pause before starting the cycle again*

Breathing Exercise #3 Bedtime/Morning Breath

Before going to bed at night, take twenty-five deep and full breaths. A deep breath might be for a count between five and ten. Feel the rib cage expand. Let each breath be conscious and complete. Do not be in a hurry. When you awaken in the morning, take twenty-five more deep breaths before you do anything else. This will get you in the habit of breathing throughout the day before your day becomes too busy.

PART THREE

Choosing
Not to Feel

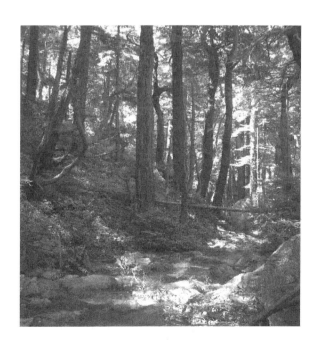

Pillar
Number
Five

Recovery
from
Addictions

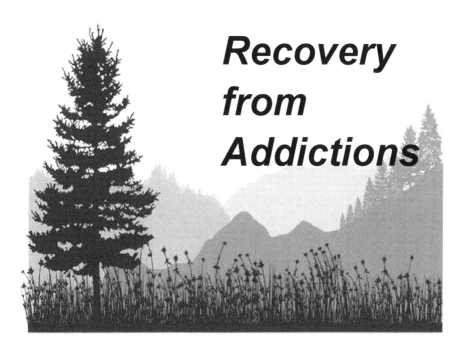

Addictions As a Relationship

You have a choice in your life to express or repress what you are feeling and experiencing. Expression leads to the natural release of energy just as a river, when left to its natural flow, will wind and turn every which way as it carves its way through the landscape. You are like the river when you are allowed to express all that you feel and experience.

When you do not express, you end up repressing and holding onto your emotions and your sensory experiences. You push down your feelings and hold on even tighter. You become like a river that is dammed up. You become stagnant and lose your flow. In this process of damming up the river within you, new ways are developed to keep everything repressed. The most critical way that you learn to not feel your sensory and emotional experiences is to create addictions. In short, addictions are the direct result of your inability to release the stress response, physical trauma and repression of emotional and sensory experiences.

There is a natural cycle at work. When you experience an event that you interpret as life-threatening, your body automatically enters into the stress response. Due to the evolution of your brain, this event could be real or imaginary. In a natural world, you complete the cycle and enter into the relaxation response when the danger has passed.

It is common to formulate false beliefs that will not allow you to complete the stress cycle and enter into the relaxation response. You create unnatural beliefs that teach you to fear your emotions and repress them deep inside. You then store the end results of stress, repression and physical trauma within your body.

As a result of this stored energy, you become agitated. You develop anxieties. You cannot relax and have a difficult time being at ease. You are stuck in a hyper-arousal state—that of stress. By not being able to relax and let go of the stress cycle, your higher brain (the cortex) has developed relationships with addictions as a way to numb out the pain that you have stored. You have addictions because you have lost your ability to feel fully.

When you are not allowed to express everything, your muscles tighten. Your joints stiffen. The fascia within your body tends to harden. It takes energy to hold on. You may feel tired all the time because your energy is being used to hold on and repress everything. This is like a giant tapeworm inside your intestines gobbling up all of the food that you eat. As a result of repression, you are irritable, tired and in pain.

You have addictions because you are in pain. You have addictions because you do not have a complete relationship with your sensory and emotional experiences. When you do not feel, you end up developing addictions as a way to make the pain go away. Addictions are a way to numb out.

When you cannot say "I hurt" or "I am in pain," you are more likely to use a host of addictions to alter your moods. You have addictions because you find it difficult to relax, normal to repress your emotions, and socially unacceptable to grieve the physical traumas that afflict you.

The following is my definition of addiction.

An addiction is a relationship with a person, object, thought,
emotion or behavior that attempts to numb out
an uncomfortable sensation or emotion.

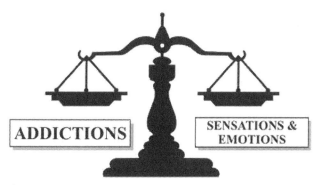

The Equation

Addictions are about relationships. When you can stop blaming a plant or a drug for your pain, then you can begin to heal the relationship that you have with that drug or plant. How you use a plant, thought or behavior is much more important than the thing itself. It is your relationships with thoughts, behavior, emotions, people, and objects that determine your addictions.

The key to understanding addictions is to uncover the relationship that you have with people, behavior, thoughts, objects and emotions in your life that prevents you from feeling your feelings. I find a very simple way to think about addictions is to put the concept into an equation. The equation would be something like this: repressed feelings equal addictions.

Your out of control eating habits are not about food; they are about loneliness. A drinking problem has nothing to do with the inability to control the amount of alcohol consumed; it is about not wanting to feel anger. Compulsive prayer is not about feeling close to God; it is about not being able to honor the sadness inside.

The problem is very clear. Most people have been working on the wrong side of the equation in order to attempt to heal their addictions. They have been working on the side of the symptoms, the aftereffects. They are trying to close the barn door after the horse has already left. The **War on Drugs** is an attempt to sweep up the glass after the vase is already broken. Detox centers and Alcoholics Anonymous (A.A.) groups are trying to fix a broken record. Until you begin to work on the source of your addictions, y*our repressed emotions and inability to relax,* you will continue to be operating on the wrong side of the equation. You will continue to try to use willpower and mind techniques to push down your connection between your addictions and your repressed emotions. As long as you refuse to heal the origin of your addictions, *repressed emotions and sensory experiences*, you will continue to fight a losing battle. Addiction is the result of an inner relationship gone astray. Addiction has very little to do with what you put into your body.

Kathy's story is an example of the "addiction equation" in practice. Kathy was a client of mine who came to me complaining of being overweight and feeling frustrated with the lack of intimacy in her marriage. It appeared that Kathy's husband, the man that Kathy was deeply in love with, had a primary relationship with alcohol. Alcohol was his best friend. How could there possibly be room for Kathy (two best friends)? Her husband, Jim, would come home from work, have a couple of drinks, and then go upstairs alone and watch television. He would give his intimacy to his two cats, which he would caress while viewing television. It appeared that Jim had primary relationships with alcohol, animals and television in order for him to numb out his feelings. Even if he were to stop drinking, most likely he would not be processing the deep feelings that had led to his addictions. He would not be working on the right side of the equation but only trying to control the aftereffects.

Kathy felt she had a deep connection with Jim, but she wanted more intimacy with him. Kathy was angry that Jim's cats and television viewing had more of a priority than she did. As with most people, Jim's primary relationships were with his addictions, not with his partner, Kathy.

What Kathy ended up doing in her frustration for more intimacy is what many people do. Kathy began to isolate herself downstairs with her own television. She began to binge eat in her isolation to numb out her hurt and loneliness. She could not understand why she kept gaining weight.

Finally, the scenario began to make sense to her. By going on crash diets or switching from watching television to "something more constructive" (like sewing or reading books), Kathy still did not begin to heal her addictions. It was only when she began to address her hurt and isolation (the feeling side of the equation) that she began to come to some resolution with her addictions.

If you begin to look at your addictions as an equation (repressed feelings equal addictions), you will come to a greater understanding of yourself. Most have been looking at the wrong side of the equation for too long. You have been trying to use willpower and switching from one addiction to the next in order to solve the problem. The only real answer is to process all of the repressed feelings, which are the source of your addictions.

Returning to nature means beginning to tip the scales in nature's favor. Your emotions and sensory experiences begin to take priority over your need to repress and hold on to these very same emotions. Once you make this shift, you begin to learn and educate yourself about your inner needs.

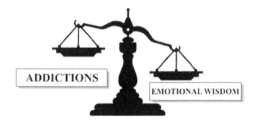

EXAMPLE OF A HIGHLY EVOLVED PERSON
The person represented by the diagram above has a high degree of emotional wisdom. His relationship with his emotions and sensory experiences is significant. Thus, there is less of a need for relationships with addictions to numb out. There is more weight placed on emotional wisdom.

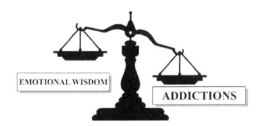

EXAMPLE OF A HIGHLY ADDICTED INDIVIDUAL
This person's primary relationships are with his addictions. He has developed very little sensory and emotional wisdom, so he relies on his assortment of addictions to get him through each day. There is more emphasis placed on ways to stay numb than on ways to feel.

Emotional Wisdom

As you look back at your life, begin to recount the years of study and learning that you have gone through. Perhaps you have achieved a high school diploma. Maybe you have even graduated from college. You might even be lucky enough to have an advanced degree, like in medicine or in business.

This accounts for a great amount of your life experience—studying and learning. However, most of what you learn in school is about memorization and rational thinking. You are taught to analyze data, recite "facts" and dates, all while striving to achieve your coveted degree. You have been educated within the Cognitive Brain world of words and intellect.

How much emotional training have you had? When was the last time you took a semester of anger work, or even an hour? Who were your role models who modeled functional emotional behavior? When was the last time a teacher in school taught you how to grieve?

Unfortunately, most people have received a poor education when it comes to their emotions and sensory experiences. They have been expected to be socially functional when it comes to their emotions, yet most were given little or no training concerning those very same emotions. We are a society that has become emotionally illiterate, favoring words and rational thought over real emotional experiences. Most of us have received far more training in how to go to the bathroom than in expressing emotions.

In general, the training has been dismal when it comes to your emotions because we live in a culture that favors control rather than expression. A young child has the ability to express her natural emotional wisdom, but that is soon repressed as she is taught how to hold it all inside. We have become a culture that is emotionally constipated. For adults, the outburst of emotion is often unskillful as only a few know how to express themselves. Emotions often come in explosions of pent up rage and sobs of misery.

While losing your natural ability to express yourself, you have found addictions instead. Addictions will numb out the feeling that you are unwilling to express and release. As you repress the energy of your emotions inside, you seek out many different addictions to help you to not feel the agitation that these feelings has created for you.

When it comes to wisdom of their emotions, most people are very *unintelligent*. They have flunking grades when they talk about educating themselves about their emotional and sensory experiences. A person with a high degree of emotional wisdom has less need to use addictions to numb out. She does not fear her emotions as painful as they might seem sometimes. She has learned to develop a comprehensive relationship with all of her emotions. She follows the laws of nature and lets out the energy of her emotions as often as she can in a safe and timely manner.

When you repress and hold on to your emotions, you are removing yourself from nature's ways. Emotional wisdom is equated with health and vibrancy. Repression and addictions keep you stuck and battling a body that is attacking itself. With emotional wisdom comes freedom from pain. Emotional illiteracy only adds to the pain that you continue to store within your body.

Addictions Are Your Best Friends

Your addictions are your most intimate relationships. When you have lost your natural guidance, addictions are what you run to for safety and comfort. Addictions are what you will protect and defend with the last ounce of strength in your body. They are as familiar to you as your best friends. In fact, your addictions are your best friends. Addictions always seem to be with you to get you out of your emotional messes. Addictions are loyal, like the family dog. Your addictions come to your rescue whenever you might need them the most. Once you begin to understand your addictions as the intimate relationships that they are, you will begin to heal yourself of them.

Your addictions are what get you through each and every day. They are a time-honored relationship. You might have a relationship with sex, food, romance, shopping, violence, power, work or exercise in order to not feel any feelings.

For you to heal, it is important to begin to establish a relationship with yourself and with your feelings. You have had a long history of a relationship with your addictions. The more you can say "No" to your addictions and "Yes" to your feelings, the quicker you will heal. You will begin to change the addiction scale so that more weight is being placed on the feeling side. The more one feels, the less of a need for addictions. When you begin to establish a relationship with yourself and your feelings, the more you will head down the path of recovery. Until then, you just keep going around and around in circles. Just as you run to be with your best friends, you will also run to be with your addictions.

You can hardly wait to see your pack of cigarettes, full plate of food or bottle of wine. Just as you might think about a loved one all day long, greatly anticipating your next meeting, the same is true with your addictions. You cannot wait to get to the bar, poker game or gym in order to numb your feelings. You begin to drool before your next shopping trip. Just thinking about the mall or what possible sales are going on really makes you anxious. You might tingle with goose bumps at the mere thought of your next meditation session. Your addictions have become your intimate relationships that you use to mask your authentic feelings.

Just like the people in your life with whom you have intimate relationships, you tend to plan your day around your intimate relationships with your addictions. You might need to plan your day around your addiction to your pets. You need to plan your weekend and nightly activities in order to not feel lonely. Perhaps you decide to rent a couple of movies, have some friends over or call a friend to go to a movie. You will do almost anything in order to not feel lonely. You spend a good part of the workday planning on how not to feel alone when you finally do arrive home.

You are consumed with thinking about your addictions. You cannot stop thinking about food. The thought, "If I only had something to eat I would certainly feel better," frequently goes through your mind throughout the day. You might be constantly thinking about sex; every woman (or man) becomes an object. Your thoughts are constantly fantasizing about having sex with this person in order to not feel your own feelings. "Isn't it time for another cigarette," or "I really need another cup of coffee," becomes your mind's rhetoric. The candy machine down the hall becomes your lover. You cannot go anywhere without your Bible. Even though you just had a piece of chewing gum, you constantly fantasize about having another one. Unless you deal with your pain, you will use whatever feels good to cover up your pain.

These thoughts of your addictions often consume your entire day. All day long, at work and at home, you might count the minutes until you can have a couple of beers at "happy hour." "Just one more hour of work and then I can go and 'relax' with a couple of drinks." "If I can just make it through the next appointment, then I can go home and sleep away my anxiety." (Yes, even sleep can be used addictively). When you are feeling fear, you might need to seduce some naive person to take away your pain. Even such simple behaviors like hand washing or locking the door can be considered part of the addiction cycle.

Arthur Janov describes the behavior of "obsessive-compulsiveness" as just another way to have a relationship with an addiction in order to mood-alter.

"Obsessive-compulsiveness is really not a special category of neurosis. It is only the way it is manifest. All neurosis is obsessive in the sense that we repeat patterns over and over again throughout our lives without being able to control them. The smoker takes a cigarette every forty minutes all day every day. The nymphomaniac or satyr is constantly in search of a sex partner. A person acts shy time and again, no matter what the circumstances. The difference is that these behaviors expand over time and are not the controlled, ritualistic, transient behaviors of the obsessive.

"The obsessive has managed to find a well-circumscribed behavior, no different from the sexual pervert who has found a ritual that offers him release. The ritual depends on two factors. The first is life circumstance-growing up with a fanatical mother who insisted that the children wash after touching the dog, the door, the chair, etc. The second is that the ritual must reflect back to a basic feeling, i.e., feeling dirty (in a broad sense of the term) and the need to feel clean constantly. An obsession that sticks is one that manages to reduce the tension level."

You will protect and defend your addictions just as you would a close friendship—even if you knew the friendship was not good for you. Just as you know that your addictions might be harming you, you will fiercely defend them. If you are addicted to religion, you might rant and rave at anyone who would propose to take this activity away from you. If you are addicted to politics in order not to feel, you will have a thousand excuses as to why your incessant politicizing is such a good thing. Just as you would fight to the death to defend your deepest friendships, the same holds true with your addictions. You become very loyal to your addictions.

Like Knights of the Round Table

Your addictions are your best friends and most intimate relationships. Your addictions are like *"Knights of the Round Table,"* and you, their king. They are extremely loyal to you. They will protect you from danger (unwanted feelings). They are always there when you need them—morning, noon and night. You know that you can count on them to serve you to numb out.

It seems like the longer an addiction has been with you, the more loyal it is. It is just like a knight in service for many years. He has proven his loyalty. Someone who has smoked cigarettes for forty years has a very loyal knight, a very loyal addiction. It is much more difficult to get rid of a knight who has served so well and so long. The same holds true with your addictions. Your loyalty to your addictions keeps them around for a long time. After awhile, you are not consciously aware of where they came from or why you have them because you have become so accustomed to them. Just like a knight of long-standing and loyal service, your addictions seem to belong with you. Who are your knights? Who are your protectors? What are your most loyal addictions?

Most Intimate Relationships

You always seem to have an extra supply on hand with your addictions. You store them away so as to never run out. You have a spare candy bar hidden in the closet or an extra marijuana joint in a shoe box—just in case. In your relationship with your addictions, you promise yourself never to be without them. You plan ahead. Addictions are your most intimate relationships and you learn to keep them close by. You know where every doughnut shop is on the way home from work or the nearest convenience store to keep you stocked with cigarettes. If you are addicted to work, then you are meticulous about your work schedule to know when you will need to find another "drug of choice" to numb out your repressed feelings.

For example, a national holiday is coming up. You will not be going to work that day. You need to find something in advance to do, to keep yourself busy. Perhaps you will go fishing or start that construction project at home. That way, if you stay busy enough, you will not have to feel any feelings that your *"workaholism"* normally numbs out. You plan ahead, think about it often and live your life for your addiction. The last thing that you want is to have a day with nothing to do and for your uncomfortable feelings to surface.

When you can acknowledge your addictions as your primary intimate relationships, it is important to understand how you came to form these relationships. In order to do this, you need to first look at how you bonded with the most important people in your life. Let us look at how you establish personal relationships.

In your primary love relationships, many times it is "love at first sight." You become overwhelmed with feelings toward someone. You can hardly contain yourself. A bond is immediately formed. This is similar to the "high" you experience when you first become addicted. Your "love" experience takes you away from all of your loneliness and uncomfortable feelings, just as the initial "high" does when you first encounter a future addiction. Cocaine, religion or alcohol might produce such a "high" that you feel as though you have "fallen in love," just like in your primary relationships with people.

In establishing relationships with other significant people in your life, there might be a common bonding experience. Your best friend might be someone whom you met at work, at a party or in school. You make a connection with someone because you find that you have something in common—a bonding experience. You might both like movies, enjoy traveling or become study partners. Your experience or interests in common are what bond you together to establish a relationship.

The way that you establish a relationship with your addictions is very similar. Initially, you might bond with alcohol at a party or during "happy hour." A friend of a friend might introduce you to cocaine. You might make a connection with workaholism when you are placed in an environment that supports and encourages this type of behavior. You might have bonded with prescription pills to take away your uncomfortable feelings when you first became depressed during your divorce. A meditation retreat gave you such a "high" that you thought you had "died and gone to heaven." You were hooked.

You can also establish a relationship with your addiction through times of crisis. Just as a natural disaster or flood will bring people together to bond in a crisis situation, the same is true with addictions. Notice how many people began smoking or drinking coffee when their lives were the most "stressed out" and life seemed unmanageable. Many men formed a relationship with heroin during the Vietnam War crisis. This is what they turned to for relief when they felt like they could not control their environment. Your many turmoils can draw you together with your personal relationships and with your addictions as well. You will bond with your addictions like army buddies going through the horrors of war together. Your pain will bring you together. The drug or alcohol habit that you form a relationship with in high school might be with you throughout your entire life, to one degree or another.

It is important to examine your relationships with your friends in order to better understand your relationships with your addictions. Each friendship has its own bond and its own purpose. For example, you might have relationships with people with whom you only work and never socialize.

This is a professional relationship. Or, you might have a relationship with a person who is only your traveling companion or tennis partner.

Perhaps you might have a group of friends who always spend their free time together. You might have certain friends who are your emotional support while other friends you enjoy going to the movies with. Begin to notice the extent of your relationships. What is the purpose of each friendship? Do some relationships have multiple roles? Are some relationships a dual relationship—professional and personal? Each friendship is its own relationship and serves its own purpose.

Now, notice the relationships that you have with your addictions. Does smoking marijuana cover up your loneliness? Is drinking alcohol a way to not feel so angry? Do you exercise yourself compulsively because of your repressed anger? Are you always traveling because you do not want to feel bored? Do you read constantly in order to avoid your sadness?

Do some of your addictions have multiple roles, like some friendships? 1) Does using cocaine numb out *all* of your uncomfortable feelings, from anger to sadness, from grief to depression? 2) Or does cocaine just help you to not feel one particular feeling? Do you have a one-on-one relationship with cocaine—a drug that numbs out one particular feeling or is your relationship with cocaine much broader—it helps you to feel nothing at all? Is religion the drug that prevents you from feeling lonely, angry or fearful? Does adrenaline addiction numb out one of these emotions or all of them?

A good deal of the time you might not know what it is that you are feeling. When asked how you are feeling, you might come up with expressions such as "okay," "blah," "down," etc. In order to understand your addictions, you need to begin to be very specific with your feelings. Instead of saying that you are feeling "down", what you might be feeling is "rejection." Feeling "worried" might really be "anxiety." Fear, terror, aloneness, peacefulness and lustfulness are all attempts to narrow down your specific feelings. Many times you might say that you are sad, but you really might be feeling depressed. When you say that you are angry, you might be experiencing fear. As you begin to be more specific with your feelings, you will begin to notice the actual relationship that you have with your addictions.

When you suffer from lack of emotional wisdom, you are stuck in a quandary. Not knowing what you are feeling puts your addiction equation on alert. If you do not know what you are feeling, you will not know how to respond to those feelings and release them. When emotionally illiterate, you most often choose the side of your addictions. This way you do not have to try to guess as to what you are feeling.

For example, you might become aware that when you are feeling anger (and not able to express it fully), you might consume peanut butter to numb out. You have a direct relationship between anger and peanut butter. However, when you are feeling lonely (and not able to let yourself feel your loneliness), you might be addicted to cigarettes. It is not just the behavior of smoking cigarettes or the nicotine that changes your mood but the feeling of having something in your mouth. Each emotion can have a specific relationship with a particular addiction. If you just say that you are feeling "down," then you have not been specific enough. You could have a handful of addictions that would attempt to cover up your mood.

It is possible to have many different addictions that numb out an individual feeling. If anger seems difficult for you to express and flow out of you, you might have five or six different addictions to cover up anger.

For Steven, exercise and food were commonly used to bury his anger, but television and sex usually numbed out his loneliness. Often, food by itself would numb out his loneliness. There are many different kinds of combinations and possibilities. Sometimes, several addictions numb out one emotion. At other times one addiction numbs out many different unpleasant feelings.

When you become more specific with your relationship with your feelings, you will begin to see what is really going on. Take the case of Jodi. Jodi was an exercise addict. She was compulsively at the gym working out. She became upset when she had to miss a day of exercise. Jodi was in great shape. Everyone complimented her on how good she looked. Let us take a closer look to see what Jodi was really addicted to.

For one, Jodi was addicted to perfection. She needed to always be fit but was rarely satisfied with the way she looked. She was always complaining about the smallest bit of flabbiness around her waist. She could never be good enough, slim enough or pretty enough.

Jodi was also addicted to movement. She was always trying to take another aerobics class, attempting to burn off any excess fat. She was on the treadmill quite frequently. She could last for hours on stair machines. You never saw her in an idle activity. She was always moving, trying to burn off more fat. Everyone commented on how much energy she had, but she really could not stop herself. Her exercise at the gym was just an example of what went on in her normal life. She did not want to slow down because she might have to feel something uncomfortable.

Let's look at why Jodi could not slow down. Why did she continue to run and exercise compulsively? In order to understand this relationship, we need to take a closer look at Jodi's childhood. Jodi was sexually abused as a child. She vowed to never let anyone violate her again. Ever since her horrible experience, she has been running (literally and figuratively). If she were to stop exercising so compulsively, she might feel like someone is going to catch her and hurt her again. Jodi's addiction to movement is about not wanting to feel fear of being out of control, and her addiction to perfectionism is about feeling dirty and shameful on the inside.

Take the case of Dale, another exercise addict. Let us look more closely at what Dale did to mask his feelings. He spent a lot of time lifting weights. He liked to pump up his body. Dale used weights to make his body feel stronger and bigger. Dale justified his compulsive weight lifting by saying that it made him feel good. What is really going on is that Dale is addicted to weight lifting to hide his anger at his alcoholic father. Dale could not feel and release his anger; he used weight lifting to prevent himself from feeling anger. Thus, weight lifting became his addiction that he regularly sought after.

Addictions can work singularly or in groups to hide either individual feelings or groups of feelings. If it is easy for you to be angry, you might not have an addiction to hide your anger. You might have other addictions to mask other feelings.

Just as you can have a person, object, thought or behavior that hides an emotion, you can also have an emotion that hides another emotion. For example, many people are addicted to anger. This is not about being able to control your anger; this is about someone who has learned that anger is a way to hide other feelings. Feelings like fear, sadness or depression are being covered up by anger. Someone who has an anger addiction has learned from childhood that anger is a normal way to act out. His relationship with anger might even begin as a healthy occurrence. When he is angry, he might feel comfortable expressing his anger. What ends up happening is that as the other feelings become more overwhelming, anger is used to cover up all the other uncomfortable feelings. Where many people have a difficult time feeling and expressing anger, someone who feels comfortable with anger might have difficulty with other feelings. It is those other feelings that are then covered up by anger. This is how one emotion can be used addictively to cover up another emotion.

Many "rageaholics" experience this equation. Most often they are not feeling anger but are using anger to cover up a deeper emotion. Many men who are unable to express and feel their fear use anger as an addictive emotion to cover up the fear. This is how one emotion can be used addictively. While these individuals might look like they are extremely angry, they are actually afraid. They are only using anger (an emotion they allow themselves to have) to cover up another emotion like fear, (which they will not allow themselves to have).

Many of these emotional addictions are culturally encouraged. For instance, your culture teaches you what it is like to be a man or woman. Many men use anger to cover up fear (because we are often told that real men should not be afraid), and many women use sadness to cover up anger, (because it is not nice for women to be angry—then you are considered a "bitch!"). Many religious or" "spiritual" people use "love" or "happiness" to hide such feelings as anger and fear.

In order to heal from your addictions, it is important to understand how you have shut off your ability to feel your feelings. You must come to understand the feeling part of yourself as a natural and normal aspect of your life. Denying your feelings is a sure recipe for creating addictions of all sorts.

In examining your intimate relationships with your addictions, it is important to recognize the degree of each relationship. Is it a deeply committed relationship or is it something that is very superficial? Rate your addictions (like your personal relationships) on a scale of 1 through 5. A level 5 relationship is a deeply committed relationship while a level 1 relationship is something that might be more superficial. Do you have a level 5 relationship with marijuana and perhaps only a level 2 relationship with food? You might use food *occasionally* to numb out feelings, but you get high just from thinking about marijuana. The amount of food or marijuana you use to numb out your feelings may not be the issue. What you are not willing to feel is the primary instigator.

The secret may be in the *intensity* of the relationship but could also mean the frequency of the activity. Are you consumed with thinking about marijuana all day long or just occasionally? This is the difference between a level 5 relationship (I can't live without it), and a level 2 relationship (I only use it occasionally to numb out my feelings).

Acknowledge the degree of your relationship with your addiction. Just as you might have some personal friendships that you are more committed to and tend to more often than others, the same holds true with your addictions. Some addictions are more significant than others, as in your personal relationships.

The following are some characteristics to help you identify the level of intimacy that you might have with your addiction. It is important to note that, just like in personal relationships, the level of intimacy might keep changing. Unless you work through the repressed emotions that brought you to your addiction, you will always have some level of relationship with it.

Levels of intimacy listed from 1-5:
1.   You seldom see each other (an occasional beer, drug or cigarette)
2.   An occasional friend (every time I go to a party, I drink; this happens once a month)
3.   Frequent friendship (late night binge eating)
4.   Close personal friend (the inner circle of friendships); (my dog is my best friend) This relationship is an ongoing occurrence.
5.   Cannot live without this friendship (the two pack a day smoker)

Exercise to determine the value that your addiction has for you
Draw five circles, one inside the other. Inside each circle place a number. Start in the inside circle and begin to number from "5" and work outward. The outer circle should have a number "1" in it. Place the most important addictions in the inner circle marked "5." The least important addictions go in the outer circle marked "1." The rest will fall somewhere between, according to your value that you place on them.

An addiction with a high priority for you is one that might take up a good "quantity" of your life. It is your most intimate friend. You spend the most time with it, thinking about it, engaging in it or planning to be with it. Just like with any personal relationship that takes up a good quantity of your energy and time, your relationship with your addiction can take up a very large quantity of your life. What type of relationship you might have with your addictions and what you expect it to do for you (which feelings has it proven to numb out) will determine how much value that addiction has for you.

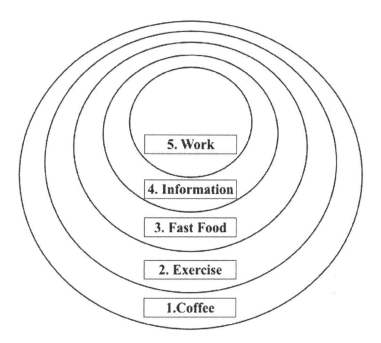

Primary and Secondary Relationships

As each friendship in your life has its own purpose and reward, so do your addictions. Your addictions, like your personal relationships with people, have primary and secondary purposes. Many times you use one addiction to numb out the effects created by another addiction.

For example, you might have a relationship with alcohol that is a secondary relationship that numbs out the pain caused by your primary addiction—work. You might have a secondary addictive relationship with busyness that numbs out your primary addiction to perfectionism. Your primary relationship with spending money addictively might be numbed out by your television viewing addiction.

A good example of this is shown in the world of exercise. Many exercise addicts are really food addicts underneath it all. There is a primary addictive relationship with food that is used to mask any or all feelings. Food is used as the lover of choice. Inability to control food intake becomes the primary problem. Bedtime snacks, binges, overeating and hiding food are all indications of this primary addiction to food. An obsession with focusing on food all of the time becomes apparent.

Exercise takes over to minimize or reduce the effects of the overeating. It may look healthy on the outside to be so passionate about exercise, but exercise just becomes a secondary addiction used to make up for the primary addiction—food.

In this manner one might be constantly trapped in the many layers of addictions. Begin to unravel the mystery of your addictions. Which are the primary addictions and which are the secondary ones? What is at the core and which addictions just support the primary problem?

Is Your Addiction a Secret?

In your relationships with the people in your life, you might have some relationships that you openly acknowledge and others that you choose not to disclose. For example, many times in your love relationships, when you are really excited about a promising partner, you are eager to have them meet your friends and family. You want to show off your prize. At other times, you might keep these love relationships a well-kept secret. You do not want anyone to know about it. You might feel guilty about being involved. You might feel ashamed about what you are doing or feel that others will not approve. Like a secretive affair, these lovers are your well-kept secret.

As with your personal relationships in your life, it is important to ask yourself about your addictions. "Am I having a secretive affair, or am I in a public relationship?" Is your addiction like a beautiful locket stashed beneath the bed that you do not want anyone to know about? Do you hide your prized possession, only to think about it constantly? Is your addiction like a jewelry box hidden in the attic? You keep checking on it daily to make sure that it will be there when you might need it.

Do you hide cookies under your bed or a bottle of vodka behind the couch? Or does everyone know that you have an eating or drinking problem? What type of relationship are you having with your addiction? What are you willing to share with the world and which of your most intimate relationships with your addictions do you keep to yourself?

In order to heal your addictions, you must bring your addictions out into the open and stop believing your own lies. It is vital to admit to yourself that you have a problem. If your addictions are a secret, you are continuing to lie to yourself. You will go on having a secretive affair with your addictions until you bring them out into the open. Your relationship with your addictions will be nothing more than your own well-rehearsed scandal.

Addictions Are Not About Chemicals

Throughout the short history of the addiction and recovery fields, there has been a widespread belief that addictions are about chemical dependency. Clinical psychologists and laboratory scientists have come to this conclusion for us. In fact, the traditional route that most people take to "heal" from their addictions is to attend a chemical dependency inpatient center for 28-days or become part of regular, life-long 12-Step meetings to learn how to control their dependency on a chemical.

Addictions are not about chemicals. Addictions are about faulty relationships. Sometimes these faulty relationships involve chemicals and other times they do not. Many times these faulty relationships are with people, thoughts, emotions or behaviors. Many people have been brainwashed into blaming a group of chemicals for their problems, when, in fact, it is their faulty relationships with their unexpressed emotions that are really to blame.

The opium poppy plant, for instance, produces heroin. The cannabis plant is the source of marijuana. The coca leaf is responsible for cocaine. Nicotine comes from the tobacco plant. None of these plants is inherently "good" or "bad." These plants are just members of nature's plant kingdom.

What has happened though is that we, humans, have found ways to use these plants to get "high" from and alter our moods. By mixing, mashing, smoking or concocting different remedies we have learned to create mood-altering drugs. The fact that these plants have chemical properties that can alter our neurobiology is the "luck" (or "misfortune," depending on how you look at it) of nature.

Chewing a mustard leaf will not get you "high." So the mustard plant is considered a "good" plant, or non-addictive. Sucking on a fennel shoot will not get you "high." The fennel plant is then thought of as a "good" plant. Smoke a little marijuana from the cannabis plant and now you have what society labels as a "bad" plant. Derive heroin from the poppy plant and now you have another "bad" plant.

It seems that many people need to blame a plant, a chemical or a drug rather than to take responsibility for the choices that they have made. In *The Truth About Addiction And Recovery,* the authors, Stanton Peele, Ph.D., and Archie Brodsky, state,

" . . . crack addiction, like every other addiction . . . is a product of the user's circumstances and expectations more than of the drug's chemical properties."

The same authors go on to add, "In reality no drug is addictive in and of itself."

One such example of how our culture wants to blame a chemical for addictive behavior lies in the rather antiquated practice of castrating a sexual predator. The belief is that by cutting off the flow of testosterone, a sex offender will automatically stop his behavior. By cutting off the testosterone, the belief is that you are cutting off his sex drive.

What is not acknowledged is that someone with a severe addiction to sexual crimes has a faulty relationship with sex and violence. This has little to do with testosterone itself. Most likely, the predator gets "high" off stalking his victim and gets "high" off the power of abusing others in order to avoid his pain.

This might be the same for the sex and romance addict. It is not the female sex hormones that keep her addicted, but the "high" she gets from "falling in and out of love" on a regular basis. She is driven by the craze to get men to want her, to be pursued, and the act of playing bait and catch games is what keeps her "high." She is addicted to the behavior of seducing men in order to not feel her pain.

Much of our dilemma regarding addictions comes from the dualistic thinking process. We often separate our understanding into black and white categories. A chemical is either "good" or "bad," depending on how it is used in society.

For instance, alcohol is considered a "good" drug in our society. It is sold openly and is in abundance. There are many national manufacturers. These manufacturers donate money to political campaigns and sponsor many sporting events. Alcohol goes with the holidays and celebrations. Alcohol and the viewing of sports are a big combination. Alcohol is "normal" for many in our culture and is commonly used to take the edge off the stress of our normal work lives.

Alcohol is a very accepted part of life and is considered a "good" chemical—as long as you can control it and not overdo it. Alcohol becomes a "bad" chemical when you use it at the wrong times—like when you are driving. Alcohol is also considered a "bad" chemical if you are a minor and not yet of drinking age. Once you pass the legal drinking age, alcohol now becomes a "good" chemical for you.

The dualistic thinking pattern leaves very little room for understanding your addictions. You are classified as either an "alcoholic" or "not an alcoholic." You are either under age and "bad" or of legal drinking age and "good." There is no middle ground. There is no acceptance of responsibility for the choices that you make. You live in an "either" "or" culture. Either you are an (alcoholic, sex addict, shopping addict, etc.) or you aren't.

Addictions are not about chemicals. Addictions are about faulty relationships used to numb out your pain. Sometimes chemicals are used in these faulty relationships. Most of the time your addictions are about other things that have nothing to do with chemicals. You will begin to heal from your addictions when you stop blaming a drug or a plant for your pain and begin to examine your relationships with your inability to feel.

Addictions As Rewards

The fallacy about addictions is their classification as chemicals that you cannot stop using once you begin and you have a genetic predisposition that attracts you to them. This is the farthest thing from the truth. Addictions are about rewarding yourself with something in order not to feel something else. *Addictive means reward.* This is the relationship that you have established with your addictions.

Heroin might be considered addictive because it rewards the brain with a pleasurable experience that makes an imprint on the brain. *Anything that rewards the brain is addictive—be it a drug, a behavior, an emotion or a thought.* Your relationships with addictions are those that reward you to take away your pain.

Thinking about your upcoming vacation could be addictive because it rewards your brain with a pleasurable experience. The thought of smoking or the thought of eating a doughnut might be enough to alter the chemistry of your brain. Running is a behavior that can be quite addictive. The "runner's high" produces an endorphin rush in the brain to reward you as a pleasurable experience. A "rageaholic" will use the emotion of rage to change the chemistry of his brain so as to not feel his pain. In this case, rage would be considered addictive because it acts as a reward to alter one's moods. Swinging a golf club, hammering a nail or watching television could all be considered addictive if they are used to reward your brain and keep you out of your pain.

Anything that rewards your brain is potentially addictive. It could be a chemical that you ingest or a behavior in which you participate. That is why addictions are not about blaming a chemical that you put into your body. Addictions are about faulty relationships in your attempt to numb out your pain.

Understanding the rewards of addiction is as simple as observing a rat in a laboratory cage. The rat is rewarded by a scientist with a shot of heroin or sugar every time he performs the correct task. It is the same as the "high" that you experience when you are addicted. The pain goes away when you are acting addictively. That is what we are all looking for, relief from pain.

There are different types of "highs" produced from your relationship with your addictions. Some chemicals ingested in the body, like cocaine, heroin or sugar, produce a rapid and euphoric state that make you want to keep repeating this behavior. The endorphins released into the brain from long distance running or frequent meditation sessions might create similar "highs" that make you want to continue to repeat them. These are ecstatic "highs" that the body stores as memories. These "highs" then become a reward system that you crave even more in order to numb out your uncomfortable feelings. The higher the "high" and the longer the high lasts, the stronger the addiction. The more frequently rehearsed, the more cellular memory becomes associated with addictions.

With such addictions to substances and behaviors like cocaine, religion or meditation, you could have a "super-high" and many times of long duration. This type of high is so mood-altering that it normally does not allow you to continue to function in your daily activities. Your body will strongly remember this experience. On the other hand, the effects of nicotine last about twenty minutes and need to be repeated frequently to get a numbing effect. With a "super-high," it is very difficult to quit the addiction because the reward is so stimulating. With nicotine, it takes a constant attempt to keep the drug in you at regular intervals and it is difficult to eliminate this habit because of the quantity and repitition involved.

Another form of reward to numb out your feelings is the steady low-grade "high." This might be experienced as the addiction to watching television or work. Where a climatic scene from a horror movie might produce vast amounts of adrenaline and a very "high" feeling, long-term television watching might produce what I would call a "low-grade high"—just a steady numbing effect to dull your uncomfortable feelings. This is a constant attempt to not feel. A low-grade "high" might be found in one or two servings of alcohol or in a medium-size candy bar. This is just enough of a mood-alteration to give you a fix and "take the edge off." The "high" associated with rewarding you for being addicted might be nothing more than a neutralizing effect.

Something as simple as turning on your car radio every time you go for a drive might neutralize the pain of always feeling lonely. You might not notice a "high" feeling, but the music addiction has served its purpose—to neutralize loneliness. The "high" produced from an addiction such as running could be something as simple as feeling free at last, invincible, indestructible, nobody is going to catch you and being alive. There are so many ways of experiencing this "high" which keeps leading you back to your addictions. This "high" does not have to feel orgasmic or "bounce you off the ceiling." The "high" only has to change your mood for it to be considered addictive. Addiction to skydiving or bungee jumping might produce a rush of adrenaline to keep you coming back for more. However, the constant effects of nicotine or compulsive reading are doing the same thing in a "low-grade" manner. They are all numbing you out, only with different levels of intensity.

Whether your addiction produces low-grade "highs" or ecstatic "highs," the results are the same—you are trying not to feel something.

Imprinting

Anything that creates pleasure will cause a biological imprint in the brain, be it sugar, sex, alcohol, reading or cocaine. The brain will remember the experience as a rewarding experience. Whenever you are in pain, your brain will call on all of the memories of rewarding experiences that you have ever experienced in your lifetime. Your addictions are nothing more than a relationship with something that has left a powerful imprint upon you to allow you to recall it and mood-alter whenever you might need to.

The authors of *Willpower's Not Enough*, Arnold Washton, Ph.D., and Donna Boundy, M.S.W., write,

"All it takes is your brain's memory, or imprint, of an experience with some activity or substance that was inordinately comforting, relief-giving, or pleasurable. Later, when you experience a high level of stress (as we all do at one time or another), you may be unconsciously compelled to seek that substance or activity again. Without your even realizing it, a vicious cycle can be set in motion."

The same authors go on to add, "Actual biochemical effects on the brain reinforce the dependency."

The author of *The Continuum Concept,* Jean Liedloff, writes about how the brain remembers the good feeling that it receives from your addiction:

"But for the sake of simplicity, let us here consider only the heroin addict. Heroin is chemically addictive in that it creates in the body of the user a demand for more, and that the effect diminishes with use so that more and more of the drug produces less and less the effect desired. Eventually, the addict seeks the drug less to experience the 'high' than to ward off the symptoms of withdrawal. Trying to keep ahead of the tightening circle of demand and use, the addicts are sometimes driven to fatal overdose.

"More often, they deliberately confront the agonies of withdrawal in order to 'get clean,' free of the increasing chemical imbalance caused by use. They free themselves of the physical dependence over and over again so as to be able not only to fight off withdrawal symptoms but again to experience the 'high.' Thus, a great deal of their suffering is in de-addicting against the current of the body's urgent demand, against the pain and violent sickness of withdrawal, so that they can start afresh to feel the 'high.' Knowing that they will have to pay for it by repeating the whole terrible cycle afterward does not deter them.

"Why? If they can break out of the so-called addiction time and again, why do they readdict themselves? What is the feeling of being high that makes it so irresistible that the mere memory of it causes hundreds of thousands of people to withdrawal, readdict, risk death, steal, prostitute themselves, lose their homes and families and all they have ever owned or cared for?

"The fatal attraction of the high, I believe, has not been understood. It has been confused with the very separate demand the drug creates in the body's chemistry, which urges it to continue and increase use once it has upset the chemical balance in its favor. But once the drug is stopped and the last traces of it are gone from the body, the chemical addiction has ceased. There remains only the memory then, the ineradicable memory of the feeling one had."

The same author tells the story of a teenage girl who was hooked on drugs.

"The girl was not too weak to go through the terrible business of stopping drug use without any help from an intermediate drug such as

methadone, nor was she in jail or in a hospital, where the unavailability of the drug might reduce the moment-to-moment strain on her will power. What she could not do was to forget what she knew, what she envied the square girl every day of her life for not knowing . . . how it feels to be high."

It is when you bond with an addiction that you feel its pleasure in taking away your pain. You then remember this experience to be used whenever your pain becomes intolerable. A reward is produced and a relationship established. Deva Beck, R.N., and James Beck, R.N. write in *The Pleasure Connection*, "The potential for addiction lies within each of us. Powerful, intrinsic biochemicals reward our bonding, learning and behavior."

All of your addictions are the result of your loss of the ability to feel and a powerful biochemical imprint on the brain. Many times this biochemical reward is the direct result of drugs that you put in your body. Other times it is your brain's own natural pharmacy that causes you to imprint an addiction. The authors of *The Pleasure Connection* write, "Endorphins can have addictive side effects. Indeed, narcotics like heroin and morphine are themselves addictive because their chemistry is similar to our natural Endorphin biochemistry." Even nicotine, which binds to your neurological receptor sights, creates a stimulating euphoria for you.

Most of your addictions have nothing to do with the drugs that you put into your body. Your brain serves as its own pharmacy most of the time. Candace Pert writes in *Molecules of Emotion*, "The brain is like a bag of hormones." The authors of *The Pleasure Connection* write, "In some instances Endorphins create euphoric pain relief that is several hundreds of times more powerful than addictive narcotics."

The act of gambling, hiking or doing needlepoint can create chemical changes in the brain that reward you to want to use these activities and ward off any pain in your life. The sight of the ocean might be all it takes to dump endorphins into your brain to create a rewarding experience and a biochemical imprint. Even the act of "falling in love" can imprint on your brain chemically.

Charlotte Davis Kasl, Ph.D., writes in *Love, Sex, and Addiction,*

"Falling in love has another little catch. Physiologically, it produces a chemical high similar to an amphetamine high. The muses of creation must have had a good laugh when they arranged for chocolate, sex, aerobic exercise, and meditation to all release endorphins from the brain, causing

feelings of pleasure and calm. Fantasizing about a sexual encounter can also create an adrenaline high in the body. This is similar to the rush you get from eating a lot of sugar and chocolate. It is no mystery why so many people lose weight when they fall in love; they switch from a sugar high to an 'in love' high."

Kasl goes on to add that "Falling in love is an altered state of consciousness." It is no wonder why a romance addict will want to keep "falling in love" week after week. She is looking for the biochemical "highs" in her brain. Her brain remembers this "high" and she continues to seek it out.

We all know the power that specific foods have over us when it comes to cravings. The author of *Food and Mood*, Elizabeth Somer, M.A., R.D., writes, "Both sugar and fat are suspected to release endorphins in the brain and produce a natural pain-killing effect." It is this craving for a reward that you continue to seek, either from what you ingest or your brain's own pharmacy.

Certain foods will create a reward effect for many people. Carbohydrates can be one of these foods that cause a pleasurable feeling by releasing serotonin in the brain. The author of *Food and Mood* writes, "Just as Pavlov's dog salivated in anticipation of food whenever a bell rang, carbohydrate-sensitive people become conditioned to crave desserts, breads, or other carbohydrate-loaded foods whenever they are tired, depressed, or anxious." Many times the mere smell or taste of a pleasure food is enough to cause endorphins to be released into the brain.

"While the serotonin response from eating carbohydrates would take some time to occur, the mere touch of sugar on the tongue produces an immediate endorphin rush. Thus, eating a doughnut produces an immediate endorphin-triggered rush followed by a lingering good mood induced by the slow-acting increase in serotonin." Food and Mood

Hot tubs, acupressure, massage, meditation, prayer, yoga, love, sex, breast-feeding and tai chi can all release endorphins in the brain. Cleaning the house or walking your dog might create the biochemical imprint on your brain to keep you "high." The authors of *From Chocolate to Morphine*, Andrew Weil, M.D., and Winifred Rosen, write,

"It is possible that endorphins and other endogenous agents are the basis of all the highs people experience, whether obtained with drugs

or without. People who get high by meditating or running, for example, may have found ways to stimulate the production or release of their own neurotransmitters."

No matter what you choose, whether it is a drug or a behavior, when you are experiencing a painful feeling or sensation, you choose a way to alter your consciousness. You have learned how to change the chemistry of your own brain in order not to feel your pain. All of your addictions help to create a biochemical reward in your brain to take you away from your pain. Every time you reach for your addiction, whether it a chemical or a thought, you are reinforcing a reward in your brain. You continue to reward your brain with the memory of a relationship that has served you for some time. Even though chemicals might be involved in some addictions, it is still your personal will that has chosen to use them. This *imprinting* of what masks our pain is the underlying relationship with addictions.

The body remembers the effects of your addictions as a reward for not feeling. Your cells store these memories. Then, as uncomfortable feelings creep into your life, your body remembers how to reward itself and not feel anything. An addiction has been imprinted. You have a storehouse of memories and past experiences on which to draw.

Arthur Janov writes in *The New Primal Scream*, "Under Stress the brain and body scan the past, both the personal and the species' past, to see what worked before. The system then digs into its archives and retrieves the behavior again."

The high feeling produced, whether it is from alcohol, sugar, chocolate, control or love, produces chemical changes in your body. These changes then numb out the uncomfortable feelings that you have chosen not to feel. As your body becomes accustomed to the chemical highs in the body, it requires more of the drug to produce the same rewards. This is called "tolerance."

Addictions are about relationships that are rewarding. As long as you have feelings that you are not free to express, you will continue to be like rats in a cage looking for the reward to numb out the pain. The higher the "high," the more intense the reward is. The higher the "high," the more you might crave the addiction. When the intensity is lower, the longer the duration is needed to achieve a numbing effect.

In order to have an addiction you must first have a bonding experience with a person, object, behavior, thought or emotion. In order for you to have a bonding experience with an addiction, you must grant the addiction permission to have a relationship with you. It is this granting permission that lets you know that it is okay to use this addiction whenever you have feelings arise that you do not want to feel. With every relationship that you have with an addiction, you have granted permission for that addiction to be in your life. In plain language, you are responsible for saying "Yes" to allowing your relationship with your addiction. You are responsible for creating your addictions. You have chosen which addictions work best for you.

You grant permission for an addiction to be in your life based on your own personal values. If you conform to the rules established by your family and culture, you are more apt to develop socially acceptable addictions like drinking, cleaning or working. If you rebel against the norm, it is more common to develop addictions that reflect a rebel attitude, like addictions to street drugs or pornography.

For instance, many people who become addicted to religion or spirituality do so in a flash. It is as if a lightning bolt hits them and they are entranced. For many, sex and cocaine have similar properties. The high experienced from orgasm or the chemical euphoria of cocaine sweep you away. It is such a wonderful "high" that you are eager to repeat it. This happens quickly, like the first time you try your favorite sugary snack food. Many of your addictions begin as lightning bolts because of the intensity of the "high" that you experience. This intensity then hooks you. You have now granted permission for this to be an addiction to numb out any pain in the future. You carefully imprint this to be used again and again.

Other addictions are more of a gradual process. Workaholism and shopping addiction are two such examples. Most people do not become addicted when they first begin to work or shop. It might require many years to become addicted to working or shopping, and to use these activities to numb out your feelings. With regard to alcohol addiction, people usually become addicts over time. They might begin by enjoying the taste of a glass of wine with a meal or the refreshing feeling of a cold beer at a barbecue. The more "acceptable" it is to have alcohol in your life, the greater the chance that you will use it to hide your feelings. This process might take time. Just as with some love relationships which begin as co-workers or friendships and develop into romantic relationships, many times this is true for your addictions. Candy or alcohol might have begun in your life as something very obscure, but gradually and overtime developed into your best friend.

You might not have smoked cigarettes in ten years, but unless you work through your feelings associated around cigarettes, you will always have a relationship with cigarettes in some form or another. You have bonded with cigarettes at one time. You have history together. You have granted permission for cigarettes to numb out your pain. You remember what it feels like to inhale nicotine-laden smoke to change your mood. It is only your willpower that keeps you away from cigarettes. This helps to explain why so many people return to their addictions after a lengthy time away. During times of stress or under the right circumstances, you subconsciously know that you still have a relationship with cigarettes because you still have not learned how to process the feelings that the cigarettes numbed out. This happens because you have granted cigarettes the permission necessary to be in your life. Without first granting permission to something, you cannot be addicted to it.

In order to better understand your relationship with your addictions, keep asking yourself what was it like to first bond with alcohol. What was your attraction to smoking? Was it a feeling, an image, a certain quality? Why did you grant permission for chocolate to have a relationship with you? Notice how your relationship with your addictions continues to evolve. At times, it might seem that you have finally licked your food addiction and at other times it keeps crawling back into your life to weigh you down. Just when you thought you had finally overcome the enormity of the addiction, why does it keep coming back? It returns because you have created a significant relationship with food in order to mask your feelings. You bonded with food in order not to feel. Food becomes more than just nourishment: food becomes a drug. When feelings arise that you do not have the ability to recognize and feel, your brain seeks out a way to numb these feelings out. Searching for an addiction is the way this is achieved.

Your relationship with food might continue to evolve. At times, you might have a significant relationship with food in order to not feel (a level 5 relationship). You might think about food in all your waking moments and even during your dreams. Food becomes your partner and your lover. Your relationship with food might continue to change (as all relationships do), and you might develop a level 2 relationship with food. Your food addiction might "seem" to be under control, which means you might be on a diet or losing weight, or through willpower are able to stop abusing food. You still have a significant relationship with food in order to not feel. The cravings just keep coming up. Through willpower or strict dieting, you have learned to control your food intake, but you have not healed your relationship with food. Diets are just a way of being addicted to "not eating" in order to mask an uncomfortable feeling. Willpower will not stop your cravings. You are still working on the wrong side of the equation. Only when you learn to experience the feelings that the cravings want to numb out is when things will change for good.

Take the case of the "reformed" alcoholic. She believes that just by sheer willpower, by not going out to bars and "partying," she will end her relationship with alcohol. She is trying to distance herself from alcohol and deny that the relationship ever existed. Unfortunately, until she processes and releases the feelings that brought her to alcohol, she will always have a relationship with alcohol. Alcohol will still be an intimate friend; only she will use willpower to not see this friend.

There is a big difference between a non-smoker and an ex-smoker. A non-smoker does not have the memory of how it feels to numb out with nicotine. There is no relationship. An ex-smoker will always have that memory of what nicotine can do for him.

Whenever you try to distance yourself from your relationships with your addictions and not attempt to heal the repressed feelings that brought you there, the addiction will still be alive, only buried a little bit deeper. In order to heal from addictions, you must first work through your pain and stop denying your relationships with your feeling experiences. Addictions are about relationships. You will heal and come back to nature when you begin to unravel the mystery of your relationships with your addictions.

There is quite a similarity between limiting your personal relationships and limiting your addictions. Think of all the things that you are not addicted to. Look at those around you. Notice somebody else's alcohol problem, or your boss's addiction to jelly-filled doughnuts. Have you ever asked yourself why you are not addicted to the same things? Why does your brother smoke and you don't?

Most likely, you have never granted that person, behavior, thought, object or emotion permission to be used to numb out any of your emotions. You might treat food as nourishment, not as a drug. Because of your value system and "how" you learned about food, you have a different relationship with food. Exercise might be taken moderately and never to change your mood. You watch little television and only when something "important" is on. You use television as a source of information or entertainment rather than as a way to become a "boob tube" zombie. You have not granted permission for these things to be in your life in an addictive way.

The Exceptions: Addictions That Are Forced On You

For most of your addictions, it is your conscious or unconscious choice to grant permission to allow them to be in your life. That particular behavior, thought, object, person or emotion is compatible with your personal history and value system. You begin to use these addictively to mask your feelings.

There are a few exceptions to the belief that we all choose our own addictions. For example, a baby born to a drug-addicted mother has no choice about the chemicals that were put in her body. She is the prey of an already addicted system. She will inherit the addiction of chemical dependency because her choice has been taken away from her. Her body will crave the drug that it is accustomed to having. The baby has not made a choice while in the womb: the mother has made the choice for the child. This is just one example of how your capacity to give permission for an addiction to be in your life can be granted by someone else. Even though the majority of times we choose our own addictions, there are a few exceptions when our addictions are forced on us.

One Addiction Leads to Another

There is a popular belief among many people in society that says if a young teenager begins smoking marijuana, he will continue on to use drugs with more life-damaging consequences (like cocaine or heroin) as his life progresses. There is a lot of validity to this statement, but for different reasons than what most people might think.

The popular assumption is that if a person begins to start smoking marijuana, he will develop or activate an "addictive personality." From here, his supposed "addictive personality" gets a hold of him and his life begins to spiral out of control. He is then doomed to be on a roller-coaster ride of addiction because he "let the cat out of the bag."

I do not agree with nor do I support this assumption. First of all, I do not believe that there is such a thing as an "addictive personality." It is too easy to blame your genes for something that you create yourself. All humans have learned how to numb out their feelings with all sorts of addictions. Smoking marijuana does not create an "addictive personality" that might cause someone to progress on to more lethal street drugs. The need for an addiction to numb the pain was already present and the marijuana was just the addiction of choice that came along at the right time.

I am very disturbed by many people's need to blame their biology for their addictions. The assumption of being able to activate your dormant "addictive personality" puts you into a blaming position instead of taking responsibility for what you yourself have created. Most people are led to believe that if you start smoking a minor street drug like marijuana, you will go on to do other harder drugs because your biology now craves it. This has nothing to do with your biology; it is about the initial drug acting as a "gateway" drug that opens the door to further drug use.

The term "gateway" first came to my attention while I was reading from a book by Avram Goldstein, M.D.'s, *Addiction: From Biology to Drug Policy*. In the book, the author credits the term "gateway" to have originated in the 1970s by researcher Denise Kandel, who " . . . showed that adolescents who become addicted to heroin or cocaine as they enter adulthood have almost always, when they were younger, used cigarettes and alcohol first, then marijuana."

I strongly support the "gateway" theory. A "gateway" drug or addiction is nothing more than an opening to a whole different world. What a "gateway" addiction tends to be is a permission slip to travel to a different place. A "gateway" drug helps to create an environment that is familiar so that other drugs and behavior with similar environmental cues and similar physiological effects can be experimented with.

Take for example the cigarette smoker who has chosen to alter her moods by inhaling nicotine laden smoke through her mouth into her lungs. Smoking cigarettes becomes a "gateway" for other similar addictions. She becomes accustomed to the ritual of smoking. The act of lighting up, carrying lighters, cigarettes and matches becomes very normal. She always needs to have her cigarettes nearby. She learns when and where to smoke. She has established cues for smoking, like after a meal or in the car. She is accustomed to smoke entering into her lungs, the act of holding a cigarette between her fingers, the association with other people who have similar addictions. Thus, smoking becomes a "gateway" as it opens up the door to other addictions that create a similar feeling. The ritual of smoking is now imprinted and has a greater possibility of leading to other smoking rituals—harder street drugs perhaps.

A person who has never smoked cigarettes before would have much less chance of smoking marijuana because he has not bonded with the ritual of smoking. A person who has never smoked might not associate with those who smoke, so the whole idea of smoking a marijuana joint would not occur to him. Someone who has never smoked might see the negative impact of ingesting smoke into her lungs (whether it be tobacco or marijuana) and rejects the idea completely.

Does smoking marijuana lead directly to the use of stronger street drugs? No, not necessarily. Smoking marijuana might only be a "gateway" drug that could encourage the use of harder drugs. Many times, though, the person does not go any further than smoking cigarettes or smoking marijuana. It depends on many factors involved. According to the "gateway" theory, a person who smokes cigarettes or marijuana is more likely to go on to use other drugs than a person who does not smoke at all.

For instance, someone who smokes marijuana is participating in something that most of society recognizes as illegal. This person has to search out a supply from a drug dealer—a person selling drugs illegally. There is a big secret around the whole affair. It is not like going to a bar and ordering a beer out in the open. Buying drugs on the streets is quite different than going to a pharmacy in plain view with your prescription from your doctor. Purchasing street drugs is a secretive affair.

A marijuana smoker usually associates with others who have a secretive, illegal drug life. Being around a group of people who are accustomed to using drugs might give someone the opportunity to try other street drugs because the environment that is created is conducive to street drugs of all sorts being available. Someone who is a tea drinker and never leaves the house except to play bingo would be less likely to find herself in an environment where these types of drugs were available.

A person who is addicted to marijuana is also used to ingesting substances that are considered by most health experts to be rather toxic to the body. Once again, marijuana smoking then might become another "gateway" drug to ingesting other toxic substances like alcohol, crack cocaine or heroin. A person who is a health fanatic would have less chance of becoming a marijuana addict or addicted to other street drugs because the "gateway" has not been opened. He might have more resistance to putting toxic products into his body. A person who is willing to abuse his body is much more likely to develop addictions to alcohol, marijuana or PCP than a person who cares for his body with appropriate nutritional and exercise regiments. There is no "gateway" in this case to allow toxins into the body.

If you are willing to ingest large amounts of alcohol with the knowledge of the apparent liver and brain damage being done, most likely you will be willing to engage in other "high-risk" behavior like snorting cocaine, driving recklessly or smoking cigarettes. If you create a "gateway" to something like "high-risk behavior" to alter your moods, similar behavior is likely follow.

Street drugs and alcohol are not the only way that you transfer one addiction for another. Adrenaline addicts might engage in all types of extreme sports like scuba diving, parachuting or bungee jumping. All of these activities are in search of the "high" produced by these activities. A person who has an addiction to adrenaline will eat, sleep and think of adrenaline producing activities in order to mood-alter. Becoming an adrenaline addict then becomes the "gateway" to other similar addictions.

An article in the *Los Angeles Times* newspaper brings to light the story of the adrenaline junkie. This article is based on the life of a woman named Marta who chases the thrills of the adrenaline rush all over the country.

"Chasing Thrills at 1,400 Feet

"For Marta, sneaking in and parachuting off radio towers and skyscrapers, gives her and other BASE jumpers an adrenaline rush. 'I need it for my soul,' she says.

"Deland, Fla.—Usually she begins at night or dawn: hopping barbed-wire fences, creeping where she can up stairwells, climbing high ladders and girders.

"Her goal is elevation, the height she can reach by sneaking onto the roof of a skyscraper or the top of a radio tower. The practice is known as 'stealing altitude': risking arrest to reach a precipice. For a moment she is still, and then she leaps off, free falling through space and parachuting down—a kind of Russian roulette played with shadows and distance and time.

"The plunge often approaches 100 mph, creating a dose of terror far more intense than she can get by skydiving. The earth is not distant and abstract; it is right there—cars, fences, trees, all flying toward her. Her margin for error shrinks to two or three seconds. In that hyper-reality, she receives a jolt of adrenaline so intoxicating that she must have it over and over again.

"'I couldn't live without it. I would die inside,' Marta Empinotti says, the words streaming out in rapid Portuguese cadences. 'In a way it's not a choice . . . like you don't choose to eat. I need it for my soul, to keep me balanced, to keep me happy . . . Everything is so alive when you jump. Every single hair of my body is alive.'

"Adrenaline junkies heavily populate the world of alternative sports; they include extreme skiers and white-water rafters, downhill mountain bikers and street-luge racers, aerial surfers who dance with clouds and ocean surfers who skim the faces of 60-foot waves."

The "gateway" theory is not an automatic process, but the likelihood of bonding with similar behaviors is much more likely though. Much of your patterns are determined by the precise qualities that you give permission to in order to mood-alter. Those qualities will be different for each individual. Many times, you keep increasing the stakes and, once the "gateway" is established, you continue to take your addiction to the next level. You need to up the ante in order to produce the next level of "high" to numb you out. This has nothing to do with your genetics but the choices you continue to make.

For instance, three teenage friends try marijuana for the first time while in high school. One ends up going on to use other street drugs because he has bonded with "high risk behavior" as a way to alter his painful moods. The second uses marijuana from time to time but does not go on to use other street drugs. He is really a work addict, and staying in control is the quality that seems to alter his moods. The third never smokes marijuana again after the initial time. He learns that being perfect or gaining high achievement is his choice of mood-alteration. Each boy's values and choices help to create a "gateway," or to close the door on similar experiences.

Drugs are not the only "gateways" that encourage you to try other addictions. There are all kinds of other "gateways" that encourage your addictions.

For instance, a person who has granted himself permission to be a rebel in his family has opened up a door for the possibility of many rebel-like addictions. If the family shows a conservative tone, he might become addicted to activities that the family does not condone (like gambling, stealing or lying). These addictions counter the philosophy of the family, and become accessible once he has established a "gateway" and subconsciously labeled himself as a "rebel" or a "black sheep."

If one is the perfect daughter, being "good" all the time becomes the "gateway" for many addictions. She might become addicted to such things as attending church, prayer, cleaning, playing sports or high achievement. The act of being "good" becomes the gateway to other behaviors that numb her feelings out.

In many eating disorder clinics, there is talk about trying to stay away from "trigger" foods. It is commonly believed that such foods like chocolate or bread can become "trigger" foods leading to binges or out-of-control eating. The "trigger" food itself has little to do with the actuality of using food addictively. The "trigger" food is really just a "gateway" that could open the door to other addictive behavior.

A "trigger" food does not cause you to be out of control with food. What a "trigger" food does is to cause you to enter into a world of using food to numb out feelings. The repressed, bottled up feelings are already there. *The significant relationship with food to alter your feelings is already present and active.* What a "gateway" or "trigger" food does is to cause a shift to happen. You shift from being "in control" around food to being "out of control." Most people believe that if they just stay away from certain foods, they will be okay. If they never touch the "gateway" food they will never have to worry again. This mentality is like our current policy on nuclear waste. If we just place all of our nuclear waste in metal drums buried in the ground, surround it with concrete and never think about it again, it will go away. We do the same in our attempts to control our "triggers."

What the "gateway" food does is cause you physical and emotional reward, making you feel better. You get relief from your pain. You might be tired of being perfect and in control all of the time. By losing control and surrendering to your "gateway" or "trigger" food, you get "high" off the act of surrender. This gives you pleasure.

For instance, chocolate might be your "trigger" food that is so powerful for you that you cannot stop yourself once you get going. You might say something to yourself like, "Why stop now. I've already blown it. I'm already out of control." You might go on to continue to eat unconsciously many types of foods from breads to sweets. In this case, "trigger" foods are just another example of how a "gateway" most often leads to the use of other addictions of similar qualities. Once you give up control, it is difficult to get control back.

When your means of numbing your feelings is to search for the highest of "highs," then it really does not much matter how you get it. A romance and sex addict has a good chance of becoming a religious addict because a similar "high" is produced. It is common for spiritual gurus to go from addiction to alcohol to spiritual addiction because the alcohol and the meditation practice are creating similar altered states of consciousness. They have just traded one altered state of consciousness for another.

One particular swami brags about his drinking escapades as a young man in one of his many books. He then goes on to say how he met his guru and "Bingo!"; the drinking was no longer important. He seemed to lose his interest for drinking only after he replaced it with the "highs" of meditation. In essence, nothing changed.

There have also been a number of incidences in the ranks of the Buddhist community of high ranking monks not being able to control their use of alcohol. This is another example of searching for a similar "high"—meditation and alcohol. There is a strong correlation between the "highs" of meditation and the "highs" of alcohol.

Referring to the similarities between the "high" associated with heroin use and the "high" of sexual orgasm, the author of *Molecules of Emotion*, Candace Pert, writes, "Biff's very first question took me by surprise. I was in his office for my weekly report when he leaned forward, looked me straight in the eye, and said in a flat, dry voice, 'Do you realize, Candace, that for a heroin addict the first intravenous injection hits the brain like a sexual orgasm?'"

Candace Pert goes on to add, "We found that blood endorphin levels increased by about 200 percent from the beginning to the end of the sex act." Is it any wonder why heroin and sex could be considered similar addictive patterns? The "high" produced by them is both very powerful.

Some of the self-proclaimed experimenters and promoters of psychedelic drugs in the 1960s and 1970s are now promoting yoga and meditation. This is another example of someone who might "appear" to have shaken his drug addiction. Unless these individuals have learned how to feel and process *all* of their feelings, nothing has changed. The repressed feelings that caused them to alter their minds with drugs may now be altered with spiritual pursuits. You do not know unless you go inside of their mind and find out if they are using spirituality as a means to numb out their feelings. Most likely they have just traded one "high" for another "high." Most likely they have just traded one altered level of consciousness for another, from psychedelic drugs to Eastern mind-altering techniques. In all probability, nothing has changed.

For instance, many heroin addicts, despite using varying amounts of heroin, usually consume large amounts of sugar as well. From soda pop to candy bars, the metabolic process of getting high on sugar is very similar to that of heroin (and that of alcohol, too, since alcohol is digested like a sugar). Heroin addicts are using the euphoric "high" produced by heroin, alcohol and sugar very similarly. They are transferring from one addiction to the next in search of the same quality of "high" once the "gateway" to that "high" has been established.

Why do some alcoholics turn to prescription pills to get "high"? This is because the "high" is familiar. It is like dating twins from the same family. You already know the family rituals, what you do for the holidays and all of the family members. It's familiar. Why do so many alcoholics and drug addicts turn to religion and spirituality? This is because it is familiar to surrender and be powerless. The "high" is the same. In this case, they just trade one altered state of consciousness for a similar one.

In the same manner, an exercise addict might bounce from tennis to golf to jogging in order to maintain the same type of relief from feelings that the exercise creates. Once you establish an opening through a gateway, similar addictions often follow.

Another common addiction in today's age is that of the information addict. She will transfer her addiction from science magazines to self-help books to television documentaries. All this is done in an effort to produce a low-grade "high" or numbing effect. Yes, even the quest for information can be used to numb out painful feelings. Her "gateway" might have been opened way back in grade school where she received attention by doing well in school and bringing home good grades. She then learned to use the quest for information as an attempt to mood-alter. Once the "gateway" was established as a means of altering feelings, it then led to other similar addictions.

While in prison, many prisoners will turn to whatever is available to create the desired "high" that they are seeking. Some turn to reading while others find their solace in weight lifting. Religion is also available and accessible as many sit locked up in their prison cell. They can pray all day long. If a person's primary relief from pain is taken away, he will find another way to mask his feelings. He will choose whatever is available to him.

If one were to remove the coffee and doughnuts from an A.A. meeting (or don't allow members to smoke), those recovering addicts might think that they were going to die. They might be so irritable that they would find it nearly impossible to sit still for too long. Everyone would show up with toothpicks in their mouths to chew on to help calm their nerves. Worry beads held between the fingers would be a common sight. It is just as common for a recovering alcoholic to transfer his addiction to caffeine or nicotine to get "high" as a workaholic transfers his addiction to a hobby or sport should he retire. Chewing gum becomes the oral substitute for those who gave up cigarettes while many people gain weight from overeating after they quit smoking. In much the same manner, a person addicted to chocolate cake will find something else to be addicted to, like television or the fantasy of romance novels, if the chocolate cake were removed.

You trade one addiction for another until you process and let go of all the underlying feelings that produced the original addiction. You transfer from one addiction to another, from a substance to a thought, from a behavior to a person, etc. You might trade your "acting out" addictions to "acting in" addictions. You do this in order to seek out a similar "high" experience to deaden your pain.

Some addictions go from one extreme to the other. For example, it is easy to go from "over-consumption" to "under-consumption." This might happen with someone who attempts to control her addiction to spending by not spending any money at all, even on what might appear to be necessities. This is called black or white thinking. She feels that if she spends even a little, she will not be able to control herself. The "gateway" to "out of control" spending will be opened and she will not be able to stop herself.

Another example of the extreme of addictions is how some sex addicts become religion addicts to hide their guilt produced by their sexual addiction. Their sexual addiction is not gone, only repressed by a stronger, more socially acceptable addiction—religion. Going from the extremes with your addictions is what most diets are all about. People are either controlling their food intake and getting "high" off control or being out of control with their food and mood-altering in this manner. The external behavior might change, but the internal addictiveness is still very much alive.

Much of your life is spent as a daily ritual with your addictions. You are seldom alone and out of your trance. Just as many people go from one personal relationship to the next, you seem to do the same thing with your addictions. You never seem to be truly alone. You always seem to be bouncing from one addictive relationship to the next. First, you might give up smoking. Then you get addicted to exercise. After a while, you get bored with exercise and then you become addicted to work. From there you get burned out with workaholism and find a hobby to bury your feelings into. This cycle goes on and on. You never end the cycle until you start to feel your feelings and release the pain within you. Until you remove the repressed pain from your body, you will continue to trade one addiction for another.

Notice how on a daily basis you bounce from one addiction to the next. You might get up and seduce yourself with your morning cup of coffee (to wake up or numb you out from being alive). You move on to the morning newspaper or early morning television news. This keeps you busy enough so you do not have to feel anything. You then travel to work where you can numb yourself out with the entertainment of morning radio disc jockeys. When you get to work, you can further numb out your feelings by escaping into your repetitive tasks and busyness.

Many escape into their fantasy world and never have to feel. You stop for lunch only to overeat because of all of those bottled up feelings inside.

You come home from work and gobble down your dinner to "fill you up." You sit down in front of the television or engage in reading a novel to give you a steady "buzz." When you finally go to bed, you might unconsciously sigh to yourself, "Ah, I've made it through another day." Then, you use sleep to numb out the pressures of the day and the feelings of always needing to be busy. It is difficult for you to sleep because your mind is still racing from a day filled with busyness and incessant negative thinking.

You might end up using fifty different addictions in one day, some one at a time and others collectively. All of this happens because you are too afraid to feel. You bounce from one addiction to the next, all day long. You go from your thought addictions to behavior addictions, to people addictions, etc. This is all perfectly orchestrated so that there will be no empty time in between to feel your uncomfortable feelings. It is like a child's game of "tag" where all the trees are "safe" and the space between the trees is the danger zone. You avoid these empty spaces in your life because you do not want to feel. Your addictions are spaced out to keep you "safe" throughout the day.

Ever notice what happens when you have empty time? You are in a doctor's office or seated on an airplane. How uncomfortable! You have to find something "to do" in order to avoid any painful feelings (like boredom, anxiety). You end up reading, watching television, staring out the window, sleeping, meditating or keeping busy in other ways.

You spend most of your days and nights trading one addiction for another. You unconsciously go from one to the next without ever questioning your choices. In order to heal from your addictions, it will be necessary to examine this part of your life. You will need to find time to feel your feelings. Unless you learn to feel and let go of the feelings that brought you to your original addiction, you will only continue to find similar addictions that produce a similar feeling of relief for you. You will transfer one addiction for the next. You will continue to be addicted and live from your lost self.

Addictions Can Be Like a Party

Many times you have an intimate one-on-one relationship with one particular addiction in order to not feel one particular emotion. You might smoke marijuana to avoid feeling your loneliness. Or, you might have one particular addiction that numbs out a host of assorted feelings. You might be a workaholic to suppress all feelings—anger, sadness, anxiety, etc. Many times when you are addicted, it is like inviting all of your best friends over for the same party at the same time. This enables you to enjoy all of your most intimate relationships together and numb out one particular feeling or *all* of your uncomfortable feelings at the same time.

Take the case of Dawn. When Dawn would be angry but unable to express her anger, she would create a host of addictions at one time. She would do the following:

1) Jump into the car and drive fast (addiction to speed)

2) Play loud music (excitement addiction)

3) Smoke cigarettes (nicotine addiction)

4) Drink a diet cola (caffeine addiction)

5) Obsessively think about someone else (codependency)

All of this was done because she could not feel her anger. Dawn had invited all of her most intimate friends to be with her at the same time. Dawn was having a party and all of her addictions were her guests.

Addictions can work in combinations or they can work alone. How often do you find smoking and drinking being acted out at the same time? This is because they complement each other. They are like peanut butter and jelly. Smoking and drinking have similar properties. They are both ingestive substances taken through the mouth. Also, they are both social activities, fairly socially acceptable behaviors, damaging to the physical body, and both are ingested toxins. Both smoking and alcohol are found in the same circle of people.

Addictions form "*mini communities*." Sports addicts find each other and hang out at the ball field. Entertainment junkies will mingle at concerts and movies. Alcoholics feel the most comfortable around other alcoholics in bars and cocktail lounges. Religious addicts will merge together as a spontaneous tribe in monasteries and convents. Technology addicts will work for tech companies and find others who are always flaunting their newest lover—the latest high-tech gadget.

You tend to bond with others like you. This applies to your addictions as well. You feel like you are not alone in the world when you can congregate with others like you. A smoker can recognize another smoker from a block away. They are kindred spirits, one and the same.

Smoking, drinking and gambling are common addictions that go together while romance addiction and codependency blend well together. Coffee and doughnuts have a unique relationship. Coffee and sugar are paired together at times. Many exercise addicts are also food addicts, either overeating or undereating. Prayer, religion and codependency are common addictions that are found together.

In healing your addictiveness, you need to begin to take them one at a time. If you are constantly having a "party" with your addictions, you might always seem overwhelmed. A beginning step is to focus your energy on one addiction at a time. You might say something like this to yourself, "When I am feeling lonely tomorrow, I will feel my loneliness for as long as I can and then I will only smoke to numb out my loneliness. I will not drink alcohol or use sex compulsively. I will only smoke." When you can do this, you can begin to take your addictions as a one-on-one relationship and not be so overwhelmed by the "party" that happens when you engage in more than one addiction at a time. Instead of having coffee and doughnuts to numb out your stress of work, begin by eliminating one at a time. Allow yourself only one of those addictions when you are unable to feel your uncomfortable feelings. In this way, you will have more focus to heal.

This process of identifying and isolating each individual addiction is not a cure for your addictiveness. This is only a *step* toward healing. This process is working on the "equation." Being "mindful" of your addictions means becoming aware of doing only one addiction at a time. Being "mindful" of your addictions means you are aware of which emotion you are numbing out with your addiction. Use only one addiction at a time. Notice the feelings that you are trying to numb out and which addiction you are choosing to use. This way you will have a little more intimacy with your particular addiction. Take it one at a time. Stop the addiction party. You will get to know your relationship with your addiction even better. That is the beginning of the healing process.

Qualities, Not Chemicals, Which Attract Us

When you start to examine your intimate relationships with your addictions, it is important to first look at the *qualities* of your personal relationships that you are attracted to. You might be attracted to your partner because of the way she looks, the fact that she has proven to be a good provider or nurturer. You might be attracted to her charm or sense of humor.

Addictions are no different. Addictions have specific qualities that appear attractive to you, which help you to bond with them. For example, a smoker might not necessarily be attracted to the effects of nicotine as much as he enjoys having something in his mouth all the time. Needing an oral fixation might be the quality that he is looking for (the primary relationship), and the *effects* of nicotine might really be a secondary relationship. The object in the mouth might be enough to create a "high" feeling, numbing out any uncomfortable emotions.

You might become addicted to such qualities as sweetness, smoothness, creaminess, cold, hot, crunchy or chewy. Ice cream bars might be your weakness, but not marshmallows. Why not? They are both sweet. The reason is because it is the qualities of the ice cream bar that you are addicted to. The smoothness, cold, frozen creaminess sliding down your throat is what causes a "high" to mask your feelings. It might be a single quality or a group of qualities with which you form an intimate relationship. It might even be a particular brand of product that you become addicted to. You might only be addicted to Dove Bars or Swiss Chocolate. Something in the name or product identity is what changes your mood. It might be the quality of the cream or chocolate that is addictive to you.

It might just be the high quality of the ice cream bar or candy bar that represents "sinfulness." You might be attracted to "sinful" rewards. You might be attracted to a certain brand of beer or cigarettes because of the image that it represents for you. "Real men don't drink lite beer" might be your motto. You might want to be like the "Marlboro man." You might be addicted to buying expensive designer clothes. If you are addicted to caffeine, you might have a primary relationship with warm beverages and a secondary relationship with caffeine. The warm, smooth liquid sliding down your throat with an aroma bubbling up in your nose is really what you might be addicted to. The commercial image that the caffeine is packaged into becomes the addiction. Not just any cup of coffee will do to alter one's mood. You might only get "high" from designer coffee like Starbucks while a cup of coffee at Denny's just does not do anything for you.

If you were *just* addicted to caffeine, you might try to get it from all sources; chocolate, colas, teas, coffees, etc. This is usually not the case. You seem to want the caffeine, but it is the package in which it comes that you become addicted to. It is usually specific qualities of your addiction that are attractive to you.

If you were just addicted to sugar, why not just buy a 5-pound bag of sugar and eat it in one sitting? This is usually not what sugar addicts do. Instead, they have a carefully thought out routine to find the sugar in the right product form. Only then will their moods be altered.

Exercise for Identifying the Specific Qualities of Your Addiction

Sit down quietly and begin to examine one of your addictions. Take out a piece of paper and be your own detective. If you have a television viewing addiction, notice the type of programs that you watch, when you watch them, and how often. Are you alone? Do you enjoy violence, comedy, informational programs, children's shows, romances, or themes of sexual nature? Can you remember when you first began to engage in this activity? Begin to make a list of the qualities about your television viewing that you are attracted to, and those programs that do not interest you. Are you addicted to "channel surfing," where you use the remote control to keep flipping from one channel to the next in order to not be bored? Or, do you just have the television turned on so that it will create background noise so you can do other things and not feel lonely?

If you have food addictions, begin to be more specific about the qualities of your food addictions. Is it only "imported" chocolate that you cannot resist? Do sweets, starches, feeling full or a combination of qualities drive you? Do particular combinations cause you to act addictively, like peanut butter and chocolate, or creamy fillings surrounded by a soft, cake-like exterior? Are you attracted to one particular brand of sweets or one really "sinful" reward? Is it Hostess Twinkies that drive you crazy or Reeses' Peanut Butter Cups? Gummy Bears might be your thing or it might be fruit roll ups. Why are some people attracted to frozen yogurt and others to ice cream? Most have been led to believe that frozen yogurt is healthier for you because it contains less fat. You can get the same "high" as with ice cream and feel that you are eating something healthier.

Are you addicted to an image that a product tries to sell to you (like Marlboro cigarettes being tough and masculine), or is it an actual physical quality that pushes your button like a chewiness or crunchiness? Perhaps, you might be addicted to what a particular product symbolizes—sinfulness, decadence, strength, wealth or sophistication? If you were raised to be a "good" boy or girl, the only way you might know how to "sin," be" "bad" or rebel might be by eating something that you would consider "sinful" in order to numb out your feelings. Is there any question why most women who consider themselves a "good girl" have such an affliction for chocolate?

What kind of "high" does your addiction create? Is the "high" a slight numbing as occurs with chewing tobacco, or moderate buzz as with caffeine or large amounts of sugar? Is your "high" an ecstatic "high" or rush as in sex addiction or thrill sports? Do you feel the "high" of closing a business deal or winning a hand at poker? Does a particular brand name bring up a certain memory for you? You might only smoke a certain brand of cigarettes (after all, isn't tobacco just tobacco?) because of the way it is packaged or marketed. Do you find yourself visiting only one particular fast food restaurant, even though there may be several nearby?

Notice your drug intake or alcoholic beverages. What do you become addicted to when you drink? A sense of freedom? A buzz? Relaxation? A total obliteration of all senses? Escapism? What is the quality that you are looking for? A Merlot or Chardonnay? Do you get excited about a fruity wine or a dry wine? Does the smell of alcohol give you a high? The warmth in your belly? The rush sensation? The temperature of a cold beer? The cool fiery feeling of a tequila sliding down the back of your throat? Do you smoke marijuana because it makes you feel "laid back," without a care, or is it the sweet smell that turns you on?

Start to become more precise with your addictions. Are you addicted to "fat free" addictions? You cannot control your eating, so you choose "leaner" meals, but even these are not satisfying. You are driven by counting calories during the daytime only to gorge yourself on "fat free" crackers before bedtime. Are you addicted to "junk food" or to greasy, fatty foods? Do you eat only the richest of ice cream? Only the best is for you. Perhaps you have an intimate relationship with only "healthy" food. Perhaps you still cannot stop yourself from overeating at healthy salad bars.

Some questions about your addiction might be to ask yourself if you use it alone or in groups. Many people who use drugs addictively claim to do so only in a social setting. Others prefer to get "high" alone. It all depends on the particular person and the drug being used. Some people are actually addicted to "socially acting out," while others are addicted to "isolationist" behavior. Most people who are cleaning addicts tend to want to be alone in their own space when their cleaning addiction takes hold. Many people who need to get "high" with drugs will only do so in a group setting.

Keep asking yourself about the specific qualities of your addiction and keep narrowing it down. What exactly are you attracted to? Are you so desperate for alcohol of any sort that you will resort to drinking rubbing alcohol if you have to, or you only get "high" from the fruitiness of mixed cocktails?

Ask yourself if you need to have something in your mouth to suck, chew or ingest. Are the chemical properties of what you put in your mouth really what give you the "high" feeling? Is the act of shopping what is addictive for you or are you really addicted to spending, owning or finding a bargain? Many business people are really addicted to "deal making." The act of negotiating a lower price can be an orgasmic experience. Are you addicted to alcohol because of the chemical high, the taste or the behavior of drinking? Are you just addicted to the image of one who drinks?

Begin to be more specific about your relationship with your addictions. Take one addiction at a time. Narrow down the exact qualities to which you are attracted. Put your addiction under a microscope and uncover the truth. It is important to become very specific about your relationship with your addictions. What are the qualities that you seek out and what do they do for you?

You choose your own individual addictions that work best for you, based on the following factors: lifestyle, cultural influences, availability, economic status, family influences and personal image. One particular factor or several can come together to help you determine the addictions that are right for you.

A Scenario: Four Different Relationships with Alcohol

The following is a scenario to show the difference between individual relationships with an addiction. Addictions are very personal. You might learn about them in your family or your culture, but you take them on as your own particular prescription for numbing out painful feelings in your life.

In this example, we will follow how four different people use alcohol addictively. I have chosen alcohol because it is fairly common in our culture and addictive behavior related to it is more recognizable. You could also substitute any addiction in its place and get similar results. In this case, four friends meet frequently after work in a cocktail lounge to socialize and relax. They all have their own unique histories and their own prescription for addiction. Here are their stories:

1) Joe: Joe has a primary relationship with alcohol. Alcohol is his best friend. Alcohol is Joe's first relationship in his life. He thinks about it constantly. He plans his day around it. He obsesses about it. He would have no problem starting off the morning with a cold beer or a Bloody Mary. Alcohol has priority over Joe's work, wife, family and personal reputation. He is married to booze.

Joe grew up as a "good boy." He was achievement-oriented and tried to do his best in school and sports. Joe was very loyal to his family. Joe's father was also an alcoholic. Joe had witnessed many episodes of his father being out of control around alcohol or being unable to get up to go to work because of hangovers. Joe just accepted this behavior as the price one pays for being a man. "Real men" drank. It seemed "normal" to be drunk. He would often laugh about it.

Joe first bonded with alcohol while still in high school. He was a very social person, and drinking alcohol at night or on weekends was a very social thing to do. He did not feel that there was anything wrong with it. Alcohol helped Joe to "relax." It seemed very acceptable. Everyone else was doing it. There was no guilt. After all, dad was a drunk. Joe was a "good boy" and followed in his father's footsteps. He needed to be able to drink with his peers. Joe learned that drinking alcohol was something that men did in his family. Joe used to think that his father would be proud of him. He would brag about how much alcohol he could consume.

As time grew on, Joe continued to drink. In fact, he could not stop drinking. He had no "off" button with alcohol. As the stress of work and family began to mount, he continued to use alcohol to numb out his uncomfortable feelings. In the back of his mind, he still believed that his father would be proud of him for being a drunk.

As Joe's alcohol began to get out of control, it soon led to other problems in his life. He and his wife had very little intimacy. How could he be intimate with another person when he was already intimate with a bottle)? His work suffered. His kids knew that they could never depend on him.

Alcohol gave Joe a tremendous "high." Ever since his first encounter with alcohol, Joe had felt a strong bond. He has developed a level 4 or 5 relationship with alcohol (very intimate). His relationship with alcohol was not a secret. Joe did not hide it. He would even be quite proud of how he could hold his liquor. Joe continued to conform to the family pattern; he was just repeating what his father had taught him. Joe looked forward to his next drink, his best friend. Joe was still trying to be the perfect son.

2) Tom: In Tom's case, alcohol is his secondary addiction. He feels that he needs a couple of drinks in order to "relax" and not feel his stress (fear). His primary addiction is that of workaholism. He uses alcohol to numb out the stress that his work causes him. He puts himself under a lot of pressure by driving himself to use work to addictively numb out his feelings and then he uses alcohol to numb his tension created by excessive working. He justifies this behavior by saying that alcohol helps him to "relax." He has a level 3 relationship with alcohol—a moderate level of intimacy.

Tom, unlike Joe, usually knows when to stop drinking. He does not want his addiction to alcohol to get in the way of his primary addiction—workaholism. Too much alcohol might ruin his image of always being productive and in control. He learned how to be a workaholic and compulsively productive from his mother's behavior. Alcohol is Tom's attempt to take the "edge off" his inability to stop working. He works long hours and sometimes even on weekends. He can always find a project to keep himself busy. Having a couple of drinks after work with the gang is the only time that he feels he can slow down and be at peace. While drinking with friends, he is thinking about what project he will complete when he gets home. He is always the first to leave. He is anxious to get busy.

Tom never drinks during work hours or when he is in the middle of something "big." He feels that alcohol might distract him from completing his task. He only drinks after work is finished and sometimes on weekends when it is safe to let down. Tom first bonded with alcohol while in college when he began feeling the pressure of trying to succeed and be at the top of his class. He formed an intimate relationship with alcohol in order to numb out the pressure that he places on himself.

3) Sue: Sue does not really like to drink much. She uses alcohol as a secondary addiction to "loosen up" and not feel so uncomfortable out in public. Sue's primary addiction is to perfection and she uses alcohol to take the "edge off." She feels tipsy after one or two drinks, but that is all she needs to finally feel "relaxed." She has a difficult time stopping her busyness and need for perfectionism. She is afraid of making mistakes. She will not begin something unless she can do it perfectly. She wants to feel more social and out-going. She is terrified of feeling abandoned and not accepted. Sue drinks to feel accepted.

Sue has a level 2 relationship with alcohol (but a level 5 relationship with her addiction to perfectionism). She seldom has more than two drinks. She enjoys socializing with the guys. She knows when to stop drinking because perfect people do not lose control and get drunk. It is more important for Sue to stay in control than to get drunk. Sue first bonded with alcohol as the demands of her job seemed to be overwhelming. The more she tried to prove how perfect she could be, the more everyone expected of her. She needed a way to "relax" and feel free. Alcohol was one of those ways. Her parents did not use much alcohol while she was growing up. She learned to use alcohol to numb out her feelings as long as she could stay in control. That was her commitment to herself. She gave herself permission to mask her uncomfortable feelings deep within her as long as she was always in control.

4) Robert: Robert is Joe's brother (the level 5 alcoholic). Robert does not drink at all. In fact, he is terrified of alcohol. Robert had many negative experiences with his father's addiction to alcohol and made a commitment to himself to never drink at all. The pain around alcohol caused him to go against the family pattern. Whereas his brother Joe became just like his father, Robert went the other direction and became very "unlike" his father.

Robert was afraid of being out of control. His father was always out of control around alcohol, and Robert saw this and it hurt. Robert's primary addiction is that of codependency. In his addiction to codependency, what Robert does is consume himself with everyone else's problems so that he does not feel his own pain. In order not to feel his aloneness or anger, he thinks about his family's problems. This is how codependency works. In his addiction to codependency, Robert tries to save his father and brother from their addiction to alcohol.

Robert comes to the "happy hours" with his brother and the rest of the gang mainly to protect his brother, Joe, who cannot control his drinking. Robert does not realize that this is what he is doing. On the surface, it looks like he is having a good time. Robert is always the designated driver, always taking care of the others. He does not drink at all and he always has a soft drink. The others kid him by saying, "What's wrong with you? Why don't you have a drink?" They do not understand his fear around alcohol. Robert feels deep down inside that he is better than others for not drinking. He has developed a superiority complex for not drinking at all and judges those who do drink as being weak or inferior. Essentially, he is terrified of alcohol.

Summary

In the previous case history, each person had a different relationship with alcohol. Each of your relationships with your addictions is based on your own personal history, values and bonding experiences. Just like alcohol, you can watch anything from food to religion, from gambling to shopping, and witness how everybody has a different relationship with it. Some might have healthy relationships with gambling, food, religion, shopping or alcohol. Others might have an addictive relationship used to mask feelings. It is important to keep remembering that it is not necessarily the food, religion, gambling, shopping or alcohol that are addictive; *it is how you use them.* By beginning to examine your own relationship with your addictions, you will undoubtedly gain new insight into your feelings and your authentic self. By denying your relationship with your addictions, you will stay stuck in the same old place—addicted and powerless.

Dr. Jekyll and Mr. Hyde

For those who are not familiar with the story of *Dr. Jekyll and Mr. Hyde*, let me brief you on it. For those of you who have heard it before, let your memory be refreshed. This is a classic story about a rather ordinary scientist who takes a magical potion that transforms him into a somewhat hideous creature. While transformed, he has little control over his life. It would seem that while under the influence of the potion, he becomes possessed. His physical appearance changes. Only when the effects of the potion wear off will he return to his rather ordinary scientist nature, unaware of the possessed other side of him.

This story is a wonderful analogy to describe addictive patterns. When your addictions take over your life, you become just like Mr. Hyde—possessed and out of control. When you are in your addictive state, the rest of the world seems fuzzy and glazed over. Your vision (literal and metaphoric) is so consumed with your addiction that you cannot see straight. When you are in your addictive state, it is very difficult to see out to the other side.

Each one of us has a trigger that sends us into our out-of-control behavior. This trigger might be a false belief in the form of a dream, memory or "imagined" life-threatening event. It is as if each addiction has its own magic potion. For example, a heroin addict might begin to feel the uncomfortable feelings associated with withdrawal (anxiety and irritability). She might not have had her fix in a while. She sweats profusely, is jittery and cannot sleep. These uncomfortable feelings and sensations might be the trigger that sends her scurrying about to find some heroin to numb herself out.

Many times a childhood fear resurfaces to send you into your addiction. Your aloneness, powerlessness, disappointment, boredom or fear might trigger you to stuff doughnuts into your mouth or to light up a cigarette. Your work pressures, financial disappointment, relationship conflicts or even anxiety over having to take an exam all trigger you to enter into your addictions. Once you enter into your addictions, you literally become blind. You lose yourself.

An example of addictions being triggered might be the following. A situation might be set up where you have made plans to meet with a friend. Your friend is committed to picking you up at a pre-arranged time. She is late. You begin to worry. Maybe she forgot. You become angry. Your body tightens up. You forget to breathe. Fears of abandonment begin to surface. You become Mr. Hyde. You reach for your addiction in order to relieve you from your uncomfortable feelings and your body contracts. You might choose any number of addictions to help numb you out; cigarettes, television, potato chips, etc. You are no longer your self. You are out of control. You are now in your addiction.

All of a sudden there is a knock at the door. It is your friend. She hasn't forgotten. She hasn't abandoned you. She just got stuck in traffic. You are relieved. Your body begins to relax. Your breath returns to normal. You no longer crave food or nicotine. You are back to being your self. You are no longer Mr. Hyde—the hideous creature. For twenty minutes you were in your addictive state. You thought that the anxiety was going to kill you.

Most of the time, you do not even realize how quickly this shift happens to you. You are not aware of how your fear and anxiety act like a magic potion to transform you into someone else. You lose your sense of values when you are addicted. You might do things that you would not normally do if you were not addicted. You might lie, steal or cheat when you have dropped into your addictive state. This is why many people are shocked when someone close to them commits an outrageous act that they never thought he was even capable of. He might be in an addictive state and his whole thinking process is muddled.

Charlotte Davis Kasl has a wonderful description of this phenomenon of how we enter into our addiction. This description comes from her book titled *Women, Sex, and Addiction*. In her book, she writes about an interview with a woman named Martha. The interview goes as follows:

"From ages twelve to fourteen I put myself to sleep at night with fantasies of being ordered to be still by several women who would fondle me. I remember some nights I just couldn't wait to get into bed and start the fantasies. I could feel myself cross over a line to this intense pleasure. It was like a click to another place and all of my loneliness was gone."

Charlotte Davis Kasl goes on to add,

"The click that Martha recalled is that of crossing the addictive line, out of pain and into euphoria. People experience the same relief by shooting heroin, slugging down a drink, or buying an unneeded article. It is so seductive because it works immediately."

When you enter into your addiction, it is like going to another place, another world. It is as if you were *Alice* and you just fell into a magical place called *Wonderland*. Your whole perspective on life all of a sudden changes. It is as if you were to put on a pair of 3-D glasses.

You might have planned an outdoor wedding for 300 guests. It begins to rain. You feel panic and a very uncomfortable loss of control. You desperately need a cigarette to numb you out or "relax," as you might prefer to say. You end up smoking several. The nicotine ends up numbing those horrible feelings of being out of control. You think that you might die because the feelings are so overwhelming. The rain passes. The nicotine worked wonderfully to numb out all of the pain. Within a short time you come out of your addictiveness. You cross back over that magical line. You do not need to smoke anymore. You are back to being your self.

When you cross over that line, from your feeling state to your repressive state, you are gone. It does not matter what you choose to use to alter your consciousness; you are still running from your pain. Whether it is books, poetry or song, you are still in your trance.

Watch how you cross over that magical line on a regular basis and at regular intervals. Notice what many cigarette smokers do with nicotine.

The first thing they do in the morning when they awaken is to smoke a cigarette. The last thing that they do before going to bed is to smoke a cigarette. Cigarettes follow meals and love making. Traveling by car is a good opportunity to smoke. In fact, about every 20 to 40 minutes a smoker might need to light up. He does not want to be without nicotine for too long. He might have an emotion or sensation that he does not want to feel. He is most often in his addiction, seven days a week.

We spend much of our lives in one addiction or another. This is because when we are in our addiction, we cannot see out of it. The trance becomes like a bubble that we are living inside. When we are in our addiction, it is the only reality we know.

A romance addict probably does not realize that she spends the whole day fantasizing about her "Prince Charming" waiting for her at home. She is unaware of how her thoughts numb out all of her fear and boredom. I remember a client of mine who would leave her body and "go to the moon." She could tell me the weather and the time of day on the moon. This was her reality for much of her life.

A sex addict has no idea that most of his thoughts throughout the day are concerned with "checking out" others, flirting or sexually fantasizing. He might be always manipulating for sex, flirting, seducing, objectifying body parts or fantasizing about having sex. Just the same, an information addict might need to check his email or text messages fifty to one-hundred times per day. Information has become the magical potion.

Specific cycles of addiction are also very common. Evenings, winters or weekends could all be enough to cause a specific pattern of addictive behavior because of the feelings that those periods bring up. Many people unknowingly have a fear of darkness. When the sun goes down they unconsciously step up their addictive patterns in order to not feel the repressed fear beneath it all.

The more time you spend as Dr. Jekyll (your natural self), the less time you will have for Mr. Hyde (your addictive self). In order to make these changes, you need to recognize when you are in it and when you are out of it. It is important to become aware of what your magic potion is that sends you into your addictiveness because once you are in it your whole world becomes cloudy. Once you begin to separate and acknowledge these parts of yourself, then you will begin to heal.

You develop identities around your addictions. You begin to label the son as the "drug addict" rather than the son who has a drug problem.

Your daughter gets labeled as the "straight-A student" because she might use her addiction to achievement as a way to not feel.

Language is important. Just as society has labeled the person who uses alcohol to avoid his feelings as the "alcoholic," you can do the same with all addictions. You could call a person who stares at other people's bodies to avoid his feelings a "lookaholic." Someone who gets "high" off nature scenes could be a "natureaholic." A person whose mood changes when she sees a baby in a stroller could be called a "babyholic." Even those who use the sight of a dog to change their mood would be referred to as a "dogaholic" and would be practicing "doggism."

You carry the symbols of your addictions with you wherever you might go. Just as a gang member might tattoo his gang's identity to his chest, you do the same with your addictions. A smoker will never leave the house without a pack of cigarettes and a lighter. This helps to identify him as a "smoker." A bottle opener on a key chain might help to identify someone as a "drinker"—or one who uses alcohol as a way to mood-alter. A religious addict will wear a religious necklace or a T-shirt that boldly says,—"Jesus loves you." A "New Age" addict will have a crystal dangling from her neck. A codependent addict might plaster a bumper sticker reading "Free Tibet" from the back of his car. A pack of gum in the pocket will identify someone who uses gum to mood-alter. She is usually recognized as the "gum chewer." The information addict will carry a newspaper into a restaurant when he sits down to enjoy his breakfast. The technology addict will always have a cell phone and lap-top computer near him. You will notice the reading addict walking down the street while reading a novel pressed close to her face.

It is one thing to have a symbol that you identify with. When you are addicted, even to such simple things as gum chewing and religion, these symbols help identify your addiction for you. The main distinction is this. An addiction is something that you cannot live without and will fight to the death to save and protect. If you are not willing to give up your crystal or crucifix, then perhaps you are addicted. *The more important the symbol, the stronger the addiction.*

Addictions create a trance to protect you from any painful feelings or sensations that you believe might harm you. When you are in your trance and have become Mr. Hyde, you are repressing the energy of your feelings and sensations. Creating additional trance states is just adding to your repression. Coming out of your trance states is the key to recovery of your natural self.

What Is Withdrawal?

Your addictions are present to reward your brain and to keep you from feeling any pain. Withdrawal from addictions will naturally lead you to pain. When you have a well-defined relationship with your addictions to numb out your pain, you will ultimately experience some sort of suffering if you remove yourself from your addiction. There are many different symptoms when the addiction is removed.

We have traditionally heard about the withdrawal symptoms associated with drug use. These symptoms might be such things as nausea and vomiting, profuse sweating, uncontrollable shaking and headaches. With some long-term drug users, the body might be so accustomed to the drug that a sudden absence of the drug might be life-threatening. The shock on the body might be so severe that the body cannot handle it all at once. In this case, the favored drug of choice must be removed gradually or in a supportive environment.

There are other types of withdrawal. For instance, a sugar addict who is removed from her sugar fix will go through the blues. She might be lethargic and depressed for a while. She might have physical withdrawal symptoms, like headaches and nausea, as her body is shocked from the absence of sugar.

Your brain is its own pharmacy. Withdrawal from a particular drug that you normally ingest is not the only form of withdrawal. Love and romance addicts will go through all sorts of withdrawal symptoms if they do not have a "love" interest that they are pursuing. The whole energy of their body collapses; they become lethargic and depressed. Phenyl ethylamine (PEA), the same chemical found in chocolate to give your brain a reward, is also produced when you "fall in love." Perhaps there is a connection between romance addicts and chocolate addicts. They are both searching for the same drug high. The romance and sex addict is so accustomed to the "high" from the fantasy of romance that she, too, suffers physiological symptoms if she does not get her fix.

A caffeine addict will experience many withdrawal symptoms, including headaches and lethargy. A gambling addict, shopping addict and information addict will all experience some form of discomfort once their addiction is removed. An information addict without a book or newspaper will go crazy with anxiety and restlessness. He will resort to pulling out used newspapers from a trash can just to get his reading fix. Anytime you remove that which rewards your brain to not feel any pain, whether it is a drug that you ingest or a behavior that you participate in, you are experiencing symptoms of withdrawal.

Much of the time, your withdrawal from your addictions only allows you to feel the pain that is already present. Withdrawal does not necessarily create pain; it only stops the masking of pain. If you smoke cigarettes to cover up your anxiety, when you stop smoking your anxiety becomes even larger. Quitting smoking did not create the anxiety. Stopping smoking only allowed you to feel what was already present.

Cravings are nothing more than your recognition of a familiar object, person, thought, emotion or behavior which has worked in the past to provide relief from your uncomfortable feelings or painful sensations that are emerging. Whenever there is a craving of any sort, what is really happening is that there is something painful that you are experiencing at the moment. Instead of focusing your attention on the object of your craving (chocolate or alcohol), begin to notice the uncomfortable feelings that you do not want to feel at the moment. This will help you to recognize the relationship that you have created in your attempt not to feel.

For instance, many people who drink alcohol do so to avoid any pain. Once someone reaches a high level of physical dependence, he may continue to drink to ward off the pain of withdrawal. He begins to drink to ward off pain and then continues to drink to ward off the pain of withdrawal. Addictions are about not wanting to feel pain. Withdrawal is about making a choice to feel your pain once the addiction has been removed. Recovery is about unmasking the relationship used to cover up sensations and emotions. Feeling the feelings of withdrawal is a necessary part of returning to nature.

Internalized Addictions

Many of us have been taught to believe that addictions are external activities that we put ourselves through every day. This might include something as simple as the addiction to alcohol or the addiction to gambling. With external addictions, something is taken internally or a behavior is outwardly visible.

While these external addictions do exist and are used to numb out our feelings and sensations, there are many of other addictions that are used that cannot be seen. These might be considered "internalized addictions." These internalized addictions are going on in your head and away from public view. Nonetheless, they are just as damaging as your externalized addictions.

Thought Addiction As a Trance

As human beings, we have evolved with a great capacity to think. Our expanded thought process has been the key to developing new medicines, advancing technology and solving many complicated problems. Yet many times it is our thinking that gets in the way of our healing. Our thoughts often keep us from feeling and keep us in a trance away from our natural self.

Being in a trance takes on many forms and appearances. Most often though, our magic potion is not a pill or a plant that we ingest. Most often, our magic potion to keep us in our trance is none other than our very own thoughts.

Many people awaken each morning in their thought addictions, and these thought patterns then carry them through the day. These include such thought addictions as fantasy, religion, knowledge, spirituality, blankness, violence, niceness, spaciness, perfectionism, suffering, goofiness, clumsiness, shame, seduction, power and many others. These altered states of consciousness are created by the thinking brain to prevent people from feeling any suffering.

Any thought or group of thoughts can be used addictively. It has been said that people have thousands of thoughts daily and yet they keep repeating most of the same thoughts. Your thought patterns are like a revolving drum in your head. Your thought patterns are like a melody in your head that keeps playing the same old tune. Just as you might find yourself humming your favorite musical tunes in the car, while standing in line or in the shower, your daily thought addictions are like this. Your thoughts keep numbing out your painful feelings and sensations. Your thoughts are ever-present and available twenty-four hours a day. You never have to run to the store or to the refrigerator to retrieve them.

A businessman might be addicted to competitive thoughts. A con artist might use thoughts of "scamming" in order to avoid her pain. A preacher might use prayer thoughts as a way to avoid his feelings. Some religious addicts remain stuck in their addictive thoughts by incessantly thinking and quoting from Biblical passages. A tantric goddess becomes addicted to the thoughts of seduction as a way to avoid her feelings

There is nothing wrong with allowing your thoughts to flow to different areas. However, when a thought is used to numb out a feeling or unpleasant sensation, then it becomes an addiction.

Thought addiction has become the primary addictive trance of our time, especially in modern information-based cultures. Thought addiction is much more prevalent than anything that you could smoke or ingest in your body. Thought addiction is always there, seldom to shut off.

Information As a Trance

There are many ways that one could be in a trance with thought addiction. A common way for this addiction to manifest itself is to watch a person who reads a lot, watches or listens to news programming frequently, and works in front of a computer all day long. His world is bombarded with information. He is seldom far from information. Thinking and information come to dominate his entire life. Whenever an uncomfortable feeling or sensation arises, he quickly turns to information as a way to eliminate those painful feelings.

After a busy day at the office thinking and sorting information he returns home to read, use his personal computer and watch the evening news. More thinking and information is at his fingertips. He is constantly numb and drugged with thinking. He is walking around in one big trance. He is drunk on information. Most often he is using his thoughts of information gathering as a way not to feel.

What does it mean to be a thinking addict? You are obsessed with thinking. Your brain never seems to shut down. Your behavior is such that you surround yourself with books and other reading material. Even without the books around, you could still manage to use your thoughts to avoid feeling. Your mind might always be racing around with a host of thoughts and you are forever making lists. You have learned to be addicted to thoughts to avoid those uncomfortable feelings that might come to the surface. Anger, depression, sadness and anxiety are your worst enemies and your thoughts do a wonderful job at numbing them out.

You probably learned how to be a thinking addict as a child. You would go into your head and into your thoughts. A math problem or a story became the tried and true method of staying numb. That way you could avoid the pain that you were feeling all around you that you did not know how to express.

Positive and Negative Thinking Trances

The types of thoughts that you use to numb out your feelings could also be very important. For instance, many people are addicted to negative thoughts as a way to avoid their feelings. This usually manifests itself as "worry." *Worry is nothing more than addiction to negative thinking as a way to avoid feeling.* All day long you spend worrying. "I hope I don't get audited this year." "I hope that my husband does not get into a traffic accident on the way home from work." "I hope that the car starts tomorrow so I won't be late for work." Most of what you are worried about does not even happen.

Your negative thinking becomes a revolving drum that you continue to play in your head. You are constantly concocting elaborate and well thought-out scenarios of what *might happen.* You spend your entire day and evening with your negative thinking. Usually you are doing this in order to avoid pain, either emotional pain or pain in your body. Your negative thinking just becomes another drug to keep you in a trance to stay numb.

You can also be addicted to positive thinking in the same manner. You might use positive thoughts as a way to avoid your self. You constantly recite affirmations and self praises. You stick positive notes and affirmations on your wall and refrigerator to remind you of your thoughts. While positive thinking can be used as a helpful tool to help to repattern your negative behavior, many times these positive thoughts are used to numb out feelings.

A good example of this comes from a woman whom I met. She had changed her name from Susan to Sunshine. She did not look like Sunshine. She was still wracked with body pain and had many layers of repression. She believed that if she kept thinking positive thoughts, she would be healed. Unfortunately, the negative thinking patterns were still buried beneath it all and that was the vibration she was offering. She kept using positive thoughts as a trance to stay numb from her pain. Her positive statements were just being used to mask her core negativity.

Unfortunately, many have mistakenly been led to believe that if you change your thoughts to positive thoughts your problems will automatically go away. You then become addicted to success thoughts or achievement thoughts. There are many New Age speakers who promote these beliefs. While attracting many followers, the story remains the same. Your thoughts, whether they are about success, achievement or positive affirmations, can be used to keep you in a trance of repression. If you do not resolve the underlying issues and beliefs, there is no amount of positive thought that can change things. It is like putting a chocolate coating over a cow turd. You still have a cow turd. Unless you learn how to stop repressing yourself and come out of your trance, then positive thoughts just become the new drug of choice. The negative vibration that you are creating will certainly override any positive thought placed on top of it.

We have come a long way in our development of our thinking. Our thoughts are not going to go away. We will continue to develop new ways to think. How we use our thoughts will need to change if we are to recover our natural self.

States of Consciousness Used As Addictions

Your brain is a very clever device that finds many ways to avoid feelings. Not only your thoughts but your states of consciousness are used as addictions. These states of consciousness become like the ingested drug, numbing you from your feeling states.

Humor is one state of consciousness that may be used to mood-alter. Someone who uses humor addictively might wake up each morning in a joking mood. In fact, the whole day might be filled with jokes. Many times this is nothing more than an addictive state of consciousness created by the higher thinking brain (cortex) in order not to feel.

The concept of "professionalism" is another such example. Many people in our modern culture develop an image around the addiction to professionalism. They use professionalism as a way to hide from their feelings. Professional people are not supposed to feel or bring their emotions to work with them. Professional people many times use their career as a place to hide from their pain. When you are addicted to professionalism, you use this state of consciousness as a drug not to feel. The addiction to professionalism then becomes your image.

Candace Snow and David Willard, R.N., write in *I'm Dying to Take Care of You,* "*Professionalization,* closely related to delusion, is another type of defense. It invites us to mask our dysfunctionality behind 'looking good,' behind being 'professional.'"

Many doctors, lawyers and psychotherapists may have addictions to professionalism. They have invested so much time and money into their image that they cannot get out of it. They might use their professional addiction just as a drug addict would use drugs to mood-alter. They might continue to keep up the image of acting professionally long after work hours are over, just as an alcoholic continues to think about alcohol long after the last drink.

The professional addict cannot separate himself from what he does. Many times, he is using his professional identity as a place to hide. *He no longer is a person who has a career, but he has become the career itself.* There is no distinction. He continues to use professional thoughts and behavior as a place to hide from himself. This could not happen unless he lived in a society that encouraged and supported this type of behavior.

A famous athlete might be addicted to the state of consciousness of "winning, winning and more winning." He will do anything to win and stay on top because this state of consciousness is really just as much of a drug as alcohol is to the alcoholic. Another way to view this is that of addiction to "*domination of others.*" The ever-present need to dominate is what keeps one "high." Several professional athletes come to mind when I think of this type of addiction pattern.

Any state of consciousness can be used as an addictive trance. For instance, it is possible for many gang members to be addicted to the gang mentality. The excitement and adrenaline rush of being in a gang and having to survive against the threat of another gang's attack is enough to create a "high" to keep one addicted. This "high" acts like a rush to try to survive each day and ultimately numbs out the hopelessness and impoverished feelings that are often found in most gang neighborhoods.

Your emotions can be used just as addictively as any substance. Sometimes you get stuck in one emotion all the time to cover up other emotions. This then creates an image for you. For instance, "niceness" or "happiness" could be used to cover up other feelings. You might have received numerous messages that it was not acceptable to display any emotion if it wasn't a "positive" emotion. When this happens, you become the "nice man" or the "happy lady." You are almost always in the addictive mindset, trying to stay upbeat and positive all the time. This image is used to cover up all of your pain. You are never real. You are always hiding from your natural self.

There are many common myths that perpetuate the New Age World. One of these is the myth that there are only two emotions—that of love and fear. This is absolutely wrong and usually propels New Agers into a state of consciousness trance.

There are essentially two states of consciousness, fear and relaxation. Fear is what we refer to as the Stress Response when we feel threatened. Relaxation occurs when we feel safe and this activates the Relaxation Response. Relaxation is not necessarily love.

Love, as well as all of the other emotions like anger, joy and grief, was designed to flow. Sometimes you feel it and other times you don't. Love was designed by nature to be a feeling, not a state of consciousness. Emotions are not designed in the natural world to be experienced in a constant state. As this concept of love and fear spreads, believers now become addicted to a "love" state of consciousness as the drug of choice in order to avoid the other extreme—fear.

Another common myth that resides in the New Age community is the concept of "feel the fear and do it anyway" mentality. This is not what it might seem. When you practice this myth, very little emphasis is placed on the "feel the fear" part. What most people end up doing is becoming addicted to a state of consciousness called "courage" as a way to numb out the fear. This then becomes another addictive state of consciousness used to stay numb and not feel what is really going on. Very little feeling of the fear actually occurs.

Fantasy as a Trance

Another way that many use thoughts to escape into a trance is through the world of fantasy. Fantasy is a normal part of a healthy, active mind. Since fantasy most often feels good, it is easy to go inside your head in order to numb out your feelings. Children learn to fantasize as a normal developmental process. Teddy Bears talk, mud pies are real, and there is always a Boogie Man in the closet. When you are not allowed to have your feelings, you learn how to numb them out with your thoughts of fantasy.

Poor grades in school might be because a child is always off in her head fantasizing instead of paying attention. Perhaps she might not have honored all of her feelings when and where they arose, and the only way that she knows how to numb out the pain caused by those feelings is to go off into her world of fantasy. The world of daydreaming can become just as addictive as a favorite chocolate bar. What begins as creative thinking quickly becomes a world of escapism.

A child learns early on that if he cannot control his external world, he sure can control his thoughts and his body. Fantasizing or learning to leave his body is often another addiction that a child learns in order to not feel and to survive what seems like death. "I just want to get away," might be the addictive mind-set that many develop in order to numb out their pain. These are thoughts that carry them into another world to keep them safe from suffering.

Addiction to fantasy can be, and usually is, just as powerful and seductive as a snort of cocaine or a bite of a chocolate chip cookie. Many live much of their lives in a trance of fantasy. They are seldom their natural self. Whether you fantasize about food, vacations, your next purchase, or romance, it does not matter. Much of the time you are using your thoughts of fantasy to escape from your emotional pain.

Spiritual States As an Addictive Trance

Any thought can be used addictively if it is used to numb out emotions or sensory experiences. This includes spiritual or religious thoughts too. Many people, when experiencing something uncomfortable, turn to religious or spiritual thoughts as a way to stay in a trance. "Don't push the river" might be the ever-present thought that is etched in your brain. This phrase then is used to avoid feeling any pain in your life. "Only the meek shall pass through the gates of heaven" becomes addictive mind chatter. These spiritual phrases become welded to your mind and can create addictive states of consciousness to keep you numb. Just as caffeine or alcohol can create an addictive state, so too can your thoughts. It is not the thought itself that makes it an addiction. If the thought is being used to numb out an uncomfortable feeling or sensation, then it becomes an addictive thought.

The following is a story of a client of mine, Rita, and how she used spiritual thoughts to go into her trance.

As I was giving her a massage, Rita kept saying, "OM NIVA SHIVAYA," whenever I would find a tender area in her body. She was using a spiritual thought to avoid the feeling of pain. She was attempting to stay in a trance using spiritual thoughts instead of feeling and releasing her painful muscles. She did not want me to know that she was in pain. She just tried to stay in her trance. The pain from her sore body was with her every day of her life. She had learned that if she was always "nice" and "happy," the painful feelings in her back would just seem to go away. She was using a thought addiction of being "happy" to numb out physical pain. Well-rehearsed clichés may be just addictive thoughts that keep you from feeling.

People who always appear happy can be using the thoughts of being happy to cover up deep, painful feelings. This is an addiction to a state of consciousness. The attempt to always appear "nice," "good," "holy" or "mindful" can be a mental technique used to cover up other feelings and painful sensations. Being in a mindful trance can be just another way to be addicted and another way to stay repressed.

A meditative state can be just as addictive as a heroin addict's "high." With this altered state of consciousness created by your thoughts, you might appear to be in a wonderland. An Indian mystic will strive for the illusive state of *Samadhi*. A Zen monk will try to achieve *Satori*. A calm and blank stare on a person's face, no matter how "spiritual" he might claim to be, is often nothing more than a state of consciousness being used to stay numb and mood-altered.

Addictiveness does not have to be to a particular drug or food. It can be a state of consciousness that one compulsively attempts to achieve. John Firman and Ann Gila, the authors of *The Primal Wound,* state,

> *"We can become addicted to anything, from the comfort of morphine to the thrill of romance, to the creative process, to the intuition and higher states of consciousness. One might say that any level of consciousness, on any spectrum of consciousness, can become grist for the addictive process."*

Thus, unless the early childhood traumas are resolved and the inability to grieve pain is restored, most will continue to be addicted. Mindfulness, "enlightenment" or even calmness many times are just addictive states of consciousness used to avoid pain.

A Zen Buddhist master can be just as addicted as a cigarette smoker. The Zen master might get "high" off a state of consciousness rather than nicotine. There is little difference. He can be passionate and fanatical about what he does. He might have an extreme or significant relationship with spiritual thoughts and behavior. He is often motivated by his fear of being "off-center." Being "off-center" might mean that he would have to feel the extremes of his pain and couldn't hide in his head any more. Arthur Janov writes in *The New Primal Scream,*

> *"New Age thinkers talk a lot about consciousness and the higher mind. They believe that you can transcend to higher levels of mind unknown to ordinary mortals. They concoct rituals to use to rise to these levels. Yet, the only way to rise to a higher consciousness is by descending to lower levels. That is the true dialectic of mind.*
>
> *"It is paradoxical. Those who claim to have achieved a state of bliss and cosmic calm come to our research laboratory, where we find a mind that is racing a mile a minute and a body in a panic state. Billions of neurons are busy in a job of repression. It works, and the person believes he is calm or has achieved nirvana. Repression's job is to deceive."*

For instance, many primitive tribes use trance states as part of their normal every day life. The people of the Kalahari Desert in Africa called "the! Kung" will dance for hours to achieve a state of consciousness called "!Kia." While new insights can be revealed, these altered states of consciousness do very little to release the patterns of stress, repression and physical trauma. An altered state of consciousness most often is just another drug of choice.

Codependence As an Addictive State
While the term "alcoholism" has been around for quite some time, "codependence" is a relatively new concept. The last thirty years or so have seen great progress in getting closer to what codependence actually is. Codependence is a critical issue in our culture, and much work has been done to bring it out in the open.

Initially, stemming out of treatment for alcohol, codependence began to emerge with its own 12-step program and its own membership. Codependents were initially thought to be those who wished to rescue an alcoholic from his addiction to alcohol. It is much simpler than that.

Codependence is a trance of thought addiction. When someone who has the addiction to codependence is experiencing a feeling or sensation that she is unable to feel and experience, she turns to a relationship with thoughts of others as a way to avoid any feelings.

Just as a workaholic will think thoughts of work to numb out and a busyholic will create endless tasks to accomplish to numb out her pain, a codependent will think thoughts of other people to keep from feeling any discomfort in her life. In the case of codependence, the mere thought of another person is enough to create a "high" feeling to numb out any pain. Many times these thoughts are of others who appear to be in trouble (like someone who is actively practicing his relationship with alcohol in order to not feel).

We have been sidetracked into placing codependence in the sickness category. We have been labeling codependence and alcoholism together as sicknesses that feed off each other. Codependence is often associated with those who are close to someone practicing numbing with substances. However, codependence is essentially its own separate way to stay numb.

A codependent addict will eventually develop an image around her disease. She will be the one who can never say "No." She will always be volunteering for something else. She is always looking for a charity to give her time to. Codependents often show signs of physical stress because they do not know when to stop. They do not take care of their own needs. They cannot stop rescuing others.

The authors of *Recovery From Addiction,* John Finnegan and Daphne Gray, write,

"Co-dependency is an addiction, as devastating to life as addiction to substances. While the alcoholic often dies of cirrhosis of the liver, the co-dependent will die of stress-related diseases."

A person with a primary codependent addiction will begin to take on some very pronounced characteristics, like the "helper" or "rescuer." Just as many people with an addiction to alcohol will work in and around the alcohol industry, the same is true for codependents. Many people with a codependent addiction will find jobs in the helping professions like nurses or massage therapists. These are people who tend to give much more than they receive. In fact, Candace Snow and David Willard, R.N., write in their book *I'm Dying to Take Care of You*, "Our experience indicates that codependence creates harmful consequences for better than 80 percent of the nursing profession."

Another well-known researcher in the recovery field is Pia Mellody. In her book *Facing Co-dependence*, Mellody writes about the five symptoms of codependence. She says that a codependent has trouble with the following:

"1) Experiencing appropriate levels of self-esteem
2) Setting functional boundaries
3) Owning and expressing their own reality
4) Taking care of their adult needs and wants
5) Experiencing and expressing their reality *moderately*"

Yes, these are definite symptoms of codependence, but they are not the root cause. How could someone have self-esteem if he is frequently thinking about others? He is probably not very aware of his own thoughts and feelings very often. How could a codependent set functional boundaries if his thoughts are merged with others all of the time? How could a codependent own and express her own reality when she is frequently thinking about others' reality? How could a codependent take care of her adult needs and wants when she spends so much time thinking about other's needs and wants? Moderation is usually hard to find when it comes to codependence addiction; it is usually all or nothing.

Terry Kellogg, who appears in John Bradshaw's video-taped series on *The Family*, tells a wonderful analogy of what it is like to live life as a codependent. He says that a codependent is someone who, while drowning in the ocean, will think about others. Even in his time of crisis, a codependent is still very "other-centered."

In order to heal from codependence addiction, it is important to begin to notice your own needs and wants. It is important to notice when and why you focus your attention on others. It is also very important to recognize how you became "other" oriented. Once these beginning measures are initialized, you can take the steps to heal from your codependence addiction and recover your natural self.

A higher degree of emotional health occurs when you spend less time in your addictive states and more time feeling your feelings. Returning to nature is choosing to remove yourself from your magic potions and come out of your trance states. Anything that continues to bring you to your Mr. Hyde state (addiction) must be removed, be it a thought of another person to numb out your pain or a substance that you might ingest.

Recovery of the natural self is learning how to release your altered states of consciousness, not to create more of them. Most traditional healing remedies have included ways to create another altered state of consciousness to cover up your natural self. These altered states of consciousness may include such things as motivational or positive thinking, spirituality or success thoughts. It does not matter. As long as you continue to create new thought patterns to cover up your repressed patterns, you are still addicted. As long as you continue to put a positive thought on top of a negative thought, you will still struggle.

Characteristics of Addictions

How Do I Know If I Am Addicted?

As a bodyworker for many years, I would often have the pleasure of giving a client her first massage. Along with explaining to her the benefits of massage and the actual process that she would be experiencing, I often joked with my client that she would become addicted to massage. The pleasure and sense of relaxation is *that* wonderful. I would add that she might resort to stealing from her children's piggy banks in order to pay for her next massage. All of this was done in a humorous and light tone.

The skepticism on my client's face when she entered was transformed into a magical glow as she departed. Frequently, the relaxed and calmed client would make the comment, "I can see how easy it would be to get addicted to massage." I believe there to be a lot of truth to this statement. Anything, including something as pleasurable and innocent as a massage, can become an addiction.

Most believe that addictions are those awful habits that other people have. We have heavy judgments about those who smoke, drink heavily or use illegal drugs. We have been taught to believe that addictions are about substance abuse. People with addictions have a problem or disease. The traditional concept of addictions seems to be focused on how to break a nasty habit.

This is only the tip of the iceberg. Your nasty habits, as you call them, are only the obvious addictions. I agree with many of the pioneers in the field of addictions, such as John Bradshaw and Fr. Leo Booth, when they suggest that addictions are at the root of most social problems. In fact, I believe that we are all addicts in one form or another. I also agree with Dr. Andrew Weil who says in his book *Natural Health, Natural Healing*, "I reject the concept of 'addictive personality' unless it includes everyone."

Only you can decide what an addiction is for you. I cannot determine your addictions. For example, one day you might come home from work and find pleasure in eating an ice cream bar. The next day you come home and cannot live without that ice cream bar. You have been thinking about the ice cream bar all day long and are obsessed with devouring it. You hardly even taste it. What is the difference? The difference is what you are feeling at the moment. The second day, the ice cream bar becomes your addiction only because of the feelings that you are trying to repress. You might have been feeling lonely or angry. You might have had a very stressful day at work. You were looking for a way to ward off those uncomfortable feelings, whereas the previous day at work everything went well and you were feeling pretty good about yourself. You did not need to repress your feelings.

Only you can decide for yourself what exactly your addictions are. This is because nobody can fully know what it is that you are feeling inside. Others can only *imagine* what it is that you are feeling, and that may or may not be your actual reality. Your behavior might help others to *imagine* your reality, but only you can decide if that ice cream bar is an addiction or a pleasure based on what you are feeling inside of you. Since it is very challenging to identify with certainty what an addiction is for each of us, I have included a set of *characteristics* of addictions. These *characteristics* have five parts. Any addiction may include all five characteristics, a couple of them, or only one of them.

1) An Addiction Has Power Over You

When you become addicted to something or someone, you enter into a trance-like state and become powerless. An example might be found in the old Superman movies. Here you have a super hero—powerful, strong, independent and dynamic. Yet, when a tiny rock called Kryptonite is placed in his presence, he crumbles. He loses his power and his strength, and becomes trance-like. He acts unconsciously and is humbled.

Addictions are just like Kryptonite; you become powerless over them. You can think of nothing else but them. Your behavior changes and you act irrationally. You become irresponsible and lose yourself.

A good example of this might be what happens in a marriage, when one person is addicted to reading the newspaper or a novel. This person *has to* have his reading material. When you try to communicate with him while he is engaging in this activity, you might find it very difficult. He seems to be entranced in his behavior. The book or newspaper seems to have power over him. He does not seem to be himself. He has become someone else. He is addicted; the Kryptonite has taken over. You somehow learn to wait until that person is finished reading or you become angry and cannot understand his behavior.

A gambling addict may be no different. Once the cards start to be shuffled and the dice begin to roll, he loses his power and is entranced. It would be difficult to pull him away from the table at this time.

It is important to distinguish here the issue of power. All addictions give you the illusion of power, but in reality you are powerless over your addictions. Many people addicted to such drugs as PCP and cocaine say that these drugs make them feel powerful. This is just an illusion. While you are in your addictive state, you are powerless over your addiction.

There is an important point to remember. Anyone, no matter how far down or how addicted, has the power to eliminate his addiction. You choose to stay in your addictions. Anyone has the power to move beyond their addictions. Anyone has the power to change. Addictions are very powerful, yet, just as Superman learned to avoid the Kryptonite, you, too, can learn to move beyond your addictions.

2) An Addiction Takes Away Your Choice

Whenever you reach for an addiction, you are acting out a well-imbedded pattern within you. Whether it is to grab a smoke or to gobble down a frozen yogurt, when you are in your addictive stage there are few choices. You tend to choose what is familiar and that is usually the closest addiction. Being addicted is like traveling the same route to work everyday. Being addicted is like a well-worn path that you continue to settle into.

Every time you sit down to watch television, is it because you choose to or because you are addicted? How do you know? Check inside. Are you feeling an emotion that you do not want to feel (boredom, fatigue?) and is this behavior a way to make you feel better? Or are you functioning unconsciously? Take a minute before you actually turn the television on and ask yourself, "Do I have a choice?" or "Is the choice being taken away from me?"

Is this substance, person or behavior something that you are unable to not have or unable to not do? When you seem driven by something, a good question might be, "Do I have a choice?"

3) An Addiction Takes Away Your Control

Many times when you are addicted, you have no control over your thoughts and behavior. Instead of having one bowl of ice cream, you might have two or three. You cannot stop yourself until you are full or physically sick. You cannot stop yourself from eating a whole box of doughnuts. You are like a tiny robot operating on automatic pilot. The internal regulating devices don't seem to be working. You appear to be possessed. You cannot control yourself from not having that next bottle of beer. Often times you are out of control when you are addicted. There is no way to stop.

Learning to moderate your behavior is learning to listen to what you want and need. When you are acting addictively, you do not know what you want. You just want the pain to go away. You are in a trance and have no means of stopping yourself.

4) Addictions Are Mood-Altering

An addiction can be a person, object, behavior, emotion or thought process that prevents you from feeling an emotion or sensation that you do not want to feel. In order to understand how and why you become addicted, you need to be able to recognize your feelings when they arrive. Many people just feel "blah" at times and do not know if it is because they are hungry, tired or angry. You need to recognize what the mood is that you do not want to feel.

It is not an addiction if you are not attempting to numb out a feeling or to change a mood that you do not want to feel. Much of the time you are attempting to numb yourself out and change your moods. This is a key aspect of addictions. They are used to keep you numb.

5) Addictions Are the Purpose of Your Life and Not Just a Part of It

Imagine what it would be like to attend 18 aerobic classes per week. You might say that a person like this is a very fit individual who is hooked on exercise, but this might not be such a healthy practice after all. The reality in this case is that this person becomes addicted to the endorphin rush or to the muscle building and exercise. Many times this becomes just another addictive process. For many people, exercise becomes the purpose of their lives. It allows them not to feel their emotions. In this case, exercise has become an addiction.

Anytime something (person, object, behavior, emotion or thought process), becomes the sole purpose of your life and not just a part of it, it has become an addiction for you. This includes what most people would consider to be extremely healthy behavior like exercise, spirituality, social work, prayer, God, love and even reading self-help books.

To be addicted does not require that you demonstrate all five of these characteristics. Sometimes only one is all that is needed to verify your addiction. For many addictions there is no loss of control. However, being addicted to control becomes the addiction in this case. For many other addictions, all five characteristics become activated. There are no two addictions alike for any two people.

For example, the state of "sobriety" is often nothing more than transferring your "acting out" behavior of drinking alcohol to change your moods to an "acting in" thought process. What appears to be going on in your head when an uncomfortable feeling begins to emerge is that instead of numbing out with alcohol or drugs, you use the thought of *not drinking* or *not taking drugs* to keep you numb. You stay numb by a thought rather than a substance. The cravings are still there because you have not yet learned how to identify and feel your feelings when they arise. You still have a relationship with drugs or alcohol. You might be able to "control" your drug or alcohol use, but you have not healed from your addiction. You will always need to be on guard so that when a craving emerges, you will have enough strength and willpower to mask it with an appropriate thought—in this case the thought of not drinking.

It is important to become honest with yourself to admit that you might have an addiction. For example, how many people would be willing to admit that their cat or dog is their addiction? Having a pet seems so normal. Yet, is your little poodle the sole purpose of your life? Can you ever leave town without your animal or are you constantly in its presence? Do you have trouble sleeping at night without your cat near your side? Do you have a choice about what kind of activities you can have, all dependent on how long you can be away from your pet? Does your mood change when you are away from your pet and do you quickly become happy again when reunited?

A good method to find out if you are addicted to a specific pleasure in your life is to listen to your body. How do you feel when you remove yourself from something that you enjoy so much, whether it is a beverage that contains caffeine or a behavior as familiar as playing cards? Are you irritable when you cannot have it and find relief when you finally get it? Do you think about it obsessively? Are you angry or restless when you are without this behavior or object that seems so important to you? Does your head hurt when you cannot have sugar or caffeine? Are you tired or depressed when you cannot exercise? All of these body signals might be telling you that you are addicted.

In order to know if you are addicted or not, it is important to ask yourself some tough questions. This is admitting your imperfections and acknowledging your flaws. This takes courage. In order to heal from addictions, you need to be completely honest about them, first to yourself and then to others. For many people, it is embarrassing to admit that they are not perfect. You need to become vulnerable enough to admit that you have a sex addiction or that you use food addictively in order to numb out your feelings. It might be difficult in the beginning to completely understand what your addictions actually are. Addictions have become so ingrained in most people's lives that they seem normal. Keep asking yourself these important questions.

Addictions are very sneaky and so much a part of your life that you might be unconscious about what exactly is happening to you. By continuing to ask yourself these tough questions, you will begin to bring your addictions to consciousness where they can be healed. Denying that you have addictions will heal very little.

Saying "Yes" and Saying "No"

When most people think about addictions, they usually think about them as behaviors that could be classified as "acting out" behaviors. You might overeat or cannot control your drinking. You exhibit antisocial behavior that is visible to the outside world (even though it might be one of your very best kept secrets). Your gambling addiction or your addiction to pornography is being displayed for the whole of society to see.

The other end of the spectrum takes you to addictions that may or may not be visible to the human eye. These addictions are commonly referred to as "acting in" addictions. "Acting in" addictions have many common characteristics. Some of these are as simple as an addiction to avoiding something. "Under-consumption" of something is also a common characteristic of "acting in" addictions.

"Acting in" with your addictions is no better than "acting out" with your addictions. You are still addicted whether you "act in" or "act out." You are using addictions because it is too difficult to feel.

Some of the distinguishing characteristics between "acting in" addictions and "acting out" addictions are as follows:

ACTING IN	ACTING OUT
DIETING	OVEREATING
SEX AVOIDANCE	SEX ADDICTION
UNDERWORKING	OVERWORKING
SOBRIETY	DRUNKENNESS
SAVING	SHOPPING

There are two main areas that you either "act in" or "act out": 1) saying "Yes" versus saying "No" and 2) over-consumption versus under-consumption.

The first way that "acting in" and "acting out" addictions come into your life occurs when you say "Yes" or say "No" to certain behaviors. When you get drunk, you are saying "Yes" to use alcohol to numb you out. When you overeat, overspend or are compulsive about anything, you are saying "Yes" to acting out. This is *surrendering* to your behavior.

You can also get "high" and have your mood-altered by controlling your thoughts or behavior. You can control your use of alcohol, your thoughts or your food intake (like an anorexic). The act of saying "No" can also change your mood. You now get "high" on *control*. You are "acting in" when you change your mood by controlling your behavior. By either "holding on" or by "letting go," you can be addictive and attempt to mood-alter. This is referred to as" *control or surrender.*

Just as you feel powerful with such things as gambling or sexually "acting out," you also feel powerful by depriving yourself. You might feel stoic and righteous when you deny yourself material possessions or your favorite after dinner treat. You feel better than others for not having something.

This thought process is just as addictive as "acting out" with your addictions. What you are really doing is numbing your feelings by depriving yourself of something. Just as you might "act out" by always needing to attend movies or parties to numb your boredom, the act of renouncing worldly things or isolating yourself often is what gets you "high" to avoid your pain. The act of renouncing things and pleasures can be just as intoxicating as a hit of marijuana or a mixed drink. This is "acting in" behavior by saying "No!"

One way that "acting in" behavior manifests itself is with someone who is a dry drunk. He is "acting in" with alcohol. He is saying "No!" to alcohol every time the cravings come up. He is using the denial of alcohol to get "high" from the uncomfortable feelings that emerge that cause him to crave alcohol. He is not necessarily resolving the root of his conflict with alcohol; he is only trading one "acting out" behavior for another "acting in" thought process. This is what is commonly called "sobriety."

When you replace the "acting out" behavior once the cravings begin with "acting in" thoughts you have done very little to heal from addictions. You have relied entirely on guilt or willpower to prevent your "acting out" behavior. There is still the battle going on inside your head. If you wanted to heal from your addictions, a better answer would be to ask yourself what it is that you are feeling when an urge arises. Why do you need to numb out that feeling and where did you first learn to have a relationship with that type of behavior?

"Acting in" by saying "No!" can be a very powerful mood changer. For instance, many people who have food addictions use the thoughts of not eating to mask their feelings. When someone has a bad day, he may really want a sweet. By saying "No!" to the sweet he stays in control. "Acting in" by saying "No!" is really about getting "high" from being in control.

Depriving yourself is a way to stay in control and being in control changes your mood. Those who take a vow of celibacy (for religious, spiritual or other reasons) are many times addicted to "acting in" behavior. They are really saying that they are better than others for depriving themselves and can mask their feelings by staying in control.

Many people get "high" from the act of deprivation, especially around money. They get "high" from not having. They hold on to everything. Many times they deny purchasing luxuries and often even necessities. They are pack rats, refusing to throw anything away for fear they might need it someday.

Some become penny-pinchers and cheapskates. They refuse to eat out because they refuse to pay for valet service to park the car. They are addicted to holding on and fear letting go of anything. They deprive themselves of pleasure because it feels good to be in control. As Donna Boundy writes in *When Money is the Drug*, "We are becoming more vulnerable to using anything as a mood-changer, including money."

Money often becomes the drug of choice, either to accumulate it or to push it away. Many become addicted to scarcity because they are still in control. They believe they don't deserve anything. Perhaps they believe they will be rewarded later (in "heaven" or in their "next lifetime"). They become addicted to "acting in" by saying "No!" and not allowing themselves to possess anything.

"Acting in" behavior is about numbing your feelings by not doing something. This is a very sneaky addictive practice because it looks so positive on the outside. What you see are the martyrs, saints, helpers and savers. What you don't see on the inside is the addictive process of deprivation and control to numb out painful feelings.

It appears that those who have been addicted to control or "acting in" behavior have written the moral code on what an addiction is and is not. Current addiction theory was created by a group of people solely dedicated to the process of addiction to control. As a consequence, they have finger-pointed and labeled those who "act out" or are out of control as "the addicts." This way they do not have to look at themselves.

Whether you are acting "out" or acting "in" with your addiction, it does not matter. You are still acting addictively and attempting to mood-alter. No matter if you are trying to control your addiction or have lost control and surrendered, it does not matter.

For example, if I were to ask you to not think of an elephant, the first thing that you would think about is an elephant and then you might mask this thought with other thoughts. The same is true with your "acting in" addictiveness when you use a thought to replace an addictive behavior.

One of the drawbacks to using "acting in" thought techniques to cure "acting out" behavior is that it is very difficult to picture yourself not doing something. The image of not eating still has food involved. The image of not smoking marijuana still has marijuana involved. Even if you substitute images in your head of not doing something, every time the cravings come up you are still being haunted by images of the prohibited item. It seems that you have to compensate for the craving to "act out" with a thought of not doing something. This is not solving the addiction problem. This is not setting you free from your addictions. Rather, it is like tying a ball and chain around your ankle reminding you to not stray too far away.

These "acting in" thought addictions are widely used mental techniques used by many drug and alcohol treatment centers. You might be taught to change the urge to drink into a vision with a negative impact. For example, you might envision that alcohol makes you sick to your stomach every time you have a craving. Imagine that each time your feelings are too painful to feel, a craving for alcohol emerges. In order to get relief from those "terrible" feelings, you might change the urge to drink to a thought of hanging your head over a toilet while vomiting. For some people this might work in preventing them from drinking, but it does not solve the problem of where the cravings come from. This is only behavior modification and treats the symptoms, but never the problem. You must forever remain on guard and disciplined enough to use this technique.

Another technique used to replace an addictive behavior with an addictive thought pattern is to use the "cancel" method. Every time you have the urge to smoke, you change the behavior by replacing the craving with the thoughts "cancel, cancel, cancel."

You attempt to eliminate the cravings by treating only the symptoms. You will never heal your addictiveness with this technique because you are just trading one "acting out" behavior for another "acting in" thought process. You might appear to have succeeded in quitting drinking or smoking, but you still have a relationship with alcohol or nicotine. You will always have to brainwash yourself to be vigilant and on guard in order not to "act out" your addiction. To the outside world, you might appear to have conquered your addiction, but in your head the addiction battle is still being fought on a daily basis. You are forever "acting in" with your thoughts whenever the cravings emerge. You will have to be eternally vigilant with your mental techniques in order to not slip back into "acting out" behavior. Many people believe that addictions are about attempts to go outside of yourself to fill your "inner longing." However, many go inside their heads with mental techniques in order to avoid their pain.

Why are there such heavy judgments on those who "act out" with their addictions, yet we praise those who seem to have everything under "control" and are really "acting in" with their addictions? It seems that society prides itself on thinkers, intellectuals and productivity. Being "in control" is rewarded much more than being "out of control."

Addiction is an inner process. No matter how you display your addictions, you are still practicing repression and still attempting to change your mood. The addictive trance comes in many shapes and forms. Whether you "act in" or "act out" you are still practicing addictions.

What Is Willpower?

Willpower has been the standard treatment choice in most addiction recovery programs. However, willpower is nothing more than attempting to deny a relationship. Willpower is always having to be on guard. You can never let down. You can never drop your attention. You can never fall asleep at your post. You can never be soft on yourself. You must remain rigid and disciplined. Willpower is knowing that there is a shadowy figure behind you. Willpower never heals addictive behavior. Some addictive behavior is stopped, but the relationship is still alive. You keep being reminded of the addiction by internal thoughts, cravings and external cues. Whenever a craving or an addictive thought emerges, your willpower attempts to rid you of it. Willpower is attempting to place a "No" on top of a well-ingrained "Yes." The relationship lives on.

In Alcoholics Anonymous, the approach is to try to deny the relationship with your addiction to alcohol. Sobriety is about always having to be on guard because you have never healed your relationship with alcohol. Just as you might have a conflict with a friend and the way you choose to deal with it is to distance yourself and stop seeing the person, neither the conflict nor the relationship ever goes away. It remains unresolved. By distancing yourself from your relationship with alcohol, drugs or any other addiction by using sobriety, willpower or 12-Step meetings, the conflict in the addictive relationship will never be resolved. Willpower or discipline might keep you from using your addiction, but you will always have to be on guard, rigid and never let down. Because the emotions have never been resolved, the cravings will continue to emerge.

The Language of Addictions

The Mind Tries to Justify Your Addiction—Mind Games

The Cognitive Brain is very clever and devious. This part of the brain will create elaborate lies to protect you from pain. Your rational brain will do whatever it can to protect you from pain, including causing you to lie to yourself. Your higher brain is responsible for creating and continuing your trance. Coming out of your trance means ending your own self-deception. When beginning the process of returning to nature, it is important to unravel these lies and alibis that you have come to rely on to protect yourself.

The mind has attempted to "justify" your addictions. Subconsciously, you have found an acceptable way to feel good about being addicted. For some addictions, your guilt is what haunts you to keep you in check. For many other addictions, there is no guilt. You have learned how to justify your way of numbing your feelings by referring to them as a passionate part of your life. You have created a storehouse of techniques to justify your addictions in order to cover up their true intent—to mask your feelings. This is your Cognitive Brain at work again.

Some of these techniques are as follows:

1. You lie. "No, I am not a drunk and have not touched alcohol recently." "No, I don't do drugs anymore." "No, I am not dating anybody else at this time."

2. You are in denial. "No, there is not a problem." "No, my father is not really an alcoholic." "It's just a nervous habit." Biting your nails could be a "habit," but biting your nails every time you are feeling fear or anxiety is most likely an addiction.

3. You live in delusion. "It is not that bad and I can stop whenever I want to." "I am not addicted because I only get 'high' on weekends." "I am not addicted because I can control my drinking." "I do not have an addictive personality and I can stop whenever I want to."

4. You joke about it. "Ha, Ha, Ha! I'm a chocoholic!"

5. You have secrets. "It is nobody's business but my own."

6. You rationalize. "A couple of glasses of wine are good for you. It helps your heart and blood pressure. It helps you to relax." "I am not addicted because I only smoke a pipe" (which still contains tobacco). "I am just under a lot of pressure right now and will stop smoking when things calm down."

7. You minimize your addiction. "I am not addicted because I don't inhale." A food addict might minimize her addiction by saying something like, "It wasn't really that much!"

Listen to the stories that you continue to tell yourself. Does alcohol numb you out or do you really enjoy the taste? Many chefs use alcohol to cook with and to season the meal. In this case, the primary purpose of alcohol is to enhance the meal. The chef does not intend to intoxicate his guests. A nice glass of wine might complement a wonderful meal. In this instance, the primary purpose of the wine is not to numb out feelings but to enhance the flavor of the meal.

If, however, the purpose of the wine is to "loosen up" or "relax," this could be a way to numb out feelings. Keep asking yourself, "What is the primary purpose of this person, object, behavior, thought or emotion? Am I being clear about what my actual intentions are or am I really lying to myself?" Discovering your actual intent will help to determine if you are using it addictively.

You might have sneaky ways of justifying your addictions. This is your Cognitive Brain protecting you from any pain. You might not realize what you are doing most of the time. You are just sabotaging yourself. When you feel the need to reward yourself with a sweet for putting in a "hard day" at work, you try to justify this by saying that you are passionate about desserts. You are still acting addictively but are calling it something else. Your mind is very clever and tricky.

When receiving pleasure motivates you, then "passion" often becomes a very worthwhile experience. You become passionate about stamp collecting, painting or reading comic books. Your passion seems to enrich you.

The other side of the coin is this. When you are motivated by your fear of pain rather than your desire for pleasure, your passion just becomes an addictive relationship with something in order to numb yourself out. Many times you have convinced yourself that your passion is a positive and worthwhile element in your life, but in reality it has become just another lie to yourself and just another way to numb out.

Part of the problem is the language that is used to keep you addicted. Addictions are a way to "cope" with the stress of life. "Coping" has become accepted as normal. "Recreation," "experimentation" and "relaxation" are many times just more words to mean addiction. Much of this wayward thinking stems from the language that is used.

For example, many people report that alcohol helps one to "relax" or to "loosen up." On the surface this appears to be a noble and truthful statement, but on closer examination, there is a very different story going on. When I hear someone say that alcohol helps him to "relax" and to "loosen up," what I hear is that alcohol helps someone to "not feel something." It might be that alcohol numbs out the pressures of work or the insecurity of being around people. Alcohol might minimize your inhibitions, making you more social. All of this behavior is really just avoiding pain. You might be numbing out the fear of being judged or the fear of not being liked.

Whatever the case, the vast majority of times when you think you are using something like alcohol in a positive manner "to relax," you might be trying to avoid some kind of pain. Relaxation means to feel safe, not numb. You are really running from your pain rather than seeking pleasure. After all, what do you need to "relax" from? Most of the time you are not relaxing *toward* something, rather you are attempting to relax *away* from something. While often labeled as "relaxation," most people who use this phrase are actually in a trance state with their addiction.

The rational mind has found numerous creative ways to try to justify your addictions. An addicted jogger might say, "Jogging helps me to relax. I can just go into my fantasy world." In this case the word "relax" is used to mean "a place to escape into." This is not really relaxation but a trance state.

What most people think of as "relaxation" is nothing more than attempting to "numb out" with their addiction. They are still in their Fight or Flight Response and still attempting to run from their pain. They use their mind to justify their addiction by saying that it helps them to "relax." A more appropriate phrase would be to say that the addiction helps one to stay numb, not to relax. The body does not lie. The body in most instances is still in a state of Fight or Flight and not relaxation. Only the drug of choice has helped to numb out these feelings.

In Tony's case this is very apparent. Tony works at a desk in an office building. Every 45 minutes or so, he leaves the building for a smoke. He says that taking his five-minute smoking break several times a day helps him to "relax." Tony is almost never relaxed. His body remains in a near constant state of alertness and is experiencing his Fight or Flight Response (Stress Response), not the state of the Parasympathetic Nervous System being activated. He does not enter into the Relaxation Response. He remains hyper-alert. What the smoking does is numb out any feelings and sensations that Tony might be experiencing. He may feel better because he does not feel anything.

Many people remain hooked on drugs (including alcohol) in order to avoid the pain of withdrawal. This could be physical pain like tremors or nausea. They could also be avoiding the emotional pain of withdrawal, like the feelings of emptiness or irritability. The drug user might claim that he enjoys "getting high." He might come off as if he has accepted his drug use as a normal, positive, well thought-out plan like marriage or going to college. To him, "getting high" are the words he uses. He has convinced himself that it is the pleasure that he seeks.

In actuality, what is happening is that he has learned how to avoid something very painful by using drugs to mood-alter. He might continue his drug use because of the fear of withdrawal or the fear of losing his best friend (the drug). He continues his addiction because of this fear of pain and learns to lie to himself by calling his drug use something that he enjoys in his life. This is his elaborate lie that he has convinced himself to believe.

A person who claims to use drugs for "recreational" purposes is most likely just lying to himself. The word "recreation" is most often meant as the avoidance of pain rather than the search for pleasure. She needs to get "high" because of something that is uncomfortable to feel. Most often this is not because of the absolute pleasure that this behavior elicits. Altering your state of consciousness into a trance is often just another excuse to run from your pain.

Many people use the term "abuse" to defend their addiction. Many people claim that they are not addicted to drugs (including alcohol) because they do not "abuse" these drugs. Their term for "not abusing" has come to mean the following:

1. Not overdoing it
2. Not causing physical damage
3. Still being able to function in society
4. Not causing pain to others

This is just another elaborate lie to justify addictions. By participating in any addiction, you are not learning how to fully function in society. You are keeping yourself medicated all the time to avoid feeling. You are learning how to "cope" in society. When you cannot express your authentic feelings to others, you are causing pain to yourself.

Two Case Histories

The following are case stories of people who have created an elaborate lie with their addiction. They have convinced everyone, including themselves, that they are not addicted.

Case # 1

Let's look at the case of Ted. Ted is a well-respected businessman, wonderful father and dedicated husband. Ted will smoke marijuana, but only on weekends. Ted claims to not be addicted to marijuana. Rather, Ted says he only uses marijuana as a "recreational" drug and only on weekends. Ted has convinced himself that his marijuana use is a positive element in his life. He claims that he enjoys the feeling that marijuana produces. Ted actually believes he is seeking out pleasure when he claims to be enjoying marijuana as a "recreation."

Marijuana is a Central Nervous System depressant. Marijuana tends to "mellow" one out and slow one's world down. What Ted does not realize is the reason why he needs to use marijuana. He claims to have a choice in whether he uses marijuana or not. Ted is really just running from all of his feelings—the stress at work, pressures of raising a family and fears of intimacy with his wife. Ted is really not seeking pleasure but is running as fast as he can from his pain. The only problem is that Ted has concocted this elaborate lie in his own head to justify his addiction. Ted does not want to know that he has a problem.

It's not about what kind of drug you use or how much of it that makes you addicted. What creates an addiction is about *why* you need to alter your consciousness by using drugs and other things. Ted has chosen to believe his own lies for some time now and accepts them as his truth.

Case # 2

Tony has a problem with sexual addiction. Tony comes home from his stressful day at work as a computer programmer. He is irritable because of his stress. When at home, Tony wants to be sexual with his wife. He has a reputation for being a romantic. This is wonderful if this is really what was going on. It is not. Tony and his wife Margo never really resolve any of the big issues. Tony avoids real intimacy with his wife by pursuing his sexuality. Tony never resolves his irritability from his stress at work. Tony just puts his pain behind his sexuality and uses the "high" of orgasm to numb out his pain. On the outside, it looks as if Tony has a wonderfully balanced sexuality. Deep down inside, however, Tony is just using his sexuality to avoid his pain.

Alexander Lowen, M.D., writes in *Pleasure:*

"The search for fun stems from a need to escape from problems, conflicts, and feelings that seem intolerable and overwhelming. That is why fun for adults is associated so strongly with alcohol. For many people the idea of fun is to get high or drink or escape their oppressive sense of emptiness and boredom through drugs. The use of LSD is called 'taking a trip,' which reveals its close connection with the idea of getting away. The drug user changes his inner reality, while the external situation remains the same."

Debra Waterhouse, in *Why Women Need Chocolate*, attempts to justify her own chocolate addiction by saying, "Food cravings are a natural part of being a woman." She claims that women need chocolate for biological reasons. Does that mean that women all over the world who have never even tasted chocolate will not survive without it? She goes on to say, "The forces that dictate our female food needs are biologically engrained. That's why cravings cannot be controlled or fought with willpower—but they can be managed and experienced with the 'will' to 'power' our bodies and minds with foods we were designed to eat." Her claim to eat whenever a craving arises is like a smoker who keeps himself loaded up by smoking a cigarette every thirty minutes. She is just trying to justify her addiction to chocolate by claiming that her body requires it. This is an example of how we lie to ourselves.

Is it possible to go through life and live without that which you are the most passionate about? If the answer is "No," then perhaps your passion is really a primary addiction. If you are passionate about music, can you allow yourself to drive alone in a car without music for long distances without suffering some form of distress? If you are passionate about reading the sports page every morning, can you not read it without suffering? If you are passionate about your pets, do you experience uncomfortable feelings when you are not around your pets? Many times your passions are really your addictions; you are trying to hide from your pain much of the time.

When people most think of the word "passion," they immediately have thoughts of excitement or exuberance. They use the term "passion" as a positive expression to indicate their complete focus and utter joy in directing their entire energy toward a single goal. However, passion can often be another well disguised name for addiction.

We Are All Addicts

Human beings have learned how to numb out sensations and feelings because of the evolution of the Cognitive Brain and because they live in cultures that honor intellect while disapproving of emotion and sensation. When you do not know how to have a relationship with your feelings, it is common to form a relationship with your addictions. It is your relationship with your addictions that keeps the feelings and sensations from being experienced and released. Because you cannot feel fully, you often learn to channel your repressed feelings into other pursuits. It is this channeling of feelings that keeps you repressed and addicted.

Many times, when you channel your pain rather than experience it and release it, you end up with some rather heroic outcomes. Unfortunately, you only look at the outcome and not the means by which you reached your goal. You see the results but miss the repression of feelings that led you along your path.

It is important to keep asking yourself about what motivates you. Do you seek pleasure in your super-achieving or are you running from pain? I recently heard an interview from a world champion figure skater. This particular skater had experienced a very traumatic childhood. His father's and brother's death, living in poverty, and fighting the daily battle of being openly gay in a sexually homophobic society were just a few of his wounds. He said that his sport was the secret place he could go to in order to forget about all of the pain. He became very good at figure skating because he had a lot of pain from which to escape.

This is what most of us do. We become good at focusing our pain into our achievements. People only tend to see the achievements but overlook the pain. Any great basketball player who came out of a ghetto life could tell you that the fear of having to live his life holed up in that ghetto is enough pain to motivate someone to seek super-achievement in his sport.

In order to understand how seemingly positive behavior can be an addiction, it is important to understand how and why you "channel feelings." When you have feelings that you cannot feel, you might choose behavior that will numb these feelings out—either positive or negative behavior.

A powerful leader might have channeled his childhood anger into a quest for power. Adolf Hitler comes to mind when I think of this example. Hitler's father reportedly beat him every day. A famous actress might channel her disappointment at not being noticed as a child by her parents into a thriving on-stage career where thousands of people see her. A New Age guru who teaches workshops might need the applause of the audience to fill him up because he has channeled all of his childhood shame into his image. All of these people are most likely just running from their feelings. "Channeling feelings" is just a polite way to say "addiction."

"How can this be?" you might ask yourself. It seems that you are being encouraged to channel your feelings into other pursuits. I have heard many people comment on how horrible their childhoods were and how they've overcome their setbacks by channeling all of their hurts into their work, religion or family. When this happens, though, not much has changed. All of the hurtful, repressed childhood feelings are still alive and running your life. You have learned how to survive by repressing your painful feelings and channeling that energy into something else in order to distract you.

Socially Unacceptable Behavior

Sometimes you channel your feelings into behavior that society has recognized as unacceptable. Smoking cigarettes, taking street drugs or engaging in gang activity might be socially unacceptable behavior into which you have learned to channel your feelings.

For example, if you are angry with your parents and you cannot feel and express that anger, perhaps that anger might become channeled into antisocial behavior. Your anger might be channeled into stealing cars or selling drugs. Many times you choose socially unacceptable outlets for your feelings like using cocaine or compulsive sex. You then become addicted because you cannot feel your pain and disappointment. If you could only teach your children to feel and to express their feelings, then there would be far fewer teenagers channeling their feelings into street drugs or cigarettes in order to numb themselves out.

Any behavior that rewards one to take away pain can be addictive, whether it is violent or mischievous behavior. Many times your socially unacceptable behavior is just another way that you have learned how to channel the feelings that you cannot express. This behavior then makes the pain go away.

Socially Rewarding Behavior

The other extreme is to channel your feelings into socially or culturally rewarding behavior. You might channel your heartache from an abusive marriage into a passion for social work. This is how heroes and martyrs are born. You might channel your loneliness into your pets. Your dog then becomes the purpose of your life because you cannot feel your feelings. On the outside you might be a loving, giving person, but you may be channeling your pain into saving others. Because you cannot feel and release your hurtful feelings, you then become addicted to helping others.

Your feelings of despair might be channeled into your religious fanaticism. You might channel your loneliness into a passion for gardening. Whatever the case, if you cannot feel and release your feelings, there is a good chance you will channel that energy into something else. You might reach great heights in your endeavors, but if you are motivated by your fear of experiencing pain, you are just expressing your addiction.

Bryan Robinson writes in his book *Overdoing It* that Gloria Steinem realized years later that much of her passion for feminist issues was used "as an anesthetic to buried childhood emotions."

"Don't feel" is the message that you are given by society and religion. After all, the Catholic Church preaches that anger is one of the "Seven Deadly Sins." To feel anger (according to Catholic tradition) is to be headed straight for "Hell." When you cannot feel you are directed toward places to channel your feelings. Society hopes that you choose socially acceptable outlets to channel the feelings that you were taught to "not feel." Work, school, sports, art, music and religion are some of these socially acceptable channels.

Religion and care taking are two of the most prominent ways that many channel their feelings into addictive behavior. Bryan Robinson writes, "Careaholics are often happy only when they're helping others. This keeps the focus off of themselves and gives them a type of high." People like Mother Teresa fit into this category. They keep themselves so busy focused on the problems of others that they can avoid their own pain. We seem to raise to sainthood those who have lost their natural self but spend their lives addicted to care taking of others. This is what society encourages you to do.

Bryan Robinson concludes with, "A nun said, 'I believe that some religious persons often seek salvation through the number of souls they save and sick they attend to: thus the more they do, the better human beings they are.'" Where do you think your busyness and caretaking addictions come from? It is these flawed messages that you might have received from religions and your culture that teach you to channel your repressed feelings into socially acceptable behavior.

People in the care-taking professions are not there by accident. Most of them get pleasure by taking care of others' needs. Most often this is in spite of their own needs not being met. Bryan Robinson writes, "A higher concentration of adult children of dysfunctional families is found in the helping fields than in other occupations: nursing, counseling, teaching, social work, psychology, psychiatry, the clergy, and substance-abuse field." They learn early on to channel their feelings into what looks like a good thing. That way they get extra "points" from a culture that dishonors the natural self and encourages care-taking addictions.

Often the message is confusing. For example, many are taught that drinking alcohol is a socially acceptable way to channel your stressful feelings into. Society also encourages violence. Movies, television and numerous contact sports are such reminders. When you channel your feelings into violence that harms another person, you have crossed over the line. Many times you do not know where the line is anymore. Whatever the case, if you cannot feel your feelings, your behavior will be the result of your channeled feelings. Sometimes it might be socially acceptable behavior and other times it will be socially unacceptable behavior.

CASE SCENARIOS

Case #1 Thomas

Thomas grew up in a world where he was taught to sit up straight, not talk back and only say pleasant things. He was never allowed to be angry. He was a good boy for all practical purposes. To the outside world, Thomas was the perfect son.

Thomas was a very repressed individual. He held a lot inside. Thomas learned to channel his pain that he could not feel into his education and his intellectual achievements. He achieved greatness in school and went on to a high paying job. According to cultural standards, Thomas was the model of achievement. Deep down inside though, he was holding on to all of the pain that he could not allow himself to express. He suffered from headaches, weight gain and insomnia because he was so bottled up inside.

Case #2 Monica

Monica grew up in a family where the boundaries were seriously eroded. There was no separation between herself and her parents and siblings. There never was any privacy. Monica ended up taking care of her seductive father and all of his needs.

Monica learned not to feel too much joy or emotion in her life. She did not want to feel guilt for having joy while others were suffering around her. She felt as if her power was ripped away from her as a young girl. Monica learned how to channel her repressed pain into seduction and flirtation as a way to avoid her pain. Everyone wanted to be around her. Monica used her seductiveness as a means of changing her mood. She was addicted to seduction as a way not to feel her repressed powerlessness. Monica learned to channel her pain into flirtation and seduction. This won her many friends and beauty pageants, but she was just practicing her addiction.

Case #3 Billy

Most people have heard the story of the skinny kid who had sand kicked in his face by the town bully only to grow up to be big and strong through committed weight-lifting routines. That is what Billy did. He developed late in his teens and always felt picked on as a child. Billy soon channeled all of his hurt into his weight-lifting routine and became very popular. He never learned how to release his stored up emotions but became a big success with his overinflated body. Billy's bodybuilding became his addiction to keep him numb.

We Are Taught to Channel Our Feelings

The more feelings you have repressed, the larger your accomplishments might appear. Most often, if you are a hero in any field, unless you have done a whole lot of "inner" work about understanding and feeling your feelings, you might be channeling your repressed feelings into something else. What is wrong with channeling your feelings? We all do it, right?

There is nothing wrong with accomplishing great things in the fields of science, business, medicine, religion, politics or even motherhood. It is the feelings that you cannot feel that will cause you to be addicted and lead to problems in your life. Unfortunately, there is little difference between a street junkie and an achievement addict. Only the method for expressing the addiction is different.

When you channel the energy of any feeling that you do not want to feel, you are addicted. Some of the nicest people in the world are the ones who are carrying around the most pain. The perfect mother might look like she has everything under control, but most likely she has channeled her repressed feelings into her role of motherhood. She might be dying of stress-related causes because she might have channeled all of her repressed feelings into socially acceptable behavior—in this case, raising her family.

On the outside, she might appear to be the greatest mother in the world, but on the inside her anger could be eating her up. She might need to stay busy with her family in order to avoid her feelings that seem so overwhelming at times. Not just mothers, but even people like artists and musicians frequently channel their repressed feelings into their work. Their accomplishment might be grand, but they are unaware of what is motivating them. Often, the act of running from their feelings is what is producing great works.

We are all addicts and because of the cultures that we live in, we have learned how to channel the feelings that we cannot express into something else. This does not mean that this is a healthy behavior—but it seems to be normal. We all channel our feelings because we are all addicted.

Whether it is in art, medicine, literature, business, spirituality, sports or raising a family, most often when you are a super achiever, you are an addict. This translates into having a significant relationship with a thought or behavior in order to escape from your feelings. According to this definition, many Nobel Prize winning scientists, "enlightened" spiritual masters and multi-millionaires are addicts. Championship national spelling bee contestants may be using their dictionary study in order not to feel something. Your achievements can be your addictions. When your achievements become the main purpose in your life, they become your primary addictions.

Over-achievement addictions usually begin in the home. A family that encourages high achievement while discouraging the free expression of emotions sets one up for the potential to use achievement as a means to numb out painful feelings. This is no different than a family that encourages the use of alcohol to numb out; only your achievement addictions are more socially acceptable.

When you are a super-achiever you have a single-minded goal. You forget about your needs. When you do not know what you are feeling, you will not know what you need. Your needs become pushed aside by your achievement. Whether you are a millionaire, scientist, housewife, saint, guru or explorer, most of the time when you are passionate about something you are addicted. When you are addicted you have shut off your feelings. You hide behind your disease of addiction, especially if it is enshrouded in a cloud of socially acceptable behavior. You have learned how to channel your pain into your achievements rather than to feel it and release it.

Heroes Falling Off Pedestals

Take a closer look at your heroes. The most highly respected heroes in the world are usually the most wounded. They have the most motivation to run from their pain in order to achieve success. An expert molecular engineer might have placed his whole life into his scientific thoughts and behavior. In order for him to rise to the top of his field, he most likely has had to be very focused on his work. A brilliant scientist might think many stimulating thoughts but might not have any training in how to feel. His feelings might get buried by his work. When this happens, he uses his work addictively in order to not feel. The more pain that he has buried inside, the more he works on his achievement. Unfortunately, society only focuses on the achievement and not the pain beneath the achievement. He keeps being encouraged to rise to the top of his field because of society's need to keep him productive. Society is not necessarily interested in the person, only the results of his work.

Our heroes are no different than you and I. They have only found a different way to hide from their feelings. Our heroes might be addicted to such socially acceptable things as sports, religion, poetry or music. It's their secrets that they are hiding that are not so socially acceptable.

I can remember learning that the great baseball legend, Mickey Mantle, was an alcoholic and was dying from liver failure. The whole country was in shock. How could our hero be just like us? We are led to believe that our heroes are beyond our pain. Most often our heroes have put so much energy and passion into running from their pain that all we can see is the shiny facade. How could someone who hits 60 home runs a season be an addict like you and I? This is the lie that we want to believe. Mickey Mantle did not die from complications of alcohol abuse. He died from his inability to feel his feelings which caused him to choose alcohol as a way to numb out his pain.

Our heroes are just like you and I. They were born into a human race that teaches them how to repress their feelings. The only difference is that our heroes have gotten much better at hiding from their feelings because they have wanted us to notice their outer achievements and not the pain they are hiding.

Whether it is in sports, politics, religion or business, our heroes have just as many addictions as the rest of us. Witch doctors, shamans, yogis, priests, presidents, movie stars and military heroes most likely are just running from their feelings if they never learned how to feel. Their "specialty" is really their addiction that keeps them from knowing themselves.

Our heroes come from the same family systems as you and I. They are not immune to childhood pain and repression of sensory and emotional experiences. Because of magical thinking, loss of the natural self and hero worship, we clamor toward those who appear to have risen above. The reality is much simpler. Our heroes have learned to channel their repressed feelings into positive, culturally acceptable pursuits like politics, acting, religion and sports. We see the glory but refuse to notice the wounds. Even the holiest of holy are addicted people. Pope John Paul II, Gandhi, Mother Teresa and the Dalai Lama of Tibet are among such ranks. Even Buddha was an addict. It is our magical thinking that keeps us from believing that a country as great as The United States of America would ever elect a president who was an addict.

The human body will tell you the energetic state of a person. If a person is free to express and release his feelings, he will have freedom of movement, good skin color and an ease about him. His muscles will be supple and his connective tissue open.

A body that is committed to repression and stuck in an addictive state of consciousness will tell you something very different, *no matter what the words are saying*. Let's take the example of Mother Theresa of Calcutta. This was a woman who was revered the world over for her charity work. Working with the poor, saving the sick, taking in homeless people all seem like honorable endeavors. This even won her the Nobel Peace Prize. However, Mother Theresa was a poster child for repression and was addicted to states of consciousness. She was a die-hard codependent, committed to others' needs rather than having to face her own pain. She was addicted to her rescuing state of consciousness. She was withered and shrunken, living in a body full of repression and angst. Her connective tissue had degenerated to a hapless state. She controlled her emotions and stored everything in her body. She had a complete loss of self.

In fact, Mother Theresa suffered a long bout of heart troubles, eventually dying due to complications of heart failure. *It would seem that Mother Theresa could not love herself.* Yet, she is one of the people who many have chosen to be their role model and crown her with the Nobel Peace Prize.

It is these addictive altered states of consciousness that can be so tricky. They are just as addictive as any street drug is. The authors of *The Primal Wound* state,

"So, having had a profound experience in which I saw through the illusion of my separate self and realized my union with Ultimate Reality, I may become addicted/attached to this particular state of consciousness. I may seek this state just as fervently as the addict seeks the needle or the alcoholic seeks the bottle. All addictions are similar at their core. The skid

row alcoholic and the obsessed spiritual athlete may be much closer than they appear, brothers or sisters in the grips of the being-nonbeing dynamic. The primal wound clearly has a quality of transcendence-immanence. It can be found in any and all states of consciousness, types of personality, and stages of development."

It is your early wounding that causes you to exist out of your survival personality. This personality will use whatever types of addictions it can to resist change and to keep pain away. The authors of *The Primal Wound* write,

"Once survival personality is revealed we can begin to be aware of how this orientation pervades our daily living, from disguised relationship and sexual addiction to habitual alcohol and drug use, from hidden spiritual pride to subtle revenge motives, from spiritual materialism (Trungpa) to compulsive service to others. As we address these tendrils of survival, we can uncover the primal wounding at their core and gradually begin to move towards authenticity."

The same authors add,
"This same type of compulsion can be seen in the person seeking an 'enlightenment' that is understood as a unitive state untouched by fragmentation and suffering in the world and, as we shall see later, it is a drive that underpins the addictive process as a whole."

Even the mythological state of consciousness called "enlightenment" can become another addictive state of consciousness used as a drug to avoid your natural self. It is about using the Cognitive Brain to repress the lower brain. So-called "higher states of consciousness" are often just "altered states of consciousness." Many times, these altered states of consciousness masquerading as higher states of consciousness are really lower states of consciousness because there is very little feeling and experiencing involved.

Whether it is a drug or a state of consciousness, repression of feelings leads to channeling those feelings into something else. Many times the ways of channeling feelings are scorned by society while at other times one is rewarded for the way that he channels his repressed feelings.

Thus the loss of your natural self during your early childhood years is the basis of the addictive process. No matter what you might do in your adulthood, unless you return to recover your relationship with nature, you will have a difficult time recovering from your addictions. The authors of *The Primal Wound* state,

>"The most powerful experiences may never ultimately touch the place from which we are operating, our survival ground of being. This is why, as Winnicott and others have seen, therapy can go on forever never reaching the core personhood. This also is why, as spiritual communities have seen, truly advanced spiritual leaders may yet be controlled by their psychological wounding."

All of us have come from a wounded family system. These wounds and the pain created ways to look for opportunities to numb out that pain. By numbing your pain, you have created many addictions. Just because many people, including your heroes, have chosen to numb their pain out with what appears to be positive, socially acceptable behavior, does not mean that they are not addicted. It means, perhaps, that they have chosen to do less harm than if they were to engage in socially unacceptable behavior. Nevertheless, they are still running from their pain and still are slaves to their past as long as they continue to choose not to feel. Only by choosing to feel and release your pain will you recover your natural self.

The Addict is "Us," Not "Them"

Many have been taught to believe in addictions as a black and white matter. You have an "either/or" mentality that tends to want to label someone as either an "addict" (a person who is out of control) or a "non-addict" (someone who is able to control his life). It appears that the definition of addiction has come to be whether or not you can stay in control. If you cannot stay in control, society chooses to label you as an "addict." This seems to be the root of the problem. Most people have a very naive definition of what addiction actually is.

Herbert Fingarette writes in *Heavy Drinking* " . . . the heart of the classic disease concept, loss of control, is a confused notion that is contradicted by a bookshelf of experimental evidence." He is referring to addiction to alcohol specifically, but this same idea can be applied across the board to describe all addictions.

Many prescribe to this black and white thinking. You have convinced yourself that it is *them*, those other people, who are addicts and not *you*. You cannot see your own problems but are quick to point out someone else who loses control. You have a distorted perception. It is as if most of you are far-sighted in your vision. You can see really well at a distance but have much more difficulty looking at what is right beneath your very own noses. The scale that you have been using to measure addictions is "control" versus "loss of control."

In fact, many people believe that addiction is about a down and out group of people living in the inner cities. An example of this type of black and white thinking is seen in *The Truth About Addiction and Recovery* where Stanton Peele, Ph.D., and Archie Brodsky believe that middle class America is not as addicted because they can control their drug use. When you look at addiction as only about illegal drug use, this might be easy to say.

The authors say, referring to worsening statistics about cocaine use in the inner cities, "These issues were sharpened in the United States in the late 1980s as more and more Americans turned away from drugs, yet addiction among inner-city Americans worsened, along with drug-related violence." Also, referring to a 1990 NIDA (National Institute on Drug Abuse) national drug survey, the authors say, "They also document our society's worsening division into two cultures—a mainstream capable of controlling its drug use and an intractable core that does not find sufficient reasons to give up its addictions."

There has been an ambitious campaign in the last couple of decades or so to help educate children about drug use. This effort is formally called the "Just Say No!" campaign. Teaching children to stay away from drugs is a noble cause, but it is not the drugs that are to blame as to why you become addicted in the first place. Addiction is just the end product of a series of steps that began with repression of what is natural. Addictions come in many shapes and sizes. Eliminating drugs will not eliminate addictiveness.

The Inner Conflict

Addiction is not an external event—it is an internal relationship. John Bradshaw refers to addictions as the "War Within." I would refer to them as the cancer of our soul. Addictions are eating us alive as if they were a fast spreading cancer.

Addiction is all about the disease within yourself and has very little to do with gambling, shopping, sex, etc. Many people tend to blame the external means that they create for themselves to express their addictions. That has very little to do with why they are addicted. It is very easy to place blame on something else.

For instance, you might like to place the blame on the tobacco companies because you have been smoking cigarettes for forty years and now have lung cancer. Perhaps you try to sue the tobacco companies because you want them to be responsible for the choices that you have made. You might believe that it is the pharmaceutical companies' fault that you have become addicted to prescription pills to mood-alter. No, it is not these or any other company's fault that you are addicted. These companies are just making a product available in a culture that promotes the use of pills and substances to mood-alter. They are not forcing their product on you. It is not the alcohol brewing company's fault that a drunk driver ran his car into your car.

Once again, this type of thinking is all about trying to blame someone else for your own individual suffering because you are unwilling to take the personal responsibility for yourself.

It seems that we live in a culture that teaches us not to take responsibility for ourselves. We have a legal system that is based on trying to hold others responsible for our own accidents, choices and misfortunes. After all, if you slip on a banana peel on someone else's property, you can sue them for monetary damages because you were not careful as to where you were walking. With this type of thinking ingrained in our culture, it is easy to see how you might not want to be responsible for the choices that you have made about your addictions.

Another example of this blame game is seen in the widely publicized "War on Drugs." This is another key example of the need to place blame outside of ourselves. We are led to believe that it is the Columbian drug czars' or the Mexican drug smugglers' fault that we have addicts in this country. Many want to blame *them* for our suffering. If we can send military troops to Columbia to eradicate the coca leaves or increase the security at our borders, then our addictions will be solved. Unfortunately, this is how we think.

The "War on Drugs" is nothing more than a "War on Ourselves." It seems that we need to have an enemy outside of ourselves to feel right in the world. This is another example of black and white thinking. If we were to look closely at ourselves, we might have less of a need for an enemy. For now at least, we have made the drug dealer the enemy. The drunk driver and the foreign drug lord are the ones whom we resent. This is where we have placed our blame because we refuse to look at ourselves.

The problem is *us*, not *them*. We demand drugs to keep us numb. It is back to the notion of supply and demand. If we did not choose heroin, cocaine and marijuana, there would be no demand for these drugs. We have chosen these as well as other mood-altering drugs and behaviors. If these drugs did not exist, we would find others. We keep searching to find other sources for our "highs." New designer drugs come on to the scene all the time (like crack cocaine and XTC).

We accept and allow such drugs as alcohol, nicotine and prescription pills into our culture. It is the "American way." It is part of big business and consumerism. Big business is not responsible for why you choose to become addicted to these products. Sure, their deceptive advertising helps to encourage you to use their products. However, they do not force you to do so. Big business is just capitalizing on your need to mask your pain. They know that you are looking for "highs." They pay handsome salaries to teams of psychologists who know just how to get you hooked on their products. They are only encouraging you to use what you have already asked for. If it weren't tobacco, pills or alcohol that you use to numb out, it would be something else. Perhaps work, relationships, entertainment or food would be your addictions of choice.

Why do you imagine that the prison population has escalated so dramatically in the past few decades? This is because of the self-proclaimed "War on Drugs." We have made it illegal to sell, manufacture or ingest a specific group of drugs (street drugs) while promoting, encouraging and tolerating other groups of drugs (alcohol, prescription pills, nicotine). Why is it illegal to use street drugs and end up in prison if caught but not illegal to use Valium or alcohol? I do not prescribe to the belief that the government is trying to protect us from any imminent harm that street drugs might cause.

Unfortunately, the prisons are filled with people who have formed a relationship with the types of drugs that our culture does not see fitting into its cultural image. These people are punished for choosing the wrong kind of mood-altering drug. If they had chosen alcohol, tobacco or prescription pills, it would have been different. They would be considered model citizens for going along with the program and supporting the economy. Then we would have to find an enemy someplace else. For now, we feel safe by locking up the "enemy" in prison. That way we do not have to look at ourselves.

Ask anyone who has lost a relative to cirrhosis of the liver caused by alcohol or lung cancer caused by cigarette smoking how the government has protected them. It seems that each culture chooses which mood-altering techniques fit best within the culture. The values of each culture are reflected in the addictions that are allowed and accepted. Alcohol and pills work well in a Christian-based, workaholic culture. Their sale and distribution can be controlled and taxed. In fact, most Christian rituals use wine and there are numerous writings in Christian texts referring to wine as being a normal way of life. A behavior like being addicted to MTV (Music Television) would not happen in a strict Muslim country. The culture would not allow it. It would be considered pornographic.

But a strict Muslim country would have its own addictive patterns. For instance, in these countries the average citizen is called to prayer five times per day. It would be very easy to become addicted to prayer in instances like this.

Alcohol and prescription pills come from large corporations. That is the heart of America. Street drugs often come from the darker side of life—back alleys and dark garages. Marijuana can easily be grown in homes, hillsides or back yards. It would be very easy not to pay taxes on something that you could grow and sell from your own home. We live in a culture that has chosen which type of drugs we consider to be acceptable. Our government and public policy have much to do with our choice of drugs.

Addiction is not about what you choose to mood-alter with, but more importantly, why you choose to mood-alter in the first place. Addiction has very little to do with which types of chemicals you might ingest in your bodies, nor the amount, nor the degree of control that you may or may not have.

Many people are stuck trying to point their fingers at specific foods, behaviors or chemicals as to why they are addicted. They are looking at the external. You will only heal when you begin to see the internal process.

We have been blaming "trigger" foods like chocolate or white bread for why we go on eating binges. We blame nicotine's mythological "addictive quality" that is supposed to lure us into becoming lifelong smokers. It is not the substances that are causing the problem. Your inability to express your feelings is the problem. We have been stuck trying to blame alcohol, tobacco, cocaine, schools or genetics for addictions. The real reason that we are addicted is because we have learned that it is just too painful to feel and we have developed relationships with substances, people, behaviors, thoughts and emotions as a way to avoid ourselves.

A common belief is that the ability to *control* your habit is what determines if you are addicted or not. No, it's about *why* we choose to numb out in the first place. It's not about ingesting a little, a moderate amount or a whole bunch of any mood-altering substance. It has nothing to do with the amount. It's about *why* you need to mood-alter.

We need to begin to change the paradigm. It does not matter whether a person drinks one glass of wine or a whole bottle of scotch at a time. The amount is not important. What determines addiction is *why* one needs to mood-alter in the first place.

The old paradigm is to judge an addict by how much he drinks or how often he takes drugs. The new paradigm is to recognize not the amount consumed but why it is used. When you stop trying to blame someone for your addiction and stop thinking in black and white terms, you will come to heal your addictions. When you stop blaming others, you are on the road to recovery. It is not about *them*; it is about *us*.

Addictions As Fads: Cultures Decide

Addictions are beliefs, objects, behaviors, emotions or thoughts that are acceptable and encouraged in each culture. Addictions are only a reflection of what each culture establishes as an available means to numb out feelings. Each culture might have a different range of addictions that are available. Each culture not only accepts addictions but attempts to direct its people to the type of addictions that are possible.

In strict Islamic cultures, for instance, alcohol is a taboo. It is frowned upon and considered evil. It would be very difficult to become addicted to alcohol in this culture because alcohol is not as available and its use is discouraged. In the United States, where there is a liquor store on many corners and beer commercials frequently run on television, it would be much easier to become addicted to alcohol because 1) it is readily available and 2) its consumption is highly encouraged at this time. If you lived in the age of Prohibition (1920-1933), it would have been much more difficult to be addicted to alcohol because alcohol was banned from public sale during this time.

A culture that does not have a heavily developed pharmaceutical industry would be less encouraging of its citizens to take pills of any sorts to alter their moods. In this case, pills would not be so readily available and the concept of pill taking to mood-alter would not exist as prevalently. Perhaps in a culture like this, addictions to herbal plants or to home remedies might be more the norm.

In a culture like America, because of advertising, a multi-billion dollar a year pharmaceutical industry and encouragement from everyone from doctors to government officials, most people not only accept the culture as a pill-popping culture but are encouraged to do so. It becomes a fad to do what your culture is encouraging you to do at the moment. Each fad helps direct you to the types of addictions that might be available and preferred.

As cultures change, so do their addictions. A culture that hasn't changed much in hundreds or even thousands of years would probably encourage the same type of addictions to alter feelings that have been occurring for generations. In such cases, religion, sex or alcohol are age-old addictions that have persisted for generations.

In a culture that is changing as rapidly as many modern cultures are today, the addictions that are specific for that culture are also changing very rapidly. This is why addictions are just fads that reflect each culture's values and availability at the moment. Addictions just reflect what is "trendy" at the moment. If it is "trendy" in a culture to pop pills regularly, then this is the type of addiction that will take hold.

For instance, in the United States during the 1960s and 1970s, there was a whole generation exposed to a new lifestyle. This was the "hippie" movement. A new, sometimes unbridled freedom, was emerging. There was a movement dedicated to exploring the deeper reaches of the mind and human sexuality. Marijuana was a popular drug at the time because it made one feel "mellow." The whole world of a marijuana user became a peaceful field of daisies. Being "mellow" was an acceptable state and a bit of a fad.

Others experimented with hallucinogens as a way to explore the mind. Taking a "trip" with LSD was a fad that was "trendy" at the time. Young people were especially encouraged to experiment with these drugs by others who were already doing so. Both marijuana and LSD were available and encouraged during this period of time. They were both very faddish. Both of these drugs are still around but their "faddishness" has continued to change.

In today's times, drugs that stimulate are more the fad. These drugs include things like cocaine, crack cocaine, Ecstasy and caffeine. The hippies of the 1960s have become the Yuppies (young urban professionals) of today. Cocaine and other stimulants provide an ecstatic "high" that is more conducive to the faster pace at which this society is traveling now. Cocaine is a CNS (central nervous system) stimulant creating unbelievable exhilaration when taken. It is a very social drug, often shared at parties. It is "fashionable," "trendy" and "faddish" to be out in public and "high on coke." It is very much a celebrity drug of choice. Dropping by your neighborhood designer coffee house for your hit of daily caffeine on the way to work is also very trendy. Being addicted to high-tech endeavors like "email" or "text messaging" are very much in style right now. As societies change, so do the addictions within them. The faster each society changes, the more the choices for addictions are available.

Each drug has particular qualities that the addict hopes to use to alter her mood. While cocaine provides an exhilarating "high" that helps people fit into a faster paced life, the effect of marijuana is to slow people down. Nicotine, for instance, has many properties. If you are feeling low, it brings you up. If you are feeling over-stimulated, it calms you down. Nicotine's effects, in essence, are to even you out. What better drug in a culture that encourages productivity? If you can keep on an even keel, you can still function at work.

In a society that hasn't changed in thousands of years, a long day of hunting might end with a quiet evening of sitting around the campfire. Smoking tobacco might become the mood-altering choice, which many indigenous populations use. As innocuous as it might seem, just staring at a campfire is enough to numb one out from one's feelings at times. The campfire might have been one of the earliest addictions. As Jon Kabat-Zinn has mentioned, perhaps the modern day trance of the campfire is now our addiction to television. Karl Marx has said that religion was the opiate of the masses. When he said this during the early part of the 20th Century, this was very truthful. Since the 1950s, when television became popular and available, we now have a new opiate to numb us out. Television keeps you numb just like a campfire and religion have for millions of years. In a society that is changing extremely rapidly, perhaps the computer and technological devices like cell phones are replacing the television as the modern-day opiate of choice.

As each society changes, so do the addictions that go along with it. The faster the changes in society, the faster new addictions are created. For instance, in many cultures that are now emerging beyond just industrialization, information orientation is the newest fad. More jobs are being created in information-related jobs than in production jobs. These new cultures where information has become the fad are creating a host of information-related addictions. The combination of the acceleration of information and technology together are creating an environment that is ripe for many people to become addicted to urgency. Faster cars, super highways, cellular phones, fax machines, pagers, televisions, computers, the "Internet," fast food and air planes all have helped contribute to and encourage many people to acquire urgency addictions. It is now a fad to do more in a shorter period of time. You can now conduct business in the car as you are driving down the highway.

Society has approved of work and busyness as acceptable drugs of choice. Many people are teaching their children to be busy addicts. It is stylish in our culture to overdo it. Fifty years ago, this would not have been so easy. Bryan Robinson, author of *Overdoing It*, writes,

"It is known by many names: overdoing it, careaholics, work addiction, fast-track living, busyholism, superwoman or superman syndrome. Whatever we choose to call it, we have become a nation that is unbalanced and out of control."

Our overdoing it creates consequences for the body. You might develop into a "type A" personality. Bryan Robinson adds,

"Type 'A' children, through their overdoing it, often become compulsive overachievers. They attempt to control others and suppress fatigue; are impatient, competitive, and achievement oriented, and have a sense of urgency and perfectionism. Health wise, this compulsive need to achieve in children is linked to such cardiovascular risk factors as fluctuations in blood pressure and heart rate."

Our addiction to work and busyness takes its toll on our bodies. What seems like healthy behavior many times is just a way to keep busy in order not to feel. Shopping malls, specialty stores and "junk mail" have all helped to encourage a growing trend toward shopping addictions. With plastic credit cards and shopping at home with catalogs and the internet, it is very easy to get addicted to shopping. Our culture is now encouraging these types of trends. Thirty years ago, these types of addictions would not be possible because they were not as available and were not very "trendy."

It seems that a whole industry has been created for "adrenaline junkies," or those addicted to adrenaline and high-risk behavior. These fads of extreme sports keep evolving faster than one can blink an eye. From parachuting, kayaking, rock climbing, wind surfing, bungee jumping, roller blading, etc., more and more ways to get "high" off adrenaline are being created. I saw a print advertisement for a Jeep Wrangler. Underneath the photograph of the car was the printed caption, "Who needs caffeine?" What this ad was implying was that this car will keep you stimulated if you were to buy it. Try it instead of your morning cup of coffee.

Just as seasoned bingo players become addicted to playing bingo, so do people become addicted to other fads that come along. In the 1980s there emerged a whole new philosophy and music called "New Age." This developed into a new fad that created many new addictions. People now became addicted to self-help books, crystals, psychic readings and tarot cards. Being addicted to psychic readings has become very popular. Many pay toll numbers have been set up by ambitious entrepreneurs to benefit from those addicted to psychic hot lines.

Designer coffee houses are as popular today as the frozen yogurt shop was in the 1980s. People stand in long lines to get their gourmet allotment of caffeine. It used to be that you would go to a coffee shop and get free refills of coffee as long as you could sit there and drink it. Now the fad has become designer coffee to go, in its own stylized container, so that you can drink it while you are on then move.

Addictions only reflect what each culture has chosen to numb out with. As long as cultures approve of (and encourage) things like prescription pills, caffeine, alcohol and television, people will continue to gravitate towards them in order to numb out their feelings. Societies do not create addictions; societies only create opportunities to become addicted. The more choices each society offers, the more the variety of addictions that becomes possible. What is fashionable today as an addiction might not be fashionable tomorrow. Just as clothing styles continue to change on a regular basis, so do addictions.

Addictions Are a Planetary Thing, a Common Thread

America is not alone in its crisis of addictions. America only stands out more because of the type of addictions that have appeared. Addictions have been around since the beginning of human beings and are present in every culture throughout the world.

Addictions are an age-old problem. The 21st Century is not filled with more addicts and more addictions. Because of our rapidly changing world, we now have more opportunities in our addictedness. Addictions have been around since the beginning of time, from the remote outback to deep within the darkness of the forests. As we enter into an age of understanding about ourselves, we now have more information and tools to explore our addictions.

Addictions are a planetary thing. In fact, addictions have appeared in such classic literature as the Bible. This one particular story recounts one of Noah's drunken episodes. The story in Genesis 10:20 goes as follows:

"Now Noah, a man of the soil, was the first to plant a vineyard. When he drank some of the wine, he became drunk and lay naked inside his tent."

The basis of addictions is to repress feelings and sensory experiences. There is no culture alive today nor has any ever existed that has not repressed feelings. As mentioned in the book *When Society Becomes an Addict* by Anne Wilson Schaef, our religions, communes, businesses and educational institutions become the dysfunctional family that we create to further keep our feelings repressed. Our authority figures, from gurus, priests, teachers to bosses all help to create addictions because they all encourage us to not feel.

For instance, a guru of Eastern "spirituality" might teach that "emotions are the enemy." A Catholic priest who follows the teachings of the church might tell you that "anger is a sin." A rigid boss at work could reprimand you by saying, "Be professional. Do not bring your feelings to work."

All of these authority figures, along with the institutions they represent, are encouraging you to repress your feelings. When you repress feelings you end up with addictions. Dysfunctional families across the globe are creating dysfunctional institutions. Churches, clubs and teams become just more places to become addicted. Anywhere in the world where people are taught to repress emotions there will be addictions. And that is *everywhere*.

A Zen Buddhist in Japan could be just as addicted as an American in Chicago or a Peruvian in the Andes. A homeless woman can be just as addicted as a suburban housewife or a business executive. A well-known authority and author of books in the self-help field could be just as addicted as a fifteen-year-old anorexic.

Addictions help people to function the only way they know how—by keeping them numb. Many societies place a high value on production and one needs to maintain productivity so that all members will benefit. In a modern society dependent on coal for energy, production might be hard pressed if all of the coal miners were to go home because they were in pain. The rest of the society would suffer. If your secretary is having a bad day, you will suffer if she goes home. In a primitive culture, if a hunter feels emotional pain and does not feel like he can hunt, the whole tribe will suffer.

Maintaining production has been a central focus for human beings for a very long time. In most cultures, the needs of the group come before the individuals' needs. We have addictions in order to maintain the needs of the group as we learn how to suppress our own individual needs. We have not focused much of our attention on our feelings, ourselves or on who we are.

With most addictions, it is quite easy to have them and function very well in society. Smoking, for instance, helps people to keep functioning the only way they know how—by staying buzzed on nicotine. Other addictions create enough disturbances where your work and family environments are in jeopardy.

Unfortunately, it is normal to be addicted because it has become normal to not feel. Human beings have not learned to accept pain. What is common among all people is that our feelings have been repressed. And this makes addictions as common as the air we breathe. Addiction has become what is normal.

For example, in Tibet, religion is not just a part of life but it is the purpose of life. Religion is infused in government, literature, ritual and customs. This easily encourages religious addiction. In America, Christianity is rooted in the cultural system. The Ten Commandments from the Bible (Old Testament) are the unofficial moral precepts that govern most lives. The Bible is used in courtrooms when a witness is asked to place his hand on it to force him to tell the truth. Through the use of fear (God will punish you if you lie), we use the Bible to obtain information. Christian prayer used to be common in all schools until recently. Even our money is tainted with religious overtones. "In God We Trust," meaning the one, monotheistic God that Christians believe in, is printed on the currency. It is easy to see how one could become a religious addict, even here in America, when religion is infused so very much into the culture.

Western industrialized cultures are not alone. Addictions are happening all over the world. As a teenage girl in New York compulsively chews gum to relieve her anxiety, a South American native chews on beetle nut to numb out. In the Middle East and in Asia, there is a predisposition to use heroin to numb out. Cigarettes are much more fashionable now in Europe than even here in the United States.

What is common and what is accepted become your addictions. Alcohol and drunkenness have been common in most major cultures for thousands of years. It has become accepted. This happens all over the planet, in cultures large and small, wealthy and poor.

Indigenous Cultures and Their Addictions

Even primitive cultures are embedded with many forms of addictions. Close-knit tribes that have not evolved very much might still be addicted to such things as religion, sex and alcohol. You become addicted to whatever is available. If your thoughts are the only means that are available, then they become your primary addictions. Thoughts such as "God," "love," "justice" and "truth" can be just as addictive as chewing gum or tobacco.

"Remarkably, indigenous peoples in all parts of the world have discovered natural products that thrived locally and that produced the ability to alter the sense of time and place and to produce visual, auditory, and other sensory distortions."

This quote comes from Avram Goldstein in *Addiction: From Biology to Drug Policy*. Native peoples have been using natural plants to change their moods for a long time. One of these intoxicants is the "ceremonial" drug called Ayahuasca. This drug creates hallucinations and altered states of consciousness. Hallucinations mimic the effects of serotonin. Ceremonial hallucinations are usually a secondary addiction, whereas religion, God or rituals are usually the primary addiction in many of the native people's lives. Just as prayer or ritual are the drugs of choice in many developing cultures, the rush of adrenaline is the drug that keeps many Westerners "high" day in and day out.

It seems that avoidance of feelings is a widespread human occurrence. Getting "high" together is also a basic human event. South Sea Islanders get intoxicated on a beverage called kava. South American Indians chew on coca leaves all day long. This is the plant that cocaine comes from. The author of *Addiction: From Biology to Drug Policy*, Avram Goldstein, writes,

"Cocaine is a natural substance found in coca leaves. Chewed by natives in the Andes highlands, the leaf was said to prevent fatigue and to increase energy for laborious physical labor."

The raw leaf only produces about 3% of the stimulating effect of the purified street cocaine, so the Indians are able to still function with only a mild buzz. This is like our modern-day caffeine buzz. Coca is a more powerful stimulant than caffeine though and produces a pleasant mood state. No wonder why millions of South American Indians have been chewing it daily for thousands of years. It is believed by many that cocaine was first used by ceremonial priests in ancient Incan rituals. These priests would chew on the leaves of the coca plant in order to heighten their religious experience.

It would seem that drugs being used addictively have occurred all over the world. Opium addiction in China was rampant until the Communists took over in 1949. In Islamic cultures, alcohol is prohibited with severe penalties, but heroin and other drugs are quite acceptable. The authors of *From Chocolate to Morphine,* Winifred Rosen and Andrew T. Weil, write,

"Some yogis in India use marijuana ritually but teach that opiates and alcohol are harmful. Muslims may tolerate the use of opium, marijuana and gat (a strongly stimulating leaf) but are very strict in their exclusion of alcohol."

The same authors add, "In ancient India marijuana was eaten for religious purposes; people used it for its effects on consciousness in socially accepted ways."

It has become socially acceptable in most cultures to mood-alter with drugs. Whether it is beer, wine, marijuana or some other exotic plant, it seems that most humans are doing it. The same authors go on to add, "In fact, drug-taking is so common that it seems to be a basic human activity."

Once again, in the book *From Chocolate to Morphine*, Rosen and Weil write,

"Tea addiction is not uncommon in England, Ireland, and Asia. Japanese people drink green tea throughout the day. In addition, they conduct tea ceremonies, elaborate rituals built around the consumption of matcha, a special powered green tea that is whipped with water into a bitter, frothy beverage. This strong form of tea was developed in Zen Buddhist monasteries to help monks stay awake during long hours of meditation."

Even something as simple as a tea ritual can become an addiction. Trying to keep oneself awake for meditation even though the body is saying that it is tired is another way to be addicted.

Addictions are happening on every continent. The national drink of Brazil is guarana. This beverage has more caffeine than coffee. Argentineans, meanwhile, drink a highly caffeinated drink called mate to keep them stimulated. There is the betel nut in Asia. Millions chew it daily. It has stimulating qualities similar to that of caffeine and is as much of an addiction as chewing gum or coffee is here in the United States. Meanwhile, Native Americans are using peyote cactus to get "high." This is justified by saying that this plant is "an aid to introspection and to making prayers more efficacious," as quoted from Avram Goldstein in *Addiction: From Biology to Drug Policy*. At the same time, a bright red mushroom named Fly Agaric has been used for centuries in Siberia and Northern Europe to get "high." While this has been going on, South American and Aztec rituals use "magic mushrooms" to alter their consciousness. The Yanomani Indians of the Amazon region blow an intoxicating snuff made from a rare tree bark into each other's noses through a long pipe. This snuff, called epena, gets them "high."

Rosen and Weil continue in *From Chocolate to Morphine,*

"New World Indians used tobacco in religious and magical rituals thousands of years ago, and some South American Indians still use strong tobacco as a consciousness-altering drug today. On special occasions they build giant cigars that men take turns inhaling. They quickly become very intoxicated. Because they do not use tobacco except on special occasions they have no tolerance to its effects and get very high. In North America today, all Indian medicine men and women use tobacco ceremonially; they believe tobacco smoke carries their prayers to the spirit world. When the Spanish discovered America, they observed the Indians using tobacco and began using it themselves."

With regard to other natural substances that have been used addictively worldwide, Rosen and Weil write,

"Amphetamine was a product of the pharmaceutical industry, a compound invented by laboratory chemists. However, a fascinating discovery of the 1970s revealed that nature makes its own amphetamine. An East African shrub called khat (also kat) contains a substance (cathinone) in its leaves that is almost identical to amphetamine, differing only by a single atom. The native populations of Ethiopia and Somalia have chewed khat leaves since ancient times, much as the Peruvian highlanders chew coca leaves. Cathinone is quite unstable, so the leaves have to be fresh and young; and cathinone is destroyed rapidly in the body. Although all the psychotropic, cardiovascular, and toxic effects of cathinone are identical to those of amphetamine, it is so rapidly metabolized that it is difficult for the khat user to establish high and sustained levels in the brain. Chewing khat is certainly addictive and potentially harmful. However, it is much safer than the intravenous use of amphetamines, much as chewing coca leaves is safer and more socially acceptable than using pure cocaine."

Alcohol is another drug that has been used addictively for a very long time. Alcohol has been around as long as people have been alive. Tropical Indians, who chewed corn to a pulp and then spit it into a bucket, made one of the first beers. The saliva would act as an enzyme to break down the starch. This would then ferment into a beer.

All over the world, people are getting "high" using thoughts, rituals and drugs (some using natural plants and others concocted remedies). Drugs are just one way that we use addictions. It is happening all over the world, whether you have justified your addictions by saying that they help you to relax or it is okay because it is a religious ritual makes no difference. We are still numbing out all over the world. Addiction is about an inner conflict; the methods by which we stay numb might be different, but the results are the same.

The Myth of Addiction as a Disease

There has been much controversy whether addiction is a disease or not. Many people believe that addiction has its origins in one's biology, while others believe that addiction is more of a personality disorder.

Addictions are real and they do haunt each of us every day. However, addiction theory is very outdated, and most people have been practicing an old mythology for quite some time. In order to understand why most people are stuck believing in a prehistoric mythology, it is important to recognize the steps that brought us to this point.

Science is a belief system that gained recognition several hundred years ago. In the Western world, before this time the "Church" was the authority on explaining most important matters. Science, through deductive reasoning and quantifiable results, found ways to "prove" things. Science soon took over from religion and became the god to be honored.

It is through this unparalleled trust in scientific theory and in the scientific community that the problem with addiction lies. Addictions are about repressed emotions and sensory experiences. Addictions are not about chemicals, genetics or any other scientific experiment. Addictions can neither be explained nor healed in a laboratory or through deductive reasoning. Addictions will only be healed by learning how to feel and release your feelings. The problem with present day addiction theory is that it comes from scientific mythology.

Let's examine how most people view *disease* in the first place. In order to understand the disease concept, it is important to comprehend how the Western culture might view disease. In a Western concept, disease is something that invades your body from the outside (like a virus) or is molecular in origin. Disease is thought to disrupt the balance or homeostasis of the body. The body is thought to be attacked by such invaders as bacteria, viruses, mutant cells or defective genes.

This ideology teaches one that mutant genes (like sickle cells) or environmental factors (like asbestos, radiation, poor nutrition, lead or even wet hair) can cause these imbalances. From a Western mind, disease is very much a physical phenomenon.

This type of Western thinking has classified even such things as pain itself as a disease. Pain has become the enemy and you must kill it. There is little scope of thinking as to try to understand the underlying causes that could be creating it. The Western concept of disease is very much geared toward trying to treat the symptoms.

The problem with a Western view of addictions rises with understanding the concepts behind Western medicine. While focusing on molecules and germs, the Western scientific methodology has been very helpful at isolating and healing such germ or molecule-based diseases like malaria or smallpox. Unfortunately, most of the diseases of the modern time are not molecular-based. These diseases are degenerative in nature or energy-based (cancer, lupus, Parkinson's, heart disease etc.). Addictions fall into this energy-based category and cannot be healed with Western medical methodology.

In hopes of understanding the dilemma as to whether to label addiction as a disease or not, we need to ask the medical profession in a Western world what they would call disease. At this point I'm not really sure that they even know. Herbert Fingarette writes in *Heavy Drinking*, referring to the work of alcoholism researcher E.M. Jellinek, "Much of the same vagueness obtains in regard to the word *disease*. In medical texts the word has only a loose, ill-defined allusive sense and is not used as a basis for rigorous scientific discussion, or in Jellinek's words: 'It comes to this, that *a disease is what the medical profession recognizes as such.'*"

The disease model of addiction from a Western perspective originated with the study of alcoholics, and the same ideology was applied to other addictions. E.M. Jellinek developed much of this thinking. Herbert Fingarette states in *Heavy Drinking,* that the "folk science" of alcoholism was created partially by researcher E.M. Jellinek, whose published work was titled *The Disease Concept of Alcoholism.*

Fingarette states, " . . . it was the inadequacy of Jellinek's data that caused much of his classic work to fail the test of later scientific scrutiny." What happened was that one man, a scientific biostatistician, helped create a myth for what alcoholism was all about. However, his studies failed to hold up under closer examination. For a culture looking for a scapegoat to blame, it worked. Most adhered to the Western concept of alcoholism and later to most other addictions as biological phenomenon. That way it wasn't your fault. It was in your biology. Your genes were now the enemy. Science could now claim its prize.

Louis Pasteur was credited with inventing the germ theory. Pasteur helped to isolate pathogens and declared that illnesses were "all" related to an invasion of germs in the body (even though he later said that the germ was nothing; the environment was everything). Out of this Western concept of disease emerged the concept of alcoholism being an "allergy." In this case, certain people were considered "allergic" to alcohol. This is just a continuation of the germ theory where it is believed that you are being attacked by your own biology. The latest advances in the germ theory make your own genes your enemies. We are treating our genes as if they were invading germs, and in the process still being a victim of our own body and biology.

In fact, it is the Western medical field that created the concept of addiction as a disease as we know it today. The American Medical Association (AMA) grabbed on to this newly forming theory and in 1957 "declared" that alcoholism was now a "disease." This model and way of thinking wants you to believe that alcoholism is a genetic monster running through your veins. It preaches that the only cure is a lifetime of abstinence, forced Alcoholics Anonymous meetings, treatment centers and the stigma of having to always carry the dreaded disease.

In fact, insurance companies will only pay for treatment in a 28-day in-hospital center if you call it a disease. They can justify the expense as a "medical condition." You are told that you have a "medical condition" and it is not your fault. You are now labeled as sick or "diseased" and you now must do what you can to control your illness. You have now entered into the Western "disease care management system."

The myth of alcoholism as genetically related can be closely associated with the myth of the magical South American city of El Dorado or the myth of Noah's Ark. According to traditional scientific understanding, this is what is currently believed.

Alcoholism theory set in motion by the medical establishment modeled an expanding belief that you are the victim of your own body and biology. This way you do not have to take any responsibility. Why is it that the very same medical establishment, (medical doctors), that wish to blame your own body for its problems, report an incidence of drug and alcohol "abuse" far greater than the national average. This according to Dr. Dean Ornish in *Dr. Dean Ornish's Program For Reversing Heart Disease.*

Much of the understanding about addictions and addiction mythologies comes from "scientific" research about alcohol. This way of thinking has been applied to other forms of addictions. If the theory starts out wrong to begin with, it will contaminate everything that it touches along the way. This is exactly what has happened to the theories about addictions. Addiction theory began in a haphazard and irresponsible fashion and has continued along those same lines ever since.

An example of this type of scientific zealousness to prove a theory and win a prestigious award comes from a book by Kathleen W. Fitzgerald, Ph.D., titled *Alcoholism: The Genetic Inheritance.* "While medical science cannot at this time assert that a particular gene, a particular enzyme, or a particular neurotransmitter actually *causes* alcoholism, there is much known about the biochemistry of alcohol addiction."

I find it ironic in the aforementioned book that the author (Kathleen W. Fitzgerald, Ph.D.) is trying to convince the reader that a gene is responsible for *why* many cannot control their alcohol intake. The author infers by the title of her book, *Alcohol: The Genetic Inheritance*, that alcoholism is attributed to an inherited gene. She goes on to elaborate in great detail throughout the book about how alcoholism is genetically related. Yet she openly states on several occasions in the book that *no gene* has ever been located.

Scientists have so far been able to tell us *what* happens to us *when* we drink. Unfortunately, they have been attempting to fit this thinking into the question of *why* we drink. They have been trying to convince us that our biology is craving alcohol. Then, this biological basis for alcohol addiction is applied to every other addictive pattern.

Genetics might help you to choose which addictions you have, but they certainly do not cause them. For instance, some people might metabolize alcohol more slowly than others. This could be a genetic factor. If you are slow to metabolize alcohol, you might become drunk more easily. This explains *what* happens to you *when* you drink but fails to explain *why* you begin to drink in the first place and continue to drink thereafter.

Joel Kramer and Diana Alstad write in *The Guru Papers*, "Thus the urge to take the first drink must come from some place other than physical need."

Science has started out with a tarnished theory that has yet to be proven. Much of this error in thinking comes from the mistaken labeling of the term "alcoholic." Scientific methodology prides itself on its very organized and accurate procedures for analyzing and collecting data. Everything is scrutinized to the core before a valid test result is confirmed. This is so that each experiment can be duplicated exactly each and every time.

In the case of the scientific study of alcoholism, there are some big mistakes that have been made. It is almost as if in their haste to try to prove a theory, scientists have begun each experiment with dirty test tubes. Thus, all the subsequent results that followed were always flawed.

This is the reason why. In many of the "scientific" studies of alcoholism, what we see is that a scientist takes a "group of alcoholics" and measures their blood alcohol levels or examines their liver enzymes or takes samples of their neurotransmitters in their brains, etc. This all sounds well and fine. The only problem is that the term "alcoholic" is not a scientific term. It is not an exact, concrete thing, like calcium, magnesium or sodium. The term "alcoholic" is a subjective term, depending on who is using it, and it cannot be measured.

For instance, does someone who drinks a half a bottle of Scotch every night but never loses control qualify as an "alcoholic?" Some would say "Yes!" while others might say "No!"

Does someone considered a "lightweight" who drinks no more than two glasses of wine at a time but loses control qualify as an "alcoholic?" Does someone who loses control on special occasions (like parties and holidays) qualify as an "alcoholic?" How about the regular drinker who consumes his usual two martinis every day at five o'clock, is he an "alcoholic?" If an "alcoholic" does not seem to disrupt his work and family life, and causes no major problems, then the drinker is labeled as a mild to heavy drinker, but not the dreaded "alcoholic;" even though she might drink the same amount as one who is labeled as an "alcoholic."

It would seem that all of the studies done on alcoholics are tarnished from the very beginning. All of the studies that supposedly measure different experiments on "alcoholics" are using a pretty big assumption—that an "alcoholic" is a specific thing that can be measured. It is not. The term "alcoholic" is a subjective term open to individual interpretation. This is unlike "objective" scientific terminology, like "hydrogen" or "oxygen," which can be quantifiably measured. Scientific studies on "alcoholics" are almost always tarnished from the very beginning because a gross false assumption is made that scientists actually know what an "alcoholic" truly is.

Science cannot understand addictions because addictions are not part of the quantifiable scientific paradigm. Addictions are about not wanting to feel. This equation is outside the scope of science. This is like asking to your car mechanic to help deliver your baby. Science is not capable of answering the addiction problem any more than your car mechanic is capable of successfully participating in childbirth.

I believe that addictions are a disease. Addiction is a disease in so far as it **is *a faulty relationship with something that is used to alter your moods***. This crosses all cultural boundaries. You develop a faulty relationship with something when you lose your natural self or relationship with your natural world. You develop a faulty relationship with chocolate chip cookies, coffee or your pets. Your glass of wine becomes your lover. Your work becomes your best friend. You keep from feeling your sadness by drowning yourself with excitement and entertainment. Whether you are in the far reaches of Thailand or the downtown streets of Chicago, you choose what is available. When you cannot feel your feelings and release them, you will find addictions as a means to numb out. This is the disease process and it has very little to do with scientific methodology.

Addiction is a disease that crosses all racial and geographical boundaries. Addiction is a disease that is part of what it means to be a human being. Because we have a brain that is capable of numbing out sensations and emotions, we have created our own disease in our addictions. Addictions are a faulty relationship with people, objects, thoughts and emotions. That is why addictions are a disease. It is not the substances or the behavior that is diseased, but how and why we use them that create our disease.

If you eliminated all of the guns, you would not stop violence. Just as if you banned all tobacco, sugar and alcohol you would not end addiction. Guns by themselves do not create violence. Alcohol, tobacco and sugar are not responsible for addictions. It is your faulty relationships with these and other things that are responsible for your addictions. Without repression, there would be no need for addictions. Repression is at the core of creating your faulty relationships.

Addiction is about what is going on inside; it is about your relationship with yourself. The types of relationships that you develop with your substances and behaviors will determine if you have a healthy relationship with something or a faulty relationship. If you get "high" off something to hide from your feelings, you have developed a faulty relationship. When you are addicted, you are not at ease with yourself because you are running from your feelings. Addiction is a disease but it is nothing more than the disease of a faulty relationship.

The Myth of the Addictive Personality

Myth: Only Some People Develop Addictions Because Only Some People Have an Addictive Personality, Most Likely Based on Their Genetic Makeup.

This statement is one of the most common myths that many have been led to believe with regard to addictions. There is no truth to this statement whatsoever, nor is there any substantial evidence to support it. This idea is nothing more than a false belief that has been passed down from generation to generation. This holds true for the assumption that specific personalities create specific addictions (like the alcoholic personality) and for the belief in the general "addictive personality" type.

Let's look at the common myth that there are addictive personality types for specific addictions. The most common myth is that there is an "alcoholic personality." In *How to Stay Sober*, James Christopher writes, "The evidence is strong that there is no such thing as an 'alcoholic personality.'" He goes on to quote J. H. P. Willis, a consultant psychiatrist at Guy's Hospital and King's College Hospital in London.

"This had led to an enormous amount of speculation, which has found perhaps its most absurd expression in the notion put forward by a number of psychologists and psychiatrists that there is a special type of personality which is, as it were, addiction-prone. Unfortunately, however, no one has ever been able to substantiate this claim in any credible way."

In fact, for a long time, the trend was to blame specific addictions like alcohol on the "addictive personality." The thinking was that a person's genes were responsible for why he or she drank alcohol. The personality was thought to be created by genetic factors. Those who hold firm to this myth want you to believe that there is a monster looming within you that is passed down from parent to child. Once you let this monster out, there is no turning back. This is the farthest thing from the truth. This is another example of victim consciousness. It seems that if all else fails to find an answer, the common practice is to blame your genes for your problems rather than to take responsibility for what you have created.

James Christopher adds in *How to Stay Sober*, "Earlier advocates of an 'alcoholic personality' have abandoned this hypothesis, and the theory of an 'addictive personality' has also been discredited by lack of supportive evidence." Kathleen W. Fitzgerald, Ph.D., adds in *Alcoholism, The Genetic Inheritance*, "There is simply no such thing as the alcoholic personality."

Your false beliefs about your addictions are not just about alcohol, but carry over into just about every type of addiction. I have heard some people say that they cannot help themselves from overworking because it is just their "workaholic personality." In this case, they are assuming that their genes are responsible for their inability to stop working as well. Others have claimed that some people have "violence addiction" based on their genes. "Oh, his father was a very violent man" is the rationale for such beliefs. Here is another example of victim consciousness at work.

Those who take this stance are assuming that the violence runs within the gene pool for that particular family, just as certain species of dogs (like pit bulls) can become violent. I have even heard some people claim that they have a "chocolate personality." These people claim that their genes are responsible for their incessant cravings for chocolate. When you think like this, you are not willing to take any responsibility for the choices that you have made.

What is actually happening is that your genes are not responsible for your addictions. You choose your addictions yourself. Addictions are a choice based on elements of your personality (values, morals, likes and dislikes). You develop a relationship with chocolate, work, violence, alcohol or something else to mood-alter. You do not have a dormant gene lying around within you waiting for you to take your first bite of chocolate or your first sip of beer. The myth teaches that once you cross over that imaginary line, you are lost forever into your world of addiction. Yes, there are certain personality types that are more prone to specific addictive patterns. However, there is no direct correlation between a specific gene creating a specific addiction.

For instance, a person who has given permission for "high risk" to be the mode of numbing out might have more sexual promiscuity addictions, more toxic ingestive substance addictions and other "high risk" behavior to mood-alter. Neither his genetic code nor his personality cause him to mood-alter. His lack of ability to feel his pain is the reason that he mood-alters. His personality only helps to direct him as to which addictions to choose.

Someone with an eating disorder that causes her to overeat might have specific patterns of behavior based around her addiction. She might hide food in the house so as never to run out of her supply. She might tend to lie or deceive herself and others about how much she is actually eating. She might plan her social life around her meals. The highlight of her day becomes her eating.

There is no substantial evidence to support the theory that a specific gene would cause a specific addiction. If this were true, then you would find all sorts of aberrant genes in your double helix of genetic material from the gambling addiction gene to the television addiction gene. The gene for codependence would be right next to the gene for addiction to fantasy. You would have hundreds and thousands of wayward genes in your body that would "force" you to be consumed by a specific addiction. This fantasy myth would be even more humorous if you thought about living in a land where there were no chocolate, alcohol or tobacco. What does this dormant gene do but harbor in your body for millions of years and hundreds of generations until some wayward explorer lands on your remote island and introduces you to tobacco, chocolate or alcohol? And then you become addicted? Hardly!

No, addictions are choices that you create with something that is readily available to you that fits into your value system and takes away your pain. You cannot become addicted to something unless it is available. You cannot become addicted to alcohol if you live in a remote area that does not have alcohol. You have to develop a relationship with that substance as a way to mood-alter in order to become addicted. Your genes have nothing to do with it. There is no specific gene for any specific addiction, whether it is a substance, behavior, thought, emotion or relationship. All of your addictions are choices.

What about the person who believes that she has a general "addictive personality" and that whatever she is involved with at the moment she becomes addicted to? She seems to progress from one activity to the next with reckless abandon. She gets 100% involved with whatever she is doing at the moment at the exclusion of everything else.

She claims that she cannot help herself. She just has an "addictive personality." What is really happening is that there is an unidentified, underlying characteristic that is her primary addiction. It is this quality that becomes her mood changer. Some of these qualities might be such things as the following; compulsiveness, busyness, perfectionism, escapism, urgency, fantasy, power, excitement or drama.

As an example, let's look at three different people who believe they have an "addictive personality." Each seems to go overboard with what he is doing. They all accept this personality quirk as" "just the way I was born."

What they do not see, though, is that what appears as a personality quirk on the surface is really a lack of awareness of the underlying issues.

Examples of the Addictive Personality Myth

1. Jeff

Jeff, for example, is always fantasizing about ways to make money. He seems addicted to his thoughts of "wheeling and dealing." He claims that it is just his "addictive personality" and he cannot help himself. He is always driven by elaborate business plans or motivated by pyramid scams. He is the first to run out and buy his lottery ticket. Jeff truly believes that it is in his blood to be driven by the lust for money.

What is really happening to Jeff is that he has a primary addiction to fantasy. He gets "high" off fantasy which he uses to mood-alter. He can never have enough fantasy. He needs to keep dreaming of his next fantasy to keep him away from his feelings. His thoughts of fantasy are really his primary addiction. While exhibited outwardly as monetary goals, his real problem is on the inside with his addictive pattern of fantasy.

2. Suzy

Suzy is another person who believes that she has an "addictive personality." It seems that whatever she touches, she goes overboard with. She can do nothing in moderation. She moves from learning tennis to taking up oil painting. She uses the same energy to study a foreign language or to embrace a "cause" of saving someone or something. She feels the utmost passion about each and every one of her activities. She burns out rather quickly and needs to move on to the next subject. She finds it impossible to slow down and relax. She is never without a project or learning something new. She performs it all with the same intensity. She just shrugs her shoulders and says, "Oh well, it's just my addictive personality at work again."

Unfortunately, Suzy is not very in touch with herself and not very aware of what her motivation is. If Suzy were to slow down long enough to examine what she is feeling inside, she might find that the qualities she is really addicted to are those of achievement, compulsiveness, busyness and perfectionism. It is these qualities that get her 'high" to alter her moods. She feels the need to be perfect at whatever she does and then moves on to the next project. Staying busy is one of her primary addictions. She keeps running from her feelings by doing, doing and more doing.

3. Sally

Sally is another example of someone who feels she has an "addictive personality." However, Sally is really just addicted to excitement. She fills her life with travel and movies, social life and sports cars. She has a string of exciting men whom she spends time with. She has lots of activities and much excitement in her life. There is drama and intensity. She seems to create a world of glamour and excitement. She believes that it is her "addictive personality" which causes so much excitement in her life.

The real issue is that Sally is terrified to be alone. She is addicted to excitement in order to avoid her feelings of aloneness. She hides behind the facade of having many friends because she is really terrified to be without people around. She does everything with such intensity because she needs the adrenaline rush to stay "high." Her labeling herself as an "addictive personality" is just an excuse to cover up her addiction to excitement.

Summary

Whether it is to a specific addiction (alcohol, sugar, tobacco, etc.) or to a host of qualities (fantasy, achievement, etc.), there are no "addictive personalities." This expression is just used to place the blame on something else. You choose your own addictions. Alcoholics choose alcohol. Sugar addicts choose sugar. Adrenaline junkies choose adrenaline. Sports addicts choose sports. These are the choices that you make in your life based on your value system and which types of addictions will fit best with your personality.

Besides, if there were such a thing as an "addictive personality," that would mean there would have to be a "non-addictive personality" as well. There would be people who were not prone to any addiction at all, from the most powerful ones to the most trivial. These would be the people who could feel, express and release every one of their feelings in the moment in which those feelings emerged. These would be people who had no need to escape from their pain.

I have never seen one of these so called "non-addictive personalities" and that is because I do not believe they exist. The "addictive personality" does not exist either. This is just society's clever way of trying to place blame and thinking once again in "black and white" terms. Society believes that only some are addicted. I believe that all of us have addictions. It is time to let go of the myth of the "addictive personality" and time to take responsibility for the choices that we all make.

The Myth of "Recovery"

The story of "recovery" dates back some sixty or seventy years. The term "recovery" has become a staple part of the everyday language and vocabulary for many people. There are millions of members who claim to participate in the "Recovery Movement." Many different offshoots have arisen out of the early days.

Unfortunately, the work in the traditional addiction recovery field does very little to help one actually recover from anything. Under present mythology, the word "recovery" means to "stay in control." Those who participate in the "Recovery Movement" are more likely to become addicted to control than to actually recover from their faulty relationship with something that helps them mood-alter. Understanding addiction mythology and language means going back to its origins.

The earliest work with regard to recovery from addictions began with the field of alcohol. Most other addiction recovery programs grew out of the alcohol recovery movement. In order to understand addiction recovery mythology, it is important to understand how recovery from alcohol came into being.

"Recovery" work began with the A.A. movement around 1936. This movement was initiated by Bill Wilson and Dr. Bob (as he wished to be known). Both men could not control their drinking and were looking for a way out of their suffering. Both were searching for a solution to end their dependency on alcohol and the pain that it was causing them. They found each other and are credited with beginning the first organized support group for addictions. Those suffering with addiction to alcohol finally had some hope.

Why did the "recovery" field begin with addiction to alcohol and not something else? This was because the time was right for alcohol to be recognized. Many people were beginning to see the dangers of alcohol. In fact, during Prohibition in the 1930s, for a short period of time alcohol was banned in the United States. As with most other cultures, alcohol had always been accepted and was readily available in this culture. It was relatively inexpensive. It came neatly packaged. Consumption of alcohol already existed in most homes. Alcohol worked very well as a mood changer. Unfortunately, it also caused the most amount of pain and destroyed many lives. The time was right.

For thousands of years, alcohol had been accepted as a normal means to escape from pain. Men were supposed to drink. Women later followed in their footsteps. Kathleen W. Fitzgerald, Ph.D., quotes well known alcohol researcher Dr. E.M. Jellinek in her book *Alcoholism: The Genetic Inheritance*, saying that alcohol " . . . comes close to being an institution in our society." Fitzgerald adds herself, "It is a value to learn how to drink, because our family gatherings, our business transactions, our recreational and sporting events, demand that one knows how to drink."

According to Stanton Peele in *Diseasing of America*, alcohol was a well-recognized part of the early American colonial period. It was just as familiar as hot dogs and apple pie are today. Peele goes on to say, "The average colonial drank several times as much alcohol per year as the current American, and even the Puritans called liquor the 'Good Creature of God.'" Alcohol was accepted, abundant and encouraged. No wonder so much of it was consumed. Peele further adds, "For many immigrant groups, liquor was the glue of life . . ."

Things began to change. All of a sudden alcohol began to be recognized as a possible danger rather than a savior. Many people were suffering from health crises after many years of drinking. Families were being ripped apart. Jobs were being lost. As the automobile became more common, there were more alcohol related accidents. The pain that alcohol was causing was beginning to outweigh its benefits.

Until recently, alcohol had been very popular in most cultures. It was easy to make. It had played a role in mood-alteration for quite some time. It was normal to use alcohol; nobody ever questioned its use. It had historic origins. Historically, being a drunk was many times a noble feat. Great kings and explorers throughout the ages were recognized for being heavy drinkers.

Mythology praised those who could let go with the use of alcohol. Unfortunately, in a modern society it had become a very difficult balancing act. As society changed, so did the way alcohol affected people. We were no longer an agricultural society. More and more people were living in cities working jobs with regular hours. We were now becoming more of a time-conscious society. Many people were finding that they could not have a healthy relationship with alcohol and still perform the daily tasks that an industrial-based society was asking of them.

Alcohol was causing too great a problem for many who were trying to remain productive, scheduled, and alert while maintaining a healthy relationship. Alcohol was becoming a curse. In the past, you could get away with spending your days sleeping off your drunken episodes from the night before. Now it was becoming more difficult. You had responsibilities and had to go to work the next day. It was no longer okay to be the town drunk. Too many people depended on you. You could lose your job if you had too much to drink the night before.

As more and more people began to look for an answer to their suffering, A.A. membership began to grow. Alcoholics Anonymous began the "Recovery Movement." A.A. began a historic worldwide trend to come to grips with addictions and end this pain. A.A. had given us the beginning.

A large degree of the early success of A.A. was due to the much-needed void in society that it fulfilled. A.A. provided a community of support for those struggling with their addiction to alcohol. For most people in our culture, communities and support groups tended to be severely lacking. A.A. provided this support. One of A.A.'s principle attractions was that it provided a safe, supportive community of like-minded people who had a similar problem.

Many people felt more comfortable around others who were like themselves. This way they were not alone in their pain. They became part of the tribe, in this case the A.A. tribe. Members could listen and learn from other's struggles. There was a regular and safe location to meet at. This might be in a church meeting hall, civic center or a rented room. In the past, the bars and bowling alleys provided the only means of support and intimacy for many people.

People felt listened to at A.A. meetings. Since there was usually no "cross talk," nobody was there to solve anyone else's problems. One could just speak and be heard. What many so desperately sought in their lives was just to be heard. Often, this is when healing occurs—during the act of being heard. Support is ongoing. Members are encouraged to pass out their telephone numbers to others. This feels good. It gives people hope. When you need support the most, you will have someone to call.

A.A. has also been instrumental in helping many to admit that there is a problem and it is affecting their lives. For many, they have lived a long time in denial of their addiction problems. They have been lying to themselves by claiming that they can stop whenever they want to or that they really do not need their drug of choice. A.A. has helped many to come out of the closet and admit that there is a problem. This is the beginning of the healing process.

A.A. has also been the cornerstone of all other "12-Step" and "recovery" programs. Adult Children of Alcoholics (A.C.A.), Overeaters

Anonymous (O.A.), Sex Addicts Anonymous (S.A.A.), Narcotics Anonymous (N.A.) and so many more groups were designed around the premises first established by A.A. No matter what your addiction happens to be, there appears to be a support group available for you. Millions of people have begun their "recovery" work because of the foundation that A.A. laid down.

The problems with Alcoholics Anonymous and the "recovery" programs were there from the very beginning. It is often said that if one bird flies in the wrong direction, the rest will follow. Alcoholics Anonymous is that one bird and it has taken us in the wrong direction.

The Problems with 12-Step Groups

Alcoholics Anonymous began its treatment campaign with a structure and a formula. This structure came to be known as the "Big Book". The formula was encased in a system called "The Twelve Steps." Unfortunately, when you misdiagnose the problem, you will seek a cure that is unlikely to heal the problem. A.A. unwittingly misdiagnosed the nature of alcoholism and addiction, and the entire formula became incorrect.

Many people expect A.A. and other support groups to be the "magic pill" to end all of their suffering. Support groups are only a first step in the "recovery" process. In the long run, A.A. and many other support groups, by their very design, end up keeping you stuck. They do very little to bring you back to your natural ways or to allow you to recover from your addictions.

Twelve-Step programs are not about recovery—they are about control. Recovery is about learning to have a relationship with all of your feelings and not having to be in control all of the time. This is not what 12-Step programs do. For most support groups, including A.A., the word—"recovery" actually means to "learn how to control your cravings and repress your feelings." Practiced in this manner, this is not "recovery."

Support groups are what get you "help." They allow you to acknowledge your addiction problem and provide support and encouragement. However, 12-Step groups never let you leave. They never allow you to graduate. It is as if A.A. invented the wheel and put it on a covered wagon drawn by four horses. It was a valiant effort to get things moving. Now A.A. and other support groups are trying to maneuver those covered wagons down modern, high-speed freeways. It is a little outdated. True recovery programs bring you back to your feeling states and allow you to graduate from the initial support group that brought you to addressing your addiction problems. In the long run, A.A. and other support groups become an obstacle to recovery.

When you enter into a 12-Step program, you are usually experiencing a fair amount of suffering in your life on account of your addictions. You are usually in pain. You are usually looking for quick relief. You are very open and vulnerable. You want relief, and any magic pill to stop you from eating, smoking or gambling yourself to death will do. Many times, your vulnerability leaves you open to a form of brain washing. You allow yourself to become overwhelmed by another authoritarian system and continue to have your personal power taken away from you.

Most people are not in a strong place when they enter into a 12-Step program. They get sucked in rather quickly and do not have time to discern as to what they are doing. They just want the pain to go away. Many times people are seduced into joining.

In these groups, you are taught how to stay in control by learning new repressive strategies. *"Recovery" is when you no longer have a faulty relationship with your addiction.* You have understood, felt and processed the painful feelings and sensations that brought you to your addiction. The cravings are now completely gone. "Recovery" is learning how to trust yourself. You understand and have a skillful knowledge of how to express any and all of your emotions. There is no longer a need to remain guarded and in control. This is not what is happening in support groups, whether they lead you to believe it or not.

It is important to reacquaint yourself with the equation of addictions. "Repressed emotions and sensations lead to addictions." In the healing process, 90 percent of the work lies in learning how to feel those uncomfortable feelings, and only 10% of the work is in developing strategies for controlling the addiction itself.

The 12-Step approach is designed to teach you how to control the addiction and to remain guarded. This is not freedom. This is not "recovery." Twelve-Step programs, while they help some to learn how to stay in control around their addiction, are very limiting. They attempt to control the symptoms of alcohol, food or a deck of cards. In essence, they are still trying to blame something external for a conflict that is essentially internal.

Addictions are much more than just stopping from ingesting something. "Recovery" is about coming out of your trance. That is why most "recovery" programs are still living in the dark ages; they do very little for actual "recovery."

Staying in Control

To better understand the "recovery" industry, it is important to understand A.A.—the grandfather of all "recovery" programs. "Recovery" programs base their treatment on a myth. This myth suggests that "loss of control" is what determines who is addicted or not. Those who learn to stay in control with their behavior or substances that they ingest are not addicted, according to this belief. If you lose control regularly, you are labeled with an ill-fated disease. Now you have become the "addict" in the eyes of society because you cannot control yourself. The myth is that "loss of control" determines who is an addict.

With this type of thinking, it is easy to see what "recovery" programs teach. Most "recovery" programs teach you how to stay in control of your cravings. A.A. teaches you how to learn to control your cravings around alcohol. O.A. teaches you to learn to control your food intake. Most 12-Step and "recovery" programs are no different.

When you mistakenly believe that "loss of control" is what makes you an addict, you will attempt to regain control in your "recovery." In the meantime, you continue to deny the relationship that you have created with your addiction. You end up denying parts of yourself.

The actual goal of A.A. is to teach you how to stay in control. You are taught ways to distract yourself and learn new coping skills in order to stay in control. In order to be part of the group, you must first give up your personal power, label yourself as sick with an incurable disease, and keep attending regular meetings for the rest of your life. You are told that this will help you in order to keep your disease in control. This is what most people are being taught. This is *not* "recovery."

What Is Sobriety?

The word "sobriety" has become very popular in treatment circles and in the general population at large. "Sobriety" has come to mean "abstinence" from that which you crave the most. You are told to "live each day, one day at a time." You pass milestones by measuring how many consecutive days you have been able to control your addiction. "Success" is generally accredited if you can survive five years or more without using your drug of choice. It is hoped that by this time, you have managed to control your cravings.

If it takes something like "sobriety" for people to end the most damaging aspects of their addiction, then I commend it. If it takes "sobriety" to have meaningful relationships, a satisfying work life and a healthy body, then I am all for it. However, "sobriety" does very little to actually heal addiction nor to "recover" your natural self. "Sobriety" is nothing more than learning how to stay in control with will power and mind control. Many people become addicted to control itself in order to feel better. They get "high" off being in control. They get "high" off being sober.

"Sobriety" is often nothing more than an addiction to staying in control. "Sobriety" can be an addiction to *not drinking or not taking drugs*. "Sobriety" is about having to continuously be on guard. Referring to sober people, Herbert Fingarette writes in *Heavy Drinking*, "For them, A.A. often becomes an alternative way of life, which is as intensely focused on abstinence as their former lives had been focused on alcohol."

"Sobriety" also helps to create "black and white" thinking. You are labeled as either sober or not sober. Alcohol and street drugs are now the enemy. You have either befriended the enemy or you are on the side of the "good" guys, those who choose to be sober.

"Sobriety" is nothing more than learning how to stay on guard for your entire life. There are no "time outs" or days off. Being on guard means there is something about you that you need to *not* think about or always have to be frightened about. It is as if there is a monster in the closet all of the time.

When you attend a social event, you must put up your walls around others who are drinking. You must remain hyper-vigilant when the food is put out at a party so as not to go on an eating binge. When you are with friends who smoke, you must learn to stay in control if you are trying to quit smoking. You must learn how to extinguish thoughts of the next drink or the next chocolate chip cookie. This is what "sobriety" is all about. This is not "recovery."

When an uncomfortable feeling arises, you have three choices. You can feel the feeling and release the energy of the feeling to completion, thus entering your relaxation response. Secondly, you can repress the feeling and choose an addiction as a way to not feel this feeling. Or, you can repress the feeling and repress the *already established relationship* with something that you have used in the past to mood-alter, using control as the way to be numb. This third choice is normally what happens to someone who is practicing "sobriety."

Many people become addicted to *not doing* something. They get "high" off denying something. Not drinking, not doing drugs, not having sex or not eating (anorexia) become the addiction. This is called "acting in." The mood changes by controlling the cravings and repressing the feelings. Many times, *not drinking or not eating* now become the central activity in your life. Staying in control then becomes your addiction.

Herbert Fingarette writes in *Heavy Drinking*, "Members join a community that fosters intense emotional bonds, provides an integrated set of values and priorities, with powerful symbols and rituals, and offers frequent social activities and an active network of communication. For regular members the A.A. campaign against alcohol comes to replace drinking as an activity central to their lives and identity."

By learning how to avoid alcohol, heroin or a "trigger" food, you are never free from your relationship that you might have with it. It is like running from the law. Even after twenty years, with a new name, new identity and new location, you will always have to look over your shoulder. That is why even someone with five, ten or even fifteen years of "sobriety" might one day "slip up" or "fall off the wagon" from time to time. As intense emotional experiences might arise, the old cravings are often sought out. When you let your guard down, anything can happen. You tend to return to a familiar pattern of pain relief. Usually, that is your addiction. This occurs because you have not yet healed your relationship with your addiction and your painful feelings which brought you to your addiction.

"Sobriety" becomes like a life raft thrown to you after your ship has already sunk. You feel a sense of hope. However, you never seem to get off the life raft and remain floundering in the middle of the ocean for the rest of your life.

Getting "sober" may be the first step toward "recovery." You cannot begin to reconnect with your natural self until you have begun eliminating the addictive substances or behaviors that have prevented you from feeling. Being "sober" means taking the first step in "recovery." "Sobriety" should not be the end goal though. One will never heal and "recover" by just being "sober." There is much work to do after you become "sober."

Addiction is not an external thing. Addiction happens inside. Now you need to begin the inner work once you have become "sober." "Recovery" is not about learning how to control any substance because it is not the substance's fault that you are addicted. You are addicted because you cannot feel your pain. "Recovery" will occur when you no longer need to be on guard or hyper-vigilant. "Recovery" will happen when you no longer have to worry about your resistance being low. "Sobriety" is a start in your "recovery," but it is not the end goal.

Specific Techniques of Support Groups

The goal of support groups and treatment centers is to teach coping skills about how to avoid your problem addictions that might be causing you so much damage. These techniques vary in their ability to keep you away from your addictions, and some are more successful than others. Once again, these techniques will teach you how to stay in control around your addictions, not how to "recover" from them. The following are some of the techniques of support groups and why they may not be the best if one wants to recover the natural self.

1. Staying Busy

Many treatment programs encourage busyness in order to avoid the addictive behavior that causes so much harm. Many times this just becomes another addiction to replace the addiction that you are trying to get rid of. This technique might be beneficial in the short-term but ends up healing very little. Many 12-Step groups encourage a busy and structured life in order to keep you away from your addiction. The belief is that if you are busy doing something else, you will not have time to think about your addiction.

For example, newcomers to A.A. are urged to attend 90 meetings in 90 days. With this kind of schedule, who has time to drink? This might help you benefit while you go through the trauma of abstinence from alcohol, but it does not heal the core issues that might come up. This might help root you in a supportive structure for the time being. However, you end up numbing out your pain by keeping busy attending meetings. Whether it is 12-Step meetings or something else, you are being taught to avoid yourself by keeping busy. In *Understanding the Alcoholic's Mind*, Arnold M. Ludwig, M.D., writes, "If they keep busy not drinking, then they cannot keep busy drinking."

Distraction might keep you away from your addiction, but it does very little to encourage your "recovery." The only way to recover is to let go of the relationship that you have between your feelings and your addiction. Learning how to control your addiction by trying to stay busy will not do that for you.

2. Mind Techniques

All sorts of association tricks are used in "recovery" groups. These techniques are designed to help you stay in control, not to heal. If you erroneously believe that addiction is about loss of control, you might keep looking for something to help you stay in control. These techniques attempt to do just that. However, addiction is not about loss of control. It is about a faulty inner relationship requiring you to mood-alter.

A. Willpower

Be strong. Have a strong will. Be disciplined. This is what you are taught and it works moderately well for those who have a great amount of discipline in their lives. When you are taught to be strong and muscle your way through your addiction, what you are really learning is how to bury the pain even deeper. This technique has a high success rate for those *who are already addicted to control*. It is much more difficult for those who are not. People who have learned to shut out feelings are much more capable of staying in control. People who feel deeply will have less success with this technique.

B. Negative Association

This technique employs substituting images in place of your addiction. Unfortunately, you are never healed and have only developed another mind game that you play with yourself. For instance, learning to substitute the image of a cup of coffee every time you crave a martini has solved nothing. You are only manipulating symbols in your head. You might have learned how to control your behavior, but you have healed very little.

It is difficult, if not impossible, to imagine yourself *not* doing something. You are still haunted by the urges. Many people imagine themselves getting sick just before they are about to take a drink of alcohol. This technique might help stop some from taking that drink, but they have healed nothing. Associating other images for your addictive cravings does not heal the reason why you have the cravings in the first place.

3. Overindulgence

Some programs require you to consume large amounts of the food or chemical that you are addicted to. You begin to associate your addiction of choice with making you feel sick rather than the normal "high" that you are used to. Many programs to end smoking are like this. You begin to create a memory of how awful it feels to smoke. This might work to cure your habit of wanting to light up a cigarette, *as long as you remember how poorly the cigarette made you feel*. However, you are still masking a primary relationship with a substance in order to alter your moods. You have just learned a new technique to try to control your cravings, not to heal the faulty relationship.

4. Trading One Addiction For Another

Dr. Bob and Bill Wilson, the founders of A.A., were both heavy smokers. In fact, Dr. Bob died of emphysema, a smoking-related lung condition. It appears that both men might have let go of alcohol, but their cigarette smoking became even more important to them. They just traded one addiction for another.

If you are not conscious of what you are doing, you might just make this type of trade. For instance, many people who attend 12-Step meetings often become addicted to the meetings themselves. The philosophy and buzzwords of A.A. for example, become the new addiction for "recovering" alcoholics. These include phrases like the following; "Be positive," "Let go and let God," "One day at a time," "Fake it until you make it," "First things first," "Keep coming back; it works."

Instead of being addicted to "stinking thinking" as it is called, you now become addicted to "A.A. thinking." This is no accident. You might feel as if you are in a better place because you have learned to avoid alcohol (or cocaine, etc.), but you have just traded one addictive thought process for another. A.A. thinking now becomes the trance that you remain in to avoid your natural self. Anything that is continuously repeated in your mind over and over can easily become addictive. Thoughts about business, religion, spirituality, or even A.A. can become addictive thought patterns.

Instead of using alcohol to mood-alter, many times you might switch to another substance to alter your mood. You might need coffee, doughnuts or cigarettes to replace your alcohol. Chewing gum might be the oral fixation that you switch to in order to satisfy your need to have something in your mouth.

These techniques of trading one addiction for another will almost always occur if you do not heal the inner relationship that you have lost. If you have not healed from your pain, you will continue to replace one addiction for another. While the new addictions might be less harmful than the previous ones, this technique should only be looked at as a step until you are ready to confront *why* you are addicted in the first place.

5. Disempowerment

A.A. and other 12-Step programs take your power away. In fact, the *First Step* in most programs is to surrender away your power. It is very difficult to heal anything when you are disempowered. These programs take away your power and keep you imprisoned for your entire lifetime. There are no graduates. There is no hope of "full recovery." There is no moving forward. You are constantly reminded of how much you need the group. You are constantly reminded that you cannot do it alone and there is no cure for your "disease." You are reminded of how sick you are but not to blame yourself because it is your body's fault that your life is so out of control. Programs like A.A. do not want you to heal. They want lifetime members. They want you to stay dependent on them.

The authors of the *Guru Papers,* Joel Kramer and Diana Alstad, write,

"Yet leading a manageable life only through believing one is unalterably sick is a very limited view of recovery. If stability is dependent on continually acknowledging one's basic powerlessness, it is seriously flawed. What remains is the undying fear that one is untrustworthy at the deepest level."

When you are down and vulnerable, it is very enticing to grab onto a 12-Step support group. This then becomes your extended family. Most often you end up buying the entire package without questioning any of it. If you are looking for something to take away your pain, this is an easy trap to fall into. In fact, for many people religious conversion happens at this time as members surrender away their power completely. Many end up becoming religious addicts as another way to mood-alter.

For many, A.A. and other support groups provide structure in a world that may appear chaotic. There are "12-Steps" and "12 Traditions." There is regularity, dogma, ritual and support. When your best friend is taken away from you (alcohol, heroin, cocaine, etc.), it is easy to grab on to something else as a means to replace it. Much of the structure of a 12-Step group acts as a placebo. The actual content of a support group might not be what is important. The fact that those suffering from addiction have *something* to grab on to *is* important. Anything that appears to be structured seems attractive because the addiction has caused so much chaos. Most people in this position are willing to do whatever they are told in order to take away their pain, including giving up their personal power. Groups like A.A. are looking for vulnerable people who are willing to give up their power.

Specific Alcoholics Anonymous Myths

Treatment centers and support groups help to promote many myths concerning many different addictions. Most often these groups are still blaming a substance or a behavior instead of taking responsibility for an inner conflict. A.A. is no exception, but rather a leader in the myth-spreading department. Here are some of the myths that A.A. and other 12-Step groups continue to spread.

1. The Myth of Alcoholism As a Genetic Disease

The traditional beliefs about addictions that most people have been taught to believe are the result of scientists in a laboratory trying to analyze and uncover a belief in a theory of biological responsibility. Scientists in lab coats have come up with a truly remarkable tale of how your genetic material is responsible for your addictions. Having nothing more to grab on to than this well-funded campaign, most people have gone along with these rather remarkable myths created by these scientists.

Even though no genetic correlation has ever been found, A.A. continues to remind its members that it is not their fault that they cannot control their drinking. The dogma keeps telling you that alcoholics are "sick." Members are not referred to as "people who have a faulty relationship with alcohol to mood-alter." Rather, they are labeled as "alcoholics" suffering from the dreaded disease of "alcoholism." They are bombarded with the myth that this "disease is passed down from generation to generation and it is impossible to control oneself around alcohol once an alcoholic takes one sip of alcohol." Abstention is purported to be the only cure if you adhere to this myth.

In fact, A.A. is at the forefront of keeping people stuck by choosing language that keeps people sick. Members are not referred to as people. They are labeled as diseased persons. This stems from the close relationship that 12-Step groups have with Western medicine. In Western medicine, the medical doctor normally treats symptoms and not the whole person. The emotional life, relationships, family, movement patterns and ease of breathing are normally ignored as the patient now becomes the disease. The person becomes the "cancer patient" or the "brain tumor." Very seldom are you referred to as Sally Smith who is suffering from emphysema. In the Western medical system, you are more likely labeled as Sally Smith, the "lung problem."

If you were to use this same method of language to describe your faulty relationships and not dare claim any responsibility for them, you would create language that goes something like this. A person who works too much is called a "workaholic" and has a genetic disease called "workaholism." It is not his fault. He inherited it from his father. It is in his genes.

Someone who uses busyness to mood-alter would be labeled as a "busyholic" and forced to attend a treatment center for "busyholism." He would be required to attend regular meetings with other "busyholics" to keep his "disease" in check. He would never be allowed to be busy again.

Another person who uses intellectual thoughts as a way to numb out feelings now has a disease of "intellectualism" and is called an "intellectualaholic." Besides attending regular meetings he is required to abstain from all reading material for the rest of his life. Books, magazines, newspapers and computers are not allowed in his home. He is forbidden from going to bookstores and libraries. He must be especially strong and on guard when he goes to a public place that sells reading material. One slip-up could send him back into his dreaded disease again.

Still another uses excitement to change her moods and is labeled as an "excitementaholic." She suffers from "excitementaholism." She is not allowed to go on roller coasters, attend concerts or do anything that might activate her supposed genetic disease of "excitementaholism." You can use this same type of mythology and language as A.A. does to describe any of your addictive patterns, whether it is reading, gardening or stamp collecting. This type of thinking keeps you stuck and does nothing to encourage your healing.

A better approach to your addictions is to let go of the mythology and to change the language. Until someone finds a gene that can undoubtedly be linked to causing a specific addiction, it is best to stop telling people that they are sick because they have this mystery gene. I do not believe that this gene will ever be found, as diligently as scientific researchers keep trying. You need to change your language to language that empowers you. You might say something like the following, "I have an addictive relationship with alcohol, sweets, work, prayer, etc. which prevents me from feeling any pain." This last statement is empowering and allows you to heal much quicker. You are not blaming your genes or your body for the choices that you have made.

2. The Myth of "Once an Addict Always an Addict" and "Once an Alcoholic Always an Alcoholic"

If you believe the myth that there is no cure, then you will stop looking and accept what you are told. You will accept the myth that you are sick and will continue to lead your life that way. This is called "victim mentality." The A.A. way is to teach that there is no cure and that you will never, ever be able to drink alcohol, nor even think about alcohol again, without relapsing. According to A.A., abstinence is the only cure.

Joel Kramer and Diana Alstad write in *The Guru Papers*, "Unfortunately, the very belief 'Once an addict always an addict' is a self-fulfilling prophecy because it ensures self-mistrust, which keeps a divided self divided." Learning to trust oneself is essential in order to heal from addictions and to recover the natural self. Unfortunately, 12-Step programs do not teach you how to trust yourself. Rather, you are forever burdened with the task of giving away your power and trusting what the dogma of the support group is telling you.

Kramer and Alstad add, "The traditional family conditions obedience to authority by undermining self-trust. It is ironic that the so-called self-help programs with their 12-Steps create an extended family that does the same thing—undermine self-trust." This is a very critical part of healing and "recovery"—learning how to trust oneself. By their very nature, A.A. and other support groups are teaching you not to trust yourself. The same authors further add,—"Self-trust is gained only by experiencing positive change through utilizing one's feedback, which begins to break the loop where mistrust breeds mistrust."

A.A. teaches that "recovery" is a life-long process and that the cravings to drink will never go away. I do not agree. If you begin to discover and release with the underlying feelings that lead you to drink, you will recover. You need to begin to trust your feelings and your experience. You need to know that you will not die if a painful feeling arises. This is learning to trust yourself through positive feedback. The more you feel your feelings, the more you will trust yourself rather than run from your pain. A.A. and other programs teach you how to cope with your problem, not to recover from it.

With these programs you will carry the stigma of the "addict" your entire life. You will be called the "food addict," "the codependent," "the alcoholic" or the "sex addict." You will live your life "sick" if you continue to mistrust yourself and put your trust in these programs. This type of thinking, "once an addict always an addict," is exemplified by Arnold M. Ludwig, M.D., in his book, *Understanding the Alcoholic's Mind*. Ludwig writes about the addiction to alcohol, "If an alcoholic truly believes that under *no circumstances*, at *no time*, at *no place*, and with *no exceptions* do they have the option of returning to drink, then the voice of seduction will be completely stilled."

This is a classic example of someone continuing to spread the myth that since recovery from any addiction (especially alcohol) is impossible, you must learn how to contain it. Even worse, since most people are already trained not to trust themselves, when they hear such myths from someone with a medical credential, they tend to believe it even more.

3. The Myth That There Is a Difference Between "Alcoholics," Moderate Drinkers, Problem Drinkers, and Casual Drinkers.

Society has a very ill-conceived definition of "alcoholism." Our society at large still believes that such things as addiction to alcohol are genetic and lead "some" people to be unable to control their drinking. According to this belief, it is a person's genetic makeup that is creating the cravings that only large amounts of alcohol can eliminate. Only "some" people are rumored to have this defective gene, according to the myth. This myth is popularized by such people as Herbert Fingarette, who writes in *Heavy Drinking*, "According to the A.A. ideology, most people can drink socially without any problem. But some people have a unique biological vulnerability to alcohol and they develop a special kind of 'allergy.'"

These particular beliefs separate people into black and white categories. On one side, you are either "sick" and have this "allergy" that is rumored to be passed down in families. It isn't your fault and your body is to blame. The other side of the coin is that you are not an "alcoholic" but just tend to get out of hand with alcohol from time to time. You know how to control your alcohol usage. This exemplifies how many people have divided up their addictive behavior. I find it interesting to note that *even* Herbert Fingarette goes on to add in *Heavy Drinking*, "Almost everything that the American public believes to be the scientific truth about alcoholism is false."

Because the definition of what it means to be addicted is so out of line, many people continue to be stalled in their "recovery." If society states that someone who loses control with alcohol or who drinks in the morning is an "alcoholic," then the real issues will never be addressed. Addiction is not about your blood alcohol level or what time of day you take your first drink. Unfortunately, it is organizations like A.A. that keep promoting these myths and keep reminding you of how sick you are.

What is actually happening is that many people have learned how to drink in their families and in a culture that supports alcohol as a mood changer. Those labeled as "alcoholics" have chosen to create a faulty relationship with alcohol. But those who do not lose control with alcohol might still have a faulty relationship with alcohol. Even those who do not drink at all might use *not drinking* in order to numb out feelings.

As most "alcoholics" might have a primary relationship with alcohol, a "problem drinker" might have a secondary relationship with it. What this means is that he might really have a primary addictive relationship with something else, like work or perfectionism, and uses alcohol to numb out the pain caused by the primary relationship. Whatever the case, he has still granted permission for alcohol to be used as a way to moderate emotions.

It does not matter whether you use alcohol or any other drug or behavior to lose control with or just to "take the edge off." If you are using it to mask your pain, you are using it addictively. The quantity is not important. Whether your body suffers from physical dependency on alcohol does not matter. What is important is to understand *why* you might drink. A.A. does not address this. A.A. continues its campaign of myth-spreading.

4. The Myth that A.A. Is not a Religious Program

Of course A.A. is a religious program and has always been from the very beginning of its creation. For those who grew up in a Western, Christian-based culture, this is a very easy program to settle into. A.A. is structured just like a Western religion with dogma, ritual, prayer and the belief that you must be powerless in order to succeed. Just "have faith" is what you are told. This is similar to what most religions do to keep you from questioning the absurdities of the religion itself. The roots of A.A. are definitely Christian-based, using Christian symbols and not Jewish, Hindu or Buddhist in most instances.

A.A. claims to be a "spiritual" program, not a religious one. One could go on and on about what distinguishes religion from "spirituality." The bottom line is this—the structure is undeniably religious. At A.A. meetings, Christian prayers are recited. There is dogma (12-Steps and 12 Traditions) and an authoritarian emphasis. "Trust in the Big Book" is what you are told. Your ability to trust in yourself and question things is taken away from you (which is what most religions do as well). This authoritarian emphasis is similar to the Christian belief to trust in the Bible (and not your own inner wisdom).

When most people come to A.A., they are desperate and usually will accept most anything that A.A. has to offer. Down-and-out drinkers are not at a place to trust themselves. What A.A. does is the same thing that most religions do. They place themselves in an authoritarian position, take away your power and keep you from trusting yourself. If you question anything, you are shamed (which is what most religions do as well).

In fact, A.A. has just as many brainwashing techniques as any modern-day cult. Such constantly repeated slogans as "Keep coming back. It works" are part of the rhetoric. Because if it really did work, then you wouldn't need to keep coming back and they wouldn't need to try so hard to convince you.

A.A. does not encourage members to be self-reliant and trust themselves. It has its own propaganda. It is not open to criticism or to the media. It has an authoritarian controlled hierarchy (the Big Book). A.A. claims to have the "truth."

Joel Kramer and Diana Alstad write in *The Guru Papers*,

"Although overtly leaderless (actually old-time members assume leadership roles), A.A. shares many features of authoritarian cults: an unchallengeable written authority ("the Word"); commandments or rules to live by; a conversion experience achieved through surrender to a super-human power; and dependency on the group, which often undermines relationships with those who do not accept the sanctity of the 12-Steps. Disagreements with any of the Steps are labeled denial or resistance. Like other authoritarian groups that manipulate fear and desire, fear of leaving is instilled by the often-repeated warning 'You can't make it without us.'"

In *Alcoholics Anonymous: Cult or Cure,* Charles Bufe comments, "In every respect, A.A. orientation passes the duck test. If it looks like a duck, waddles like a duck, and quacks like a duck, it's probably a duck. In this case the "duck" is A.A.'s religious nature."

It seems that A.A. is popular with people who already have a religious background. James Christopher writes in *How to Stay Sober*,

"A.A. does reach religious persons, especially during this era of religiosity, and many are helped, if they buy A.A.'s rigid party line of turning their will and lives over to the care of God 'as they understand Him.' Unfortunately, neither willpower nor the belief in God will end our relationships with our addictions, no matter how much A.A. and similar groups lobby for such ideas."

In *Alcoholics Anonymous; Cult or Cure,* the following is one testimonial from an A.A. member. "It was a sort of magic formula of prayers, meetings, and shallow talk that was 'keeping me sober.'"

It is no secret that the founders of A.A., Dr. Bob and Bill Wilson, had strong religious affiliations. The probability of the two of them being religious addicts is very high. They went on to construct a religiously based self-help program that later came to be known as A.A. They both stopped using alcohol and started using religion as a means to mood-alter.

These were the beginnings of A.A., an ultra-rigid religious organization called the Oxford Group. In fact, Bill Wilson believed that alcoholism was the result of "sin." The concept of "sin" was a Christian concept, just like "karma" is an Eastern spiritual concept. What better way to relieve the guilt that your drinking was causing than to turn to religion as a means to deaden your pain?

5. The Myth of A.A.-Based Treatment Centers

As A.A. mythology continued to spread, treatment centers began to spring up all around. With the backing of famous celebrities and politicians' wives (most notably Betty Ford of the Betty Ford Center), these centers became very popular.

Insurance companies will pay for your "treatment" because you are labeled as being "sick" and now have a medical condition. Alcohol treatment alone has become a billion-dollar-a-year industry. These 28-day "treatment" programs as they are called, help you go through the physical pain of withdrawal from your regular drug of choice in a medically supervised environment. (That means the staff can give you medication if needed.) Some attempt at behavior modification is employed, and a minor exploration at uncovering the feelings that got you there in the first place is part of the program. However, the problems with "treatment" centers are many.

One problem in the traditional 12-Step group or 28-day detox centers is that the myth-spreading continues. Participants are still treated as people who are sick with an incurable disease. There is no responsibility placed on the choices that each individual has made as a way to mood-alter. Teaching participants to feel their feelings is altogether ignored. Detox centers have become institutionalized in our culture just like the Library of Congress and Disneyland.

The following are just some of the myths continuing to be spread by detox centers.

1. The blame is placed on the drug for the person's problems. Alcohol or drugs are not the problem; they are the symptoms. Being "clean" for 28 days will help very little in the long run to help you "recover" your

natural self. Treatment centers are still blaming a drug for your problem because they are coming out of the A.A. mentality and trying to cure you using medical science.

2. How do you teach someone to feel his feelings in 28 days who has been shut down and numb his entire life?

3. Many cross their fingers and hope that each person who is sent back into the world has developed enough addiction to control in order to stave off his "out-of-control" addiction. This is not "recovery." Outside the treatment facility, the real world can be an emotionally challenging place for many people. Keeping your fingers crossed is more like witchcraft and magic potions than verified "recovery." Why do you imagine that so many people slip up and wind up back in the program again?

4. The body and its holding on to frozen energy is all but ignored in most of these centers. How do you expect someone to stop smoking if she is in so much physical pain from the energy that she has stored over her lifetime? Sitting around in a group and talking will not release the years of repressed energy stored within the body that might initiate one to reach for her addiction as a way to numb out.

Summary

There is a heavy emphasis placed on "recovery" programs these days, from alcohol, sex, food, gambling, etc. These programs keep growing and expanding as the demand for them seems to increase. You often hear about celebrities and star athletes attending in order to "cure" their addiction. We continue to cross our fingers and hope that it works for them.

For millions of people, these programs have been a blessing and have rescued many lives from utter despair; but support groups and treatment centers are only the first step and should not be regarded as the goal in itself. They should be referred to as the first step in the "recovery" process. In and of themselves, they do very little to help one "recover" his natural self. Instead, these programs teach coping strategies that attempt to keep control over the addiction. Until you are willing to face your pain, you will need to continue to develop coping strategies. You will need to be on guard all of the time.

Addictions are not about the chemistry of your body but about faulty relationships. This is not a scientific question. The answer must come from someplace else. The answer will happen when you learn how to feel and express fully that which you are feeling in the moment. The answer will not come in a laboratory while watching a group of mice. The answer will come when we teach our children and ourselves how to feel our feelings fully. The answer will come when we begin to honor our relationship with nature.

The Myth of Positive and Negative Addictions

Society will help determine for you which addictions are more appropriate than others. Society says that it is better for you to be addicted to exercise than to drugs. Society praises you for your religious addiction yet scorns you for your gambling addiction. You are encouraged to sit in front of your computer for long hours and become information addicts, yet you are shamed if you have an addiction to food and cannot control your weight. Any addiction, whether regarded as positive or negative in the eyes of society, will lead to a loss of your natural self. That is why *all* addictions are damaging.

What are "negative" addictions and "positive" addictions? A negative addiction is believed to be something that goes counter to the values of society and brings shame and finger pointing. This might be something that you would try to hide. A negative addiction might cause a scandal.

How could a respected politician be caught on tape using all of those drugs? How could the president of the company be caught having an affair? An example of a negative addiction causing a scandal is when a well-known television evangelist gets caught in a sex scandal. His sexual addiction gets hold of him, and when this becomes public the whole Christian movement is stirred up. "How could this happen?" people ask. A favorite television star for children's programming is caught masturbating in an X-rated movie house. Another scandal is created. What, nobody ever masturbated before? No, but public figures are supposed to be able to stay in control of their addictions, or so we are taught. Whether it is sex, drugs, food or violence, a negative addiction is something that society frowns upon and might create a public scandal.

A positive addiction, on the other hand, would be something that society rewards you for having. Prayer, religion, caretaking, exercise and intellectualism are all behaviors that modern Western society rewards and could be used addictively. Each one of them also leads to a loss of the natural self when used addictively.

For instance, in our culture, you are encouraged to spend rather than to save. We live in a consumer society that supports spending. You are encouraged to spend and to be in debt to increase your credit rating. It is easy to see how one could use spending as a way to change his moods because the culture is rewarding him for doing so.

In the meantime, another positive addict would be the busy addict. He is productive and on the move all the time. He is accomplishing great things. He is also suffering from his inability to slow down. His immune system is broken down and he frequently gets sick because he does not know how to relax anymore. He sleeps poorly because his body is in distress. He does not eat right and uses many pills and nicotine to keep him on the go. He is headed for disaster.

In the same manner, the information addict has created quite a lifestyle around his information addiction. He spends long hours in front of his computer screen, including weekends and evenings at home. This leads to eyestrain and chronic neck stiffness. He does not know how to relax without seeking more information. He no longer is aware of his body because he spends so much time in his head.

Every addiction has harmful consequences. It does not matter if society rewards you or shames you for having that particular addiction. Society approves of some addictions and disapproves of others. Some consequences of your addictions are more damaging than are others. Some addictions may be hardly noticeable because there appears to be no outward or obvious harm done.

Many times feelings of guilt remind you of your addictions. You might spend addictively or cannot control your drinking once again. You are reminded by the moral code of your culture how low and despicable you are. Guilt keeps you in check that you might have a problem.

Addictions provide relief, comfort and a "high" feeling. Non-guilt producing addictions do the same thing, except you are rewarded to continue them. Whenever you are angry, you might go out and garden to numb out your anger. Whenever you are sad, you might listen to music to change your mood. You are highly encouraged to mask your feelings with what appears to be "positive" behavior. It is very enticing to be addicted to such positive things. This is especially true when there is no guilt attached to them.

Many people refer to non-guilt producing addictions as positive addictions. Many of these addictions are like a runaway freight train—there is no stopping them. For many people, guilt is like the brake on that runaway train. Without the guilt, the addictions are just free to race downhill at their own pace. You feel so proud when you are addicted to such things as religion, work, spirituality or rescuing others. Not only is there usually no guilt involved, but you are often highly rewarded. Addictions that produce little or no guilt are usually the hardest to heal from because there is no obvious reminder that you might have a problem. Yet those people with positive addictions rewarded by society can be suffering from just as much emotional pain as those with negative addictions.

We live in a society that encourages us to be addicted. Most people have a whole assortment of addictions, some viewed as positive and others viewed as negative (many times our secrets). Society hopes that you will choose those addictions that fit into the value system of your society. Those are the ones labeled as positive. A negative addiction is frowned upon because it goes against the values of society. If addiction is a "disease of a faulty relationship," then it seems that society tells you which diseases are okay for you to have and which ones are not.

Dr. Stanton Peele and Archie Brodsky (along with Mary Arnold), write in *The Truth About Addiction and Recovery,* that addicts come from people who have a low self-esteem. I disagree. Addicts come from people who cannot feel and release their feelings. That includes all of us. The authors claim that shopping addicts, gambling addicts, alcoholics and drug addicts all have a low self-esteem. These people have chosen an addiction that society looks down upon. However, even those with a high self-esteem are themselves addicts, maybe even more so because they deny that they even have a problem. These people are those addicted to what society wants them to be addicted to: perfectionism, overachievement, control and intellectualism. They might even be addicted to writing self-help books.

Many addiction "experts" believe that instead of filling yourself up with gambling, drugs or sugar, you should instead fill yourself up with poetry, literature, positive virtues and spirituality. This might be a step in reducing some of the harm done by other addictions, but you just become addicted to things that society values. This does not end the inner conflict of why someone becomes addicted in the first place.

Positive and negative addictions are just the labels that society places on your behavior based on the values that each culture feels are important. No matter what the case, addiction is still addiction, whether your culture approves of the addiction or shames you for having it. The following is an example of a positive addiction that is just as damaging as a negative addiction:

ORTHOREXIA NERVOSA

Many of the most unbalanced people I have ever met are those who have devoted themselves to healthy eating. In fact, I believe some of them have actually contracted a novel eating disorder for which I have coined the name, "orthorexia nervosa." The term uses "ortho," meaning straight, correct, and true, to modify "anorexia nervosa." Orthorexia nervosa refers to a pathological fixation on eating proper food.

Orthorexia begins, innocently enough, as a desire to overcome chronic illness or to improve general health. But because it requires considerable willpower to adopt a diet that differs radically from the food habits of childhood and the surrounding culture, few accomplish the change gracefully. Most must resort to an iron self-discipline bolstered by a hefty dose of superiority over those who eat junk food. Over time, what to eat, how much, and the consequences of dietary indiscretion come to occupy a greater and greater proportion of the orthorexic's day.

The act of eating pure food begins to carry pseudospiritual connotations. As orthorexia progresses, a day filled with sprouts, umeboshi plums, and amaranth biscuits comes to feel as holy as one spent serving the poor and homeless. When an orthorexic slips up (which may involve anything from devouring a single raisin to consuming a gallon of Haagen Dazs ice cream and a large pizza), he experiences a fall from grace and must perform numerous acts of penitence. These usually involve ever stricter diets and fasts.

This "kitchen spirituality" eventually reaches a point where the sufferer spends most of his time planning, purchasing, and eating meals. The orthorexic's inner life becomes dominated by efforts to resist temptation, self-condemnation for lapses, self-praise for success at complying with the chosen regime, and feelings of superiority over others less pure in dietary habits.

This transference of all of life's value into the act of eating makes orthorexia a true disorder. In this essential characteristic, orthorexia bears many similarities to the two well-known eating disorders anorexia and bulimia. Where the bulimic and anorexic focus on the quantity of food, the orthorexic fixates on its quality. All three give food an excessive place in the scheme of life.

Stephen Bratman, M.D.
Yoga Journal, Oct. 1997

Addictions come in many shapes and sizes. Unfortunately, each society will try to sway you as to which addictions are more appropriate to benefit the society. These are then labeled as "positive" or "negative." If you wish to heal entirely, you will need to address all of your addictions, including those that society encourages you to have.

Recovery from Addictions

Steps to Healing from Addictions

Healing from addictions can take many steps and much time. It is seldom a quick fix; it has to be a long-term goal. Healing from addictions is about healing from addictiveness and is not just about learning how to control a behavior or substance. Healing is about ending the cravings entirely and changing the faulty relationships that you have created in order to mood-alter. Healing is about getting to the root of the problem, individually and as a species.

In order to begin to recover your natural self, you must first remove the drug from your life that keeps you in your trance. Whether it is something that you ingest into your body, a behavior, a thought or a person, recovery of the natural self is impossible if you are still drugged. Healing from addictiveness is about being willing to face your pain. The following are some necessary steps required in order to heal from addictions.

1. Admit That You Have a Problem

The first step is to recognize that you might have a problem. Until this moment arrives, you will continue to live your life in denial and delusion. For some, this moment comes when the alcoholic wakes up in the gutter and finally realizes that alcohol is destroying his life. For others, it is when a relationship addict recognizes that she cannot live without a man in order to avoid her aloneness. It is when a gambling addict loses the house and car, and he finally wakes up to the fact that he has a problem. Until this time, you will continue to lie and deceive yourself.

By admitting that you have a problem, you are beginning to change what *normal* is. Until now, being addicted was normal. Running to the bar after a stressful day at work was normal. Binging on food when you are angry has come to be normal for you. Planting yourself in front of the newspaper when you feel depressed has been a regular part of your life. It has been normal for you to be addicted because you did not know any different.

It is also very important to name the problem. If you do not name it, then it will own you. However, if you give it a name other than what it actually is, then you will be heading off in the wrong direction. For instance, I have heard a number of people say that the root of their suffering is their *"spiritual emptiness."* I personally do not believe that such a thing exists. This is a very naive statement. What I notice is that the people who say this are not very aware of what they are feeling. Most likely they are feeling their fear of being alone or their shame of not being good enough. They give their "disease" the wrong name, so they seek out the wrong remedy. They go off in search of their spiritual "highs" when instead they should be learning how to feel their aloneness and their shame, two things that are distinctly very human. Coming out of denial means calling your addiction what it is. Stop calling your addictions your little vices or your spiritual bankruptcy. You need to own your faulty relationships with your own feelings and the addictions that you have created in order not to feel these feelings.

Many times it takes a good deal of pain to recognize that you might have a problem. You might look in the mirror and are aghast in horror as you finally notice your bulging waistline. The pain and reality might finally hit you. You now recognize that you have a problem with your relationship with food. Your pain has been a powerful motivation for you to change.

Recognizing that you have a problem and giving it the correct name are important steps in your recovery. Now you have something tangible to work with; your addiction is no longer some illusive monster that you cannot see. It now becomes something very real that you can begin to change. Naming your problem with the proper name helps to come out of your denial and accept yourself rather than live in a state of denial. You also now have a way to communicate with others and share your pain. This will help you to learn from others who have had a similar experience.

2. Accept the Consequences

Every addiction has consequences. One addiction might be damaging to your body while another addiction might put you in financial risk. Another addiction jeopardizes your personal relationships. The toxic chemicals that you have been putting into your body might be beginning to take their toll on you. Your lungs might be finally giving up due to the cigarette smoke that you continue to inhale. The alcohol might continue to eat away at your liver. You fall further and further into debt because you cannot control your spending that you use to numb yourself out. Your weight continues to climb because you cannot control your binging on food.

Whatever the addiction, the consequences of your addictiveness have begun to add up and are causing you to suffer. Recognizing the consequences of your addiction is a motivating factor to make you want to change. This will start to stir you into waking up. These consequences will start to cause you pain. When the pain is great enough, you might begin to make some changes. Until you can accept the consequences of your behavior, you will continue to act as a victim. Once you wake up and accept what you are doing to yourself, you will have a better chance at recovery.

3. Make a Commitment to Heal

In order to begin to heal, you need to first make a commitment. Recovery has to be something that you must want more than anything else. The type of commitment you make will help to determine what kind of actions you will follow. Is your commitment to make the pain go away or is the commitment to work through your pain?

Before you can change your commitment, you have to recognize the commitment that has already governed your life for so long. You have been committed to addiction and to running from your pain. Your previous commitment has been to keep you from feeling. It has been normal to be addicted and to run from your feelings. You have been committed to protecting your pain and to being comfortable. Your new commitment must be something that is not normal.

Whether you realize it or not, your commitment to yourself continues to run your life. When you go through traumatic events, you make commitments to never have to feel this pain again. For example, a child who feels isolation and aloneness might make a commitment at a very young age to never let anyone get close to her because it hurts too much. This commitment then continues to dictate her life. As an adult, she cannot understand why she cannot have a satisfying relationship. She does not remember the commitment she made as a child, but it is buried very deep within her and is still running her life.

Another child might experience the alcoholism in his family while growing up as a very scary and violent reminder. This pain and confusion might be so great that he makes a commitment to never touch alcohol and to never let go of control. This commitment then becomes part of him although it lies buried very deep within. As an adult, unaware of this earlier commitment, he cannot understand why he feels so different. He never likes to drink or be around others who drink. He feels anxious at parties with people "letting go" and being wild. He feels like he will get hurt if he lets go. He does not feel safe in these situations.

The same thing happens with your relationship with your addictions. You might make a commitment not to experience your pain and create an addiction to take its place. Most of this is all unconscious. You are committed to your chocolate doughnuts and your sports on television to numb out your feelings. You are committed to your computer games to numb out your loneliness before going to bed. You are committed to your workaholism by taking your work home and working any chance you can. You have made these commitments to yourself to not feel your boredom or loneliness. You have chosen to be committed to your addictions.

In order to recover from your addictions, you must make new commitments. By making a new commitment, whether a conscious statement to yourself or not, you begin to reverse the addiction trend. You need to make the choice to face your pain rather than to run from it when it comes up. You need to commit to wanting to heal.

Acknowledging the old commitments and where they came from is an important step in healing. Once you can begin to become aware of your actual commitment, you gain even more clarity in the types of steps needed in order to heal. You cannot change something until you accept it first. This step is important in taking notice of what your commitments are and then having the courage to make new commitments.

4. Seek Support

It is very difficult, if not impossible, to heal alone. Many people begin to recover from addictions by first entering a 12-Step support group, whether it is for alcohol dependency, drug use or food addictions. Others seek private therapy. Some choose to go away to an in-patient detox facility as a means of cleaning themselves out.

You all have to start somewhere. Unfortunately, a 12-Step group, private counseling or a detox center is only a beginning step in the healing process. It can be very important, nonetheless. You need to remove yourself from your drug of choice before you can begin to do your recovery work. You need to take a first step in a different direction. Unfortunately, most people never move beyond this first step. Many have a very misguided belief about recovery programs or detox centers. Most people believe that if they attend a group once a week, they will have their addiction licked. This is not recovery.

For instance, many people hold the myth that if they only get to a treatment center and the "treatment" holds, they will be "fixed" for good. Enough will happen in those 28 days for them to go home cured and able to go on with their lives. So the myth goes. A common phrase heard in Southern California, referring to a well-known treatment center, is, "Oh, he went to Betty Ford. He's okay now." Unfortunately, this is also a myth that many want to believe. It is not that simple.

Twenty-eight days at a detox center with physicians and counselors is only a quick fix. During this short period of time, you do not even come close to getting to the source of your pain. Nor do you fully learn how to feel your feelings. After the 28-days are over, then where is the support in your daily life? You might receive education about drugs, stress management, medication and relaxation techniques. What happens when you go out into the real world? When you are overwhelmed by your feelings after having a bad day at work, then what happens to you? Your feelings might feel as if they are going to kill you.

Most treatment centers are aimed at cleaning out your body for 28-days and hoping that you will acquire new coping skills. Detox centers and 12-Step groups still want to blame a drug for your addiction. Cleaning a drug out of your body *may* be an important first step for some people. Once you have decided to remove yourself from your primary drug of choice, whether it is alcohol or prayer, then the real work begins.

Addictions are much larger than chemicals. You must take what you learn and begin to apply it to your daily life. Finding support is a critical first step. A detox center, private counselor or support group are helpful beginning steps. Just having supportive family members or friends can greatly help you in your recovery. Often, these are the people whom you are closest to who will support you even when the times are rough. Your friends and family might offer you long-term support, which is essential. Short-term support, like a counselor or 12-Step group, will help you through the beginning crisis of transition to a healthier self. Long-term support will carry you through on the darkest of days.

5. Have a Plan

In order to change your addictive lifestyle, it is important to develop a strategy or a plan that you can follow. Do you quit "cold turkey" or do you remove yourself from your addictions in stages? For many addictions, it is necessary to stop completely in order to begin the healing process. For other addictions, a gradual withdrawal is more effective. For some addictions, where total abstinence is not possible (as with some food addictions), learning how to stay in control might be the first step to recovery. Each person will create a different strategy for each addiction.

For some, quitting smoking is best accomplished by going "cold turkey." Put down the last cigarette, throw away the pack and be done with it. You might have to muscle your way through the withdrawal symptoms. For these people, a strong will helps them to stop their addiction. Many times, this type of person will trade the "high" of smoking for the "high" of staying in control. A person who uses the "cold turkey" approach usually will use distraction techniques. He finds other hobbies or vices to distract himself from the addiction that he is attempting to quit.

For others, a gradual approach to addiction elimination is more effective. This method reduces the shock and produces smaller amounts of discomfort at a time. For instance, you might gradually reduce your cigarette consumption down to less and less until you eventually smoke no cigarettes at all. You might use nicotine gum or a nicotine patch until you slowly wean yourself off nicotine altogether. You then might begin a vitamin, herb or nutritional program to cleanse your body of all nicotine.

For some addictions, such as alcohol, it is difficult to begin the process of healing until you have completely removed yourself from your addiction. This is an important process because many of your addictions cause unclear thinking and you cannot begin the inner process until you have halted the outer process. For other addictions, it is possible to continue with the behavior as you begin to heal the inner relationship.

For example, with an addiction to food, you cannot stop eating. Eating still needs to happen for your survival. In this case, a plan must be installed that would allow you to continue eating as you begin to heal your inner relationship with food. You might need to learn how you can control food as a short-term goal as you learn how to feel your trapped feelings inside of you as a long-term goal. For some, *Weight Watchers* or *Overeaters Anonymous* become the short-term support while they begin to process why they continue to use food to mood-alter.

In order to recover from addictions, you must be committed and develop a healing strategy. You must make a commitment to follow that plan. This will give you structure and guidelines in order to follow and measure your progress. It will help if you can measure your progress. You might look to see that you only smoke 5 cigarettes a day rather than three packs of cigarettes. You might recognize that you can eat a carrot rather than a candy bar in order to stave off your hunger. This is progress.

Delaying the time period from when you become overwhelmed by your feelings and when you reach for your addiction will demonstrate progress for you. For instance, if you encounter a situation that causes you to be angry, you might want to reach for your addiction, whether it is a romance novel or brownie to quench your anger. If you delay reaching for your addiction for as long as possible, you will demonstrate progress. The more time you can sit with your feelings, the more growth you can measure, even if it is only five minutes at a time. This might be part of your healing strategy. Your strategy then might become to see how long you can experience your uncomfortable feelings before you reach for your addiction of choice.

Take one addiction at a time. It is overwhelming to be stripped of all your coping skills at one time. You might begin with the one that seems to be the most damaging. If your addiction to relationships with people seems to be the most damaging to you, then you might begin there. If your rage addiction causes you the most harm, then that might be a good place to start. It is important to take one addiction at a time so that you are not so overwhelmed. Begin by listing all of your addictions so that you can recognize them and eliminate the ones causing the most damage.

Whatever course you take in your healing, it is important to have a plan. You need to follow a set of guidelines to mark your progress. For some, the plan will be to eliminate your addictions in stages. For others, an abrupt stoppage will work better for you. No matter what approach you may take, it is important to follow a plan to help guide you along the way.

6. Reduce the Damage: Harm Reduction

All addictions cause damage as emotional energy is repressed and there is a loss of the natural self. Some addictions cause further damage as well. One step in the recovery process is to use the "harm reduction" technique. An important step in the healing process is to begin to reduce the damage, physical or otherwise, done by your addictions. This technique never heals you from your addictions but helps to lessen the damage caused by them. It is a step in the right direction.

For instance, if you eat sweets in order to numb out any pain or uncomfortable feelings, then you might find yourself substituting a carrot stick or other raw vegetable in its place. If sweets are causing you damage (tooth decay, sluggishness, excess weight gain, etc.), the raw vegetable will help to alleviate some of the damage done by the sweets. The carrot stick, however, might be just a short-term solution that keeps you chewing on something until the fear or loneliness subsides. You are still using food as a mood enhancer. However, you are practicing a "harm reduction" technique. The source of the addiction has still not been addressed, but some of the damage has been curtailed.

Another example of a "harm reduction" technique would be if someone got off drugs only to replace them with exercise as a way to mood-alter. This might be a much healthier addiction for the body and in the eyes of society. This could be a beginning step because you are now doing less harm to the body. This is an example of how a positive addiction is used to replace a negative addiction with the "harm reduction" strategy.

There has been a widespread program in effect for some years to help heroin addicts remove themselves from heroin. These drug addicts are given an oral dosage of a drug called methadone, which has a similar chemical make-up as heroin. Methadone keeps the heroin addict from feeling any physical or emotional pain associated with the withdrawal symptoms, but he does not get chemically "high" as he would with a heroin injection. This is another method of "harm reduction" because it helps keep addicts from sneaking around in alleys, possibly sharing needles and spreading infectious diseases.

Wearing a nicotine patch or chewing nicotine gum are other examples of "harm reduction" techniques. Instead of suffering the harmful effects of introducing nicotine into the body by way of the lungs, you are now ingesting nicotine into the body through your skin. You are eliminating the harmful effects of cigarette smoke into your lungs (and perhaps saving your lungs and your life), but you are still using nicotine as a mood changer. Nicotine patches spare smokers the effects of bronchitis, lung cancer and emphysema while still keeping the body toxic with nicotine.

In *Addiction: From Biology to Drug Policy*, the author, Avram Goldstein, M.D., writes,

"If a person who is smoking 30 cigarettes daily reduces that to 29, and maintains the new level, that smoker has actually accomplished a 3% reduction in the health hazards of the addiction. Then if even a single additional cigarette is removed permanently from the repertoire each week, in four months the health hazards will be reduced by half. Such a program requires self-conscious analysis and modification of one's own behavior. One conditional association trigger at a time has to be eliminated, by repeatedly skipping the cigarette associated with that trigger; that is the classic method of extinguishing a conditional behavior."

David Krogh writes in his book *Smoking: The Artificial Passion* about how nicotine gum is used to replace addiction to cigarette smoking.

" . . . *smokers will often become dependent upon the fix they obtain from the gum and will remain attached to it for many months. Still, if it breaks the ritual of smoking, it is worth the dependency.*"

The authors of *From Chocolate to Morphine*, Andrew Weil, M.D., and Winifred Rosen, write,

"*Tobacco addicts who give up smoking by becoming compulsive joggers may not be any freer, but they may live longer, be healthier, and feel better about themselves.*"

If this is true, then what many are willing to do is to become dependent on something else in hopes of reducing the damage done by the original addiction. Unfortunately, unless you get to the heart of your bottled up feelings, you will not resolve your addictiveness. You will just be trading one addiction for another. This can be a valuable step to reduce the damage caused by your addictions, but it should not be the ultimate goal.

Is it better to be addicted to television, exercise, reading, shopping, eating or working? You are the only one who could know how much possible harm each addiction is causing you. A compulsive runner may be causing more harm to herself than a cigarette smoker. (This is apparent when you notice the worn out joints of a compulsive runner). Choosing an addiction that does less harm is not the ultimate answer, but it might be a step in the right direction.

A step in your healing is to begin to reduce the harm done by your addictions. Reducing the damage that you are causing to yourself and others is important for the progress of your recovery.

Learning Control and Behavior Modification

Part of the harm reduction strategy is to learn to control your addiction if it is causing harm to you or to others. Learning how to modify your behavior is an important component in this process. By reprogramming your behavior, you are taking a step in the right direction, but that step in itself is not enough to heal. It is only a beginning in reducing the damage. The ultimate goal is to heal the faulty relationship, not to learn to stay in control. Sometimes you must first learn how to control your addiction before you can go on to heal.

Unfortunately, many people have been taught to believe that learning to control their addiction is the goal. It is not. Willpower and sobriety are just measures that keep you trying to control your addiction. It is almost like trying to muscle your way through your addictions. You then become (or already have been) addicted to control in order to not feel.

Attempting to control your addictions is the "dry drunk" approach. You might have ceased the behavior of drinking alcohol but you still think and act like an alcoholic. Unfortunately, most people have learned how to control their addiction under the most ideal conditions. When your stress level is elevated, you tend to have a more difficult time controlling your addictions. However, you rarely have ideal conditions.

Control and reprogramming do not heal addictions, but might be a step in reducing the harmful effects of addictions. Recovery from addictions is not about learning how to stop a craving from happening; it is about understanding why you have those cravings in the first place.

The following is an example of a woman who attempted a behavior modification technique to rid herself of her chocolate addiction. She attended a Shick Center and was administered a low-level shock while being forced to eat lots of chocolate. She was made to spit out the chocolate while watching herself in the mirror. She soon developed a revulsion for chocolate.

This is an example of a behavior-modification technique. Her cravings for chocolate might have diminished, but she never healed from the unresolved feelings that made her crave chocolate in the first place. In her particular case, she stopped craving chocolate as she just transferred one addiction for another. She later found yet another addiction to numb out her pain because she never went inside of herself to heal where the pain was coming from. She says in *From Chocolate to Morphine,* "I suppose I could get hooked again if I worked at it, but even though I test myself occasionally, my indifference to it remains the same." But she goes on to add, "The only problem now is, I am now addicted to cake (though somewhat less severely)."

It is important to begin to reduce the damage that your addictions are causing, whether it is reprogramming, control, sobriety, behavior modification or changing from a negative addiction to a positive addiction. These are methods of harm-reduction techniques, and while a step in the right direction, they should not be the ultimate goal. Unfortunately, most people who attempt to do something about their addictions never make it past this step.

7. Reduce Sabotage

In order to recover from your addictions, you must make a commitment to want to change and make a concerted effort to do so. For this to happen, you must reduce your own attempts to sabotage your healing.

The mind is very sneaky and cunning. The mind believes that it is in control. Most people attempt to play games with themselves much of the time. Sometimes you appear to be committed to healing, but your real agenda is something else. Many times you set yourself up to sabotage your recovery unless you make a conscious choice to heal.

For instance, when you are trying to eliminate your sweet addiction, you might continue to buy your favorite sugary snacks and hide them all over the house. These are "just in case" you cannot stand the cravings anymore. When you do this, you are just setting yourself up to fail at your recovery.

Another way that you might try to sabotage your recovery while trying to eliminate your addiction to alcohol is continuing to go by the "old watering hole" from time to time to visit your old drinking buddies. You might just plan on having a soft drink or two. Just being in this familiar place with a familiar crowd might be enough to set off your drinking again. You are setting yourself up for sabotage and are creating a world of temptation.

Your addiction is linked to specific cues. A person addicted to alcohol might be drawn to drink at the smell of alcohol or just by being around a familiar drinking group. Addictions form mini-communities and well-rehearsed cues. In order to be successful at recovery, you must remove yourself from the people, places and ideas that go along with your addiction. This might mean that you would have to change your friends, central activities, and social circles. Your whole lifestyle might need to be disrupted. If you are true to yourself about wanting to heal, to be effective it is important to surround yourself with others who have a similar goal. Otherwise, you are just setting yourself up for sabotage.

You must stop stockpiling the sweets or alcohol in case you get an urge. You must remove yourself from any temptation. Your traps and self-deception need to be eliminated. Up until this point, much of your time, energy and thoughts have been consumed with your addiction. Your addiction has been a major investment in your life. In order to heal, you might need to refocus all that time and energy in a different direction. You may need to seek a different group for support. You may need to start a hobby or exercise program to refocus your energy while you learn to heal your inner feelings that have remained blocked for some time. You must make an effort to begin to feel the feelings that have drawn you to wanting to be numb.

Recovery is not flawless; we all have slips. Most people have a tendency to return to what is normal (their addictions) when the emotional pain is unbearable. The more time you spend away from your addictions, the more foreign they will feel to you. After a while, you may not even want that glass of wine or that jelly doughnut anymore because it does not feel right. What begins to feel right is the time you spend with your feelings.

In order to arrive at this place of empowerment, it is important to reduce as many temptations along the way as you can. For some people, recovery might seem like two steps forward and one step backward. It is important to keep taking the steps, reducing the risks of sabotage and remaining pointed in the right direction.

Recovery often is like a balancing scale. The more work you do in recovering your feelings, the more the scale tips away from addiction and toward recovery of the natural self. The more experience you have with recovery, the more weight is added to your scale to tip it in your favor. Reducing the risks of sabotage greatly helps in the recovery process.

8. Cleanse the Body

For some addictions, your body pays a heavy price. Many people create physically debilitating conditions and ingest large amounts of toxins. In order to get to the deeper inner work, it is important to begin to cleanse the body of harmful toxic residue created by your addictions. It is important in these cases not only to stop using the harmful substance but also to begin reversing some of the damage that has already been caused.

Some of the ways to begin a cleansing program utilize herbs, vitamins, massage, nutritional awareness, yoga or exercise. The way you cleanse your body will tend to vary from person to person and from addiction to addiction. In order for you to address your deeper-feeling issues that have led to your addictions, you will need to detoxify your body and help to clear your mind.

Herbs are important because they can use nature's own healing power to cleanse the liver, lungs and other important organs, glands and body systems to bring you back into balance. If the body is not too far out of balance, most often it can repair itself with the right treatment.

Vitamins can be very important also. They help you to begin the repair work on necessary organs that have been affected by your addictions. Many substance addictions deplete your body of the necessary vitamins that you need. When reversing the harmful effects of your addiction, it may be helpful to take additional vitamin supplements to help speed up this process. A healthy diet will provide most of the vitamins that your body will need to function properly and to repair the damage.

Your liver or other organs may need to be strengthened because of years of alcohol poisoning. Your lungs might need to be cleansed because of the cigarette smoke that has damaged them. Your immune system might need to be rebalanced because your addiction to busyness has wreaked havoc on your adrenal glands.

Massage therapy is another important remedy to help reduce the negative consequences of your addictions. Massage helps one to relax and counters the ill effects of stress, which is how most people become addicted in the first place. Massage therapy also helps to increase circulation, improves lymph flow to carry away toxic-waste products and creates an overall sense of well being. If you are feeling good in your body, it is much less likely that you will reach for an addiction.

Many substance addictions help deplete your body of essential nutrients. Improving your diet is essential too. For instance, many alcoholics do not eat correctly. Their bodies are lacking many nutrients. A healthy nutritional program is essential to recover from your addictions, especially from substance addictions. After years of neglect, your body may need a nutritional program to strengthen and repair the damage.

Yoga or movement therapy is important to bring you back into awareness of your body. Yoga, for instance, helps you to breathe better, increases your energy and helps to create more flexibility so that you may have joy in your movement. This is important because your body may have been very toxic for a long time. An exercise program will help you to improve your body tone, heart rate and confidence about yourself. It is important for you to keep moving your body while you recover from your addictions.

Cleansing your body further enhances your recovery. It will help your mind to be clearer so that you can address the deeper issues that you will need to face. You will feel better about yourself and have a stronger foundation in which to continue your recovery.

9. Come Out of Your Trance

When you are acting addictively, you are in a trance; you are not your spontaneous and natural self. Most of your addictions have become very unconscious because they are part of your normal routine. You can perform them with your eyes closed.

For instance, you might come home from a stressful day at work and you immediately sit down to read the newspaper and have a drink. You use the behavior of reading and drinking to numb out any repressed feelings associated with your stress. This behavior is very automatic. You do not even realize that you are doing it.

Most people eat, work, shop and have sex most of their lives very unconsciously. They do not stop to ask "why?" anymore. Addictions have become what seems to be a normal trance that they continue to fall into.

Your trance is an altered state of consciousness. It is a state that you create in order to avoid your pain. It is important in your recovery to recognize the trance that you are in and to bring yourself out of it. Your trance helps to dictate your addictions and it is where you spend the most time. You might have a trance where you spend most of your time in your head, thinking of songs to sing. You could be in another trance of always making up and rehearsing jokes in your head so that you are thinking in jokes all the time. Your trance might be a mantra that is constantly repeated in your head. In order to bring yourself out of your trance, you must learn how to feel your feelings.

Unfortunately, over the course of human history, many people were led to believe that altered states of consciousness are a virtue to be sought after. Any state of mind can be used in order to keep you away from your natural self. When your states of consciousness are nearly always the same without fluctuations, they are most often being used as an addiction to avoid a feeling.

In order to heal from addictions, it is important to come out of your trance. Most of the time you do not even realize that you are in a trance. When you are truly acknowledging your feelings, you are being real. When you are being addictive, you are running from your feelings into a trance state. When you can recognize that you are not in your addiction trance, you will have an important reference point in which to work from.

10. Notice the Type of Addiction That You Are Using

When learning how to heal from your addictions, it is extremely important to recognize what type of addiction you are using—whether it is a thought, behavior, feeling, object or a person. It is also important to notice which feeling you are attempting to numb out. Is it loneliness, fear, anxiety or grief? When you can do this, you can establish your faulty relationship between your feelings and your addiction.

Up until this stage, you have been very general about your addictions. Now you need to become much more specific. Are you addicted to everything that is made of chocolate or just certain kinds of chocolate? Does anything that is sweet and chewy change your mood or is it more specific than that? What are the qualities of your addiction? Do you light up a cigarette only after meals or only in the car? Do you only drink alcohol on weekends? Can you not live without your *People* magazine?

Begin to be more specific with your addictions. Are you addicted to all sweets or only chocolate? Is shopping an addiction for your or only shopping for clothes? Do you just buy expensive clothes or are you addicted to bargain shopping? Is the act of buying shoes something that gives you a "high"? (Imelda Marcos, the wife of the former president of the Philippines, was rumored to have 5000 pairs of shoes.) Notice the qualities about your addictions as if you were noticing a lover. What is so attractive to you? What bonds you to your addiction? What keeps you coming back for more?

Notice the different categories of addictions. Begin to be more specific.

a) People Addictions: Are you addicted to a particular person? A relative? A celebrity? A lover? A child?

b) Object Addictions: Drugs, alcohol, cigarettes, food, cars and baseball cards. You name it. Any object can be used addictively.

c) Behavior Addictions: Which behaviors do you use to hide your feelings? Sex? Gambling? Sports? Codependence? Work? Religion? Gardening? Control?

d) Thought Addiction: Begin to notice your thoughts that you use to mask your feelings. Do you think about children when you are sad? Do you think about spiritual thoughts in order to not feel your loneliness? Are you always thinking about another cause to save in order to not feel your anger? Are your addictive thoughts in the past or in the future? Do you constantly think thoughts that are outside of yourself (like of nature), or are you drawn to thoughts within yourself (like observing the breath traveling through your nostrils)?

e) Emotion Addiction: Do you use anger to hide fear or sadness to mask anger? Do you constantly feel fear when you are really depressed? When you feel anger and hate, do you try to change it into love and compassion? Do you use one emotion to mask another emotion?

Begin to explore your relationship with your feelings. Are you a person who is uncomfortable in expressing your feelings? Were you taught to believe that it was not okay to have feelings? Are some feelings acceptable to feel while others are taboo?

Stop the secrets. Stop lying to yourself about your addictions. Acknowledge that you have a problem. Tell someone about it. Seek therapy or a support group. If you keep your addictions a secret, even to yourself, you remain trapped.

Take note about how often you think about your addiction throughout the day. See how your addiction has become your best friend. You are willing to do anything for your addiction. Become curious of how you are willing to defend your addiction at all cost. "No, I'm not an alcoholic," or "I only eat a little sugar!" Notice how you hide your addiction as if it were your own secret stash.

It is also important to recognize what triggers your addiction. Does feeling rejected by a lover cause you to race for the refrigerator? When your boss yells at you, do you run outside for a smoke? Is it an actual event, memory or a negative thought (worry) which first triggers your addiction?

Begin to recognize your addictions as the faulty relationships they are. Addictions are nothing more than a faulty relationship that you develop in order to avoid your pain. Notice what it is like to have a healthy relationship with food, for example. You automatically know when to stop eating. You only eat when you are hungry. A faulty relationship with food occurs when you continue to eat and never feel filled up. Recognize the pain that you are trying to hide with food.

Do you have a healthy relationship or a faulty relationship with exercise? Do you head for the gym when you are feeling lonely or angry instead of learning how to feel your feelings? Do you shop for what you need or shop to change your moods?

Do you have one particular addiction that you spend more time with than others?. Notice how much time you spend with your addictions. Notice how familiar you are with your addictions. Pay attention to patterns of when your addictions are more prevalent for you.

Make friends with your addictions. Acknowledge their existence. Turn your guilty feelings into a positive relationship. Thank your addictions for helping to keep you from feeling pain. Say, "Thank you Mr. Potato Chip for not letting me feel lonely today." Be grateful for the act of meditation to numb out your anger. See how addictions have helped you to survive in the world. Make contact with your addictions and let them know that you do not just want to survive anymore—you want to really live. Thank your addictions for the job they have done, because you will be seeing less of them.

Notice when you are feeling addicted and when you are not feeling addicted. Give yourself praise when you are not addicted and forgive yourself when you are using something addictively. Notice when you are being addictive and when you are not. Praise yourself when you make good decisions and forgive yourself when you make poor decisions.

11. Trace the Origins of Your Addiction

In order to better understand how you develop faulty relationships with your addictions, it may be helpful to try to remember when and where your addiction first began. Perhaps you started smoking in high school when you were feeling very angry and controlled. Your addiction to fantasy may have begun as far back as grade school when you learned that if you fantasized during class, all of your emotional pain would go away. Your addiction to animals may have begun when you were feeling the most alone, perhaps feeling isolated growing up or after the death of someone close to you. What type of pain were you in when you first began your addiction?

By piecing together when and how you developed your addictions, you will be better able to understand what your addictions mean for you. Notice if the addiction is a primary addiction or a secondary addiction used to cover up something else. Your addiction might be something relatively new or a very old friend in your life. Notice if you just transfer one addiction for another. Perhaps by giving up cigarettes, you became addicted to exercise in order to numb out your pain.

Your addictions recall the story of your life. They are as broad and wide ranging as there are people. No two people's addictions are alike as no two people have the same story. The history of your addictions is the history of your inability to express your feelings. Tracing this path back to where and when it started could be very helpful in healing.

12. Take Responsibility and Stop Blaming

Healing from your addictions begins when you take responsibility for yourself and stop blaming others. You heal when you change your thinking about your addictions. Addictions are not just about chemicals or self-destructive behavior. Addictions are about inner relationships that need to heal.

You heal when you stop punishing others for the addictions they have chosen. This helps to stop the finger pointing and begins the process of looking at yourself. You heal when you stop calling your addictions a character defect or a genetic inheritance. In the Middle Ages, addictions were called a "sin" and people were punished for having them. Many continue to punish others for having addictions. Those who use street drugs are called criminals because they have chosen an addiction that society does not support. Society has an unusual way of punishing you for some addictions while rewarding you for others. The healing process involves being willing to accept your addictions as your own. Nobody gave you any addictions nor caused you to be addicted. You did it to yourself. When you can begin to accept this and take responsibility for your addictions, you have taken a very big step in your recovery.

13. Practice Feeling

There is really only one way out of addictiveness—learning how to feel and release your feelings. It takes a courageous person who is willing to feel and acknowledge his inner world, something that is still not completely socially acceptable. Just as you are engaged in the outer world with jobs, families and relationships, you also have the same depth of relationship with your inner world. By practicing your feelings, you will begin to tip the scale of addictions in your favor.

EPILOGUE

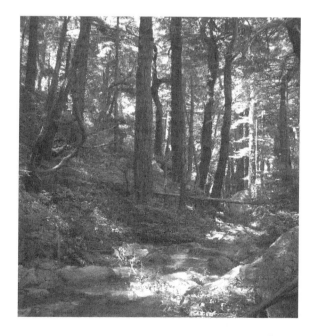

Putting It All Together

Many of you will be charting very unfamiliar territory as you begin the recovery of your natural self. You might want to know what each one of **The Five Pillars of Healing** looks like and how much success others have had with them.

Each person will place the emphasis where it is needed. If you are in extreme physical pain, you might start with a commitment to recovery of the body and receive regular bodywork. Others might start to eliminate some of the most damaging addictions in their life. Everyone will begin at a different place in hopes of achieving the same results—the recovery of the natural self.

Recovery is a dynamic process. It is a process of unraveling the mystery of who you are as a human being. Recovery teaches you about your passions as well as your dark side. When you enter into the process of recovery, you begin to understand all of who you are. Recovery is the journey of understanding your self.

We are living in a dynamic time of change. Up until this point on the planet, our species has been concerned with just trying to survive. We have spent much of our energy and time fighting off disease, harsh weather and wild animals. For many people, this is beginning to change. We now have the time, energy and freedom to delve deeper and to begin to reclaim the natural self. Recovery work is impossible if you are still trying to meet your survival needs.

In trying to describe what recovery is, you need to identify what it is that you are trying to recover from or what was lost. Essentially, through the process of your birth, your childhood and your upbringing, you have lost your natural self. The self that nature intended is gone. You have lost your ability to be spontaneous with your feelings. You have lost your voice. You have lost your freedom of movement. You have lost your breath. You have become stiff, rigid and compacted. Numbness has become the standard way to experience the world. Feelings and sensations have become your most bitter enemies. You have lost your relationship with what is natural.

Recovery of the natural self is about learning how to unblock the repression that you have created to keep yourself locked up. I have heard it said, "If you can survive your childhood you will spend the rest of your life recovering from it." There is a lot of truth to this, but I do not believe that it has to be the rest of your life if you make a concerted effort.

Recovery is *not* about learning to stay in control of your addictions or to be sober. Recovery is not about attending any group for the rest of your life because someone has labeled you as being *sick*. Recovery is not about continuing the same old patterns. Recovery is about growing and making real changes. Recovery is about dismantling the coping mechanisms that have held you tight. Recovery is not needing to be on guard anymore because you are terrified of the power a substance has over you.

Recovery of the natural self is a very dynamic process. There are many aspects to recovery and many pieces that need to be addressed. Recovery can be a very methodical, step-by-step process, which one employs to regain his relationship with nature. It is this process that can be regarded as the life journey; to regain what has been lost. There is no greater journey than to begin the journey of recovery.

Recovery Is About Learning Self-Responsibility

Most often, someone did not come and take something away from you. It was not your parents' lack of knowledge of your needs that created your lost natural self. Your teacher did not cause you to repress your feelings when he hit you with the ruler. Yes, most of us were assaulted, attacked and physically or emotionally abused in one way or another. It is your responsibility to release the energy of these assaults, set clear boundaries and expand in your growth.

You created your own repression and learned how to hold on even tighter. It was you who caused your breathing to become shallow. It was you who learned how not to move. It was you who learned how to hold your muscles tight and keep your mouth clamped shut when you were in fear. You did it, and you did it for a very good reason. You did it in order to survive.

Yes, things happened to all of us. We all experienced abuse. We all have experienced trauma. We all had injustices done to us. We all have had heartaches, disappointments and pain. We all have had to feel suffering at one time or another. There is no one to blame. Placing blame on someone else will get you nowhere. People who are hurting and repressed end up hurting and repressing others. It is a vicious cycle that has gone on for too long. This is not to say that it is okay to let others hurt you or abuse you. No, that is not acceptable. You need to set boundaries with others and protect yourself from further wounding. It is not okay to just forgive someone without first grieving the hurt that was done to you. This is an act of denial. It is this inability to grieve your losses and let go of them that is the source of most of your pain. It is not about blaming anyone else. Recovery is about learning to take personal responsibility for yourself and move on.

Addressing False Beliefs

Recovery means learning to unravel the mystery of your false beliefs. What is a natural belief and what is a false belief? Nature created natural beliefs. Humans created belief systems that in turn created false beliefs. Recovery means taking the responsibility to take back your belief systems. Governments, churches, militaries and gender roles have taken away many of your natural beliefs only to replace them with false beliefs. It is these false beliefs that led to your stress, repression, and addictions.

Recovery means being willing to confront the source of these unnatural beliefs. Being told that crying is for "sissies" is an unnatural belief. Recovery means being courageous enough to change this belief for yourself. Being told that idleness is "sinful" is an unnatural belief. Recovery is challenging this belief system and returning to what is natural. Living life as a victim no longer becomes acceptable. If your role in life has been to be the surrogate wife for your father and to mother your brothers and sisters, then recovery means to stop playing that role and establish healthy boundaries.

Recovery of the natural self is a process of beginning to identify which false beliefs cause the stress in your lives. Is the stress an actual life-threatening event or is the stress an imaginary life-threatening event based on a false belief that you have about yourself?

You might feel as if you are swimming upstream when you first begin to address these false beliefs and those institutions that created them. Recovery is not always going to be an easy journey. Your false beliefs have been with you for a very long time and seem like the only sense of normalcy for you. One of the qualities of a repressive system is its resistance to change. There are challenges ahead; replacing your false beliefs with natural beliefs may be one of these challenges.

Reclaiming the Body

A repressive system creates repression in the body. You lose your ability to breathe fully. You lose your ability to move freely. You are contracted in your stress response or you have left your body behind entirely. Recovery of your relationship with nature is learning how to reclaim your body. It is about learning to unblock the dams that have kept you frozen.

Muscles and tendons need to be relaxed and softened because of years of contraction and stiffness. Connective tissue requires a warming and lengthening as the energetic body begins to change. The pain in the body as a result of your fears and repression will begin to soften and disappear if you make the effort to heal your body.

Recovery is not "stress management." This is an important point to keep in mind. Stress-management techniques do very little to actually recover your natural self. These techniques are beneficial for reducing the effects of stress, but that is all. Stress-management techniques are designed to minimize the pain created by stress and repression. Recovery is about learning to go to the source of the repression, feeling the feelings, and then releasing them at the source. While stress-management techniques may be employed in the process of the recovery of the natural self they are not the goal. Managing your stress is not the same as recovery from that which causes your stress, namely your beliefs about yourself.

Commitment to Feel

A big step in your recovery is learning to identify your commitments. When you are repressed you are committed to your addictions and to holding your body tightly. When you are repressed, you are committed to not feeling any pain.

When you do not know how to feel, you find ways to hold on to the pain of suffering and addictions to numb out that pain. Recovery is being willing to learn to have a relationship with pain and learning that it is okay to have emotions in your life.

Pain is not a disease; it is merely a messenger. You need to learn what the messenger is saying. Most have developed an aversion to pain. Because of your lost relationship with nature and your false beliefs, you believe that all pain will kill you. That is not so. When you cannot feel and release the pain that you experience, you end up storing it within you and creating a host of addictions to numb it out.

Understanding your commitments will tell you where you are. If you are terrified of being alone and will do anything not to feel your aloneness, then you are not in recovery. If you say that you have an issue with aloneness and it terrifies you, and you are committed to feeling this aloneness until you know that it will not kill you, as painful as it gets and for as long as it takes, *then* you are in recovery. Recovery is about making a commitment to face your biggest fears. Recovery is about being willing to face and accept your pain. Without this commitment to feel pain and release it, there is little hope for recovery. You will still be holding on tightly.

Until now, many people have been searching for a scientific answer to explain why we have addictions. We have been steadfastly looking for the "illusive addiction gene." We have been formulating "magic pills" in the laboratory. We have been increasing our psychological approach—the science of the mind. Yet we are becoming even more addicted each and every day.

The reason for this is very simple. Science cannot heal you from your addictions. There is not a pill or vitamin that will take away your addictions for you. Yes, science can help you learn ways to control your addictions a little better. However, science cannot heal you. You cannot talk or read your way out of this. There is no workshop that will move you out of your addictions.

Science is a mythology that occasionally coincides with nature. This might happen with the rare germ or errant gene leading to a molecular-based disease. Most often though, science does not coincide with nature. In fact, science is famous for attempting to conquer and overpower nature. This is why addictions cannot be healed from scientific methodology; addictions are not about science.

In order to truly heal from your addictions, you must feel your way out of them. You must want to heal more than anything else. For that to happen, you must make a commitment to want to feel your pain.

What is needed is a new branch of learning and understanding. In order to teach us about our feelings, we need to develop programs and institutions that give us as much emotional knowledge as we receive in intellectual experiences. Imagine taking courses in "emotionality" that are taught by certified "emotionologists."

The reason that you have addictions is to protect you from pain. Throughout your life, you have made a commitment to not feel. As you begin to shift your focus from learning how to control your addictions to learning how to feel your feelings, the real changes will begin to happen. Your bottle of scotch, television program, brownie or computer game will no longer be your best friend. Your pornography, cigar or soap opera will cease to be your daily lover.

When you begin to make your feelings your best friends, then all of this will change. Your feelings will become your priorities. Your addictions will gradually become less important. You will begin the process of recovering your natural self.

Joseph's Story

In the past we have had some very repressed and stressed out role models that have attempted to teach us about our natural self. If our role models are teaching and practicing the myths they believe, they will pass those myths on to those who follow. What is needed is a positive role model. This role model is one who is rooted in nature, honoring the natural cycle and practicing wellness. While such role models might be rare at this time, you can certainly watch pieces of the recovery process being displayed by many who have had the courage to face themselves.

The following is the story of Joseph, who has made a bold commitment change in his recovery process.

Joseph works very hard at his job as a computer programmer. When he arrives home at night from a busy day at work, the first thing he wants to do is to run to the refrigerator and stuff himself full of food. Joseph feels this way not because he is particularly hungry but because he has a faulty relationship with food that he uses to mood-alter. In other words, Joseph is addicted to food. He constantly battles his weight. He feels ashamed for not being able to control his food intake. This shame makes him want to eat even more.

Joseph has decided that he wants to change things. He wants to heal his faulty relationship with food and find out why he has such a difficult relationship with food. He wants to actually heal his addiction and not just learn how to control it.

First Joseph seeks a support system where he can share his feelings. He has chosen his close friends for this. He expresses his problem and his desire for support. If he is going to experience his pain, he will need to have people around him who can listen to his pain as he learns to listen to himself and be there for himself. Joseph develops a nurturing support network as if he were planting a garden. The next step that Joseph makes is to actually begin to change his commitment to feel his pain. The old message that runs his behavior states, "All pain is bad and will kill me. I will do whatever I can to avoid this pain." The new commitment that Joseph makes reads like this, "I am now listening to and learning from my pain."

With this new commitment in hand, Joseph begins his healing process. Most of our lives are spent with a very crushing, critical inner dialog that fears all pain. When you change this to a supportive dialog that accepts pain, real change begins to happen.

Up until now, the message in Joseph's mind has been, "Pain equals death. I need to run and hide from this pain." Joseph's pain has felt like a death sentence that he has attempted to avoid.

Joseph, in his recovery, is attempting to create a supportive inner dialog. He may choose to use the tools of the Inner Child program. This would help create a structure for him to follow. He may choose another means, perhaps by checking in frequently with his feelings. Whichever techniques Joseph chooses to use, it is critical that he learns to know what he is feeling, and develops the inner dialog with himself that supports him and reassures him that he will not die for experiencing his feelings. Joseph has made a new commitment to let these times of discomfort be a time of learning and of change.

The new behavior for Joseph is the following. Joseph comes home from work and immediately wants to head for the refrigerator. He stops himself and begins to do his inner dialog, remembering his commitment to learn from his pain. "Am I hungry or am I feeling something else?" he asks himself. Most likely he is not hungry but is trying to numb out some type of pain. "What am I feeling?" continues Joseph's dialog to himself. "How does this feeling manifest itself in my body?" "Is there tightness around my eyes or forehead?" "Is some part of my body contracted when I experience this feeling?" Just saying, "I'm feeling stressed" is not enough. His awareness of which feeling is causing him to be addicted is very important.

Joseph continues to dialog with himself until he knows exactly what he is feeling, why he is feeling it and how this feeling becomes trapped within his body. This may not happen the first time he tries this process. Instead, he may take weeks or months of repeating this procedure until he knows exactly what it is that he is feeling and how his food addiction attempts to create a "high" feeling to numb out the pain that is in his body.

Seeing a professional therapist from time to time is a great boost for Joseph. He is able to get some outside feedback on his progress and help in identifying areas that he has difficulty processing himself. It is always good to know that there is someone there to support him as he continues to learn how to trust his own feelings.

Joseph needs to be his own detective. It is important for him to begin to trace his cravings for food. Do these cravings start at work, on the way home from work, or the minute he walks in the door? If his emotional needs *are met, does he still get the same cravings? Admitting his fear of his own aloneness is a big step for Joseph; the addiction equation looks like this:*

"My fear of my aloneness equals viselike pressure around my scalp and eyes and an insatiable craving for food that gets me 'high' to numb out the pain."

In Joseph's case, he turns to food in order to numb out his inner aloneness. Deep inside this mature adult lies a little boy who is terrified of being alone. This fear stems from a childhood wounding experience in some form of abandonment, not being able to grieve his pain fully, and then abandoning himself and his ability to trust his own feelings. Joseph uses food in order to avoid his painful feelings of aloneness. Joseph feels as if his aloneness will kill him.

As Joseph continues to honor his new commitment to feel his pain, he is becoming emotionally intelligent and is developing a supportive inner dialog that chooses healing over suppression of feelings. Joseph sits with his painful feelings as long as he is able to. In the beginning, this might only be for a few minutes. He might work himself up to an hour of being with his pain. The longer he keeps his food addiction away and learns from his pain, the more he will heal. Of course, if he chooses another addiction, like talking on the telephone or watching television, he will learn very little about his addictive relationship with food. Joseph might have to go through a "death experience" as he sits with his pain. He must be reassured time and again that his pain will not kill him. He must get the pain out of his body. After a while, it will be normal to want to experience his pain. He will have a hard time choosing to be addicted as he teaches himself how to feel and release his pain.

Joseph also is learning how to move in an expansive way. Yoga and other regular expansive movement practices continue to change his body. Joseph is much freer in his movement. He breathes deeply and receives regular bodywork treatments. His regular bodywork sessions continue to break up the hardened muscle tissue and rigid fascia from so many years of fear and contraction. He is releasing the pain that is stored within his body. As he learns to recover his relationship with nature, Joseph grows strong and courageous. He has more control over his life. He is finally able to make choices rather than his pain making the choices for him.

Joseph now has a new commitment to feeling and identifying the sources of his pain. He has a working plan in place that he uses to continue to expand and to grow. Joseph's recovery is not perfect and may not be as quick as he would like it to be. He still falls into dark holes from time to time but he continues to move in the right direction. The greatest joy that Joseph will ever know is when his addictions no longer have power over him and the pain is gone from his body. With courage, patience and determination, each day brings Joseph one step closer to his recovery of his lost self and his relationship with nature.

AUTOBIOGRAPHY IN FIVE SHORT CHAPTERS
by Portia Nelson

I

I walk down the street.
There is a deep hole in the sidewalk.
I fall in
I am lost . . . I am helpless.
It isn't my fault.
It takes me forever to find a way out.

II

I walk down the same street.
There is a deep hole in the sidewalk.
I pretend I don't see it.
I fall in again.
I can't believe I am in the same place
but, it isn't my fault.
It still takes a long time to get out.

III

I walk down the same street
There is a deep hole in the sidewalk.
I see it is there.
I still fall in . . . it's a habit.
my eyes are open
I know where I am.
It is my fault.
I get out immediately.

IV

I walk down the same street.
There is a deep hole in the sidewalk.
I walk around it.

V

I walk down another street.

RESOURCES

RESOURCES

Ackerman, Diane, *A Natural History of the Senses,* Vintage Books, New York, 1990 Armstrong, Thomas, *Seven Kinds of Smarts*, New York, Plume, 1993

Adams, Carol J. and Donovan, Josephine, editors, *Animals and Women*, London, Duke University Press, 1995

Adams, Francis V., M.D., *The Breathing Disorders Sourcebook*, Lowell House, Los Angeles, 1998

Beck, Deva R.N., and Beck, James R.N., *The Pleasure Connection,* Synthesis Press, 1987

Becker, Robert O., M.D., and Selden, Gary, *The Body Electric*, New York, Quill Press, 1985

Block, Joyce, *Family Myths,* New York, Simon and Schuster, 1994

Booth, Father Leo, *When God Becomes A Drug*, New York, Tarcher/Perigee, 1991

Boundy, Donna, *When Money is the Drug*, New York, Harper Collins, 1993

Bradshaw, John, *The Family*, Florida, Health Communications, Inc., 1993

Brooks, Gary R, Ph.D., *The Centerfold Syndrome*, San Francisco, Jossey-Bass, 1995

Bufe, Charles, *Alcoholics Anonymous: Cult or Cure*, San Francisco, See Sharp Press, 1991

Burton Goldberg Group, *Alternative Medicine; The Definitive Guide,* Puyallup, Washington, Future Medicine Publishing, Inc., 1994

Callahan, Lisa, M.D., *The Fitness Factor,* Guilford, Ct., The Lyons Press, 2002

Carnes, Patrick, Ph.D., and Moriarity, Joseph M., *Sexual Anorexia*, Minnesota, Hazelden, 1997

Carnes, Patrick, Ph.D., *Don't Call It Love*, New York, Bantam, 1991

Chetanananda, Swami, *The Breath of God*, Cambridge, Mass., Rudra Press, 1988, and, *The Logic of Love*, Cambridge, Mass., Rudra Press, 1992

Chopra, Deepak, M.D., *Quantum Healing*, New York, Bantam, 1989

Chopra, Deepak, M.D., *Ageless Body, Timeless Mind,* New York, Harmony, 1993

Christopher, James *How To Stay Sober*, Buffalo, New York, Prometheus Books, 1988

Claire, Thomas, *Bodywork*, New York, William Morrow and Company, Inc., 1995

Conger, John P. *The Body in Recovery*, Berkeley, California, Frog, LTD., 1994

Coulter, H. David, *Anatomy of Hatha Yoga*, Honesdale, Pa., Body and Breath, 2001

Diamond, Harvey and Marilyn, *Fit For Life II*, New York, Warner Books, 1987

Dobson, Dr. Justine, DC., LMT., *Baby Beautiful*, Carson City, Nevada, Heirs Press, 1994

Epstein, Donald M., *Healing Myths Healing Magic*, San Rafael, Ca., Amber-Allen Publishing, Inc., 2000

Farhi, Donna, *The Breathing Book*, New York, Henry Holt and Company, Inc.,1996

Firman, John, and Gila, Ann, *The Primal Wound*, Albany, New York, State University of New York Press, 1997

Feltman, John, *Hands-On Healing*, Rodale Press, Emmaus, Pennsylvania, 1989

Fingarette, Herbert, *Heavy Drinking*, Berkeley and Los Angeles, California, University of California Press, Ltd., 1988

Finnegan, John, and Gray, Daphne, *Recovery From Addiction*, Berkeley, Celestial Arts, 1990

Fitzgerald, Kathleen W., PH. D., *Alcoholism: The Genetic Inheritance*, Whales' Tale Press, 1996

Fox, Stuart Ira, *Human Physiology*, Second Edition Dubuque, Iowa, Wm. C. Brown Publishers, 1987

Glasser, William, M.D., *Positive Addiction*, New York, Harper and Row, 1976

Glendinning, Chellis, *My Name Is Chellis & I'm in Recovery from Western Civilization*, Boston, Shambhala Publications, Inc., 1994

Griffin, Susan, *Pornography and Silence*, New York, Harper and Row, 1981

Goldstein, Avram, M.D., *Addiction: From Biology To Drug Policy*, New york, W.H. Freeman and Company, 1994

Goleman, Daniel, *Emotional Intelligence*, New York, Bantam, 1995

Grof, Christina, *The Thirst for Wholeness*, San Francisco, Harper, 1993

Hample, Stuart, and Marshall, Eric, *Children's Letters to God*, New York, Workman Publishing, 1991

Hanh, Thich Nhat, *Cultivating the Mind of Love*, Berkeley, Parallax Press, 1996

Hart, Dr. Archibald D., *Adrenalin and Stress,* Dallas, Word Publishing, 1991

Hendrick, Gladys West, *My First 300 Babies*, Goleta, Ca., Hurst Publishing, 1964

Heller, Joseph, and Henkin, William A., *Bodywise*, Oakland, Wingbow Press, 1986

Hitchens, Christopher, *The Missionary Position*, London, Verso, 1995

Hopfe, Lewis M., *Religions Of The World*, Second Edition, Encino, California, Glencoe Publishing Co., Inc., 1979

Jampolsky, Lee, Ph.D., *Healing The Addictive Mind*, Berkeley, Celestial Arts, 1991

Janov, Dr. Arthur, *The New Primal Scream,* Wilmington, DE, Enterprise Publishing, Inc., 1991

Johnson, Don Hanlon, *Body, Spirit, and Democracy*, Berkeley, North Atlantic Books, 1994

Johnson, Don, *Body*, Boston, Beacon Press, 1983

Jordan, Peg, *The Fitness Instinct*, Emmaus, Pa., Rodale Press Inc., 1999

Jordan, Michael, *Encyclopedia of Gods*, New York, Facts On File, 1993

Juhan, Deane, *Job's Body*, Barrytown, New York, Station Hill Press, 1987

Kabat-Zinn, Jon, *Wherever You Go There You Are*, New York, Hyperion, 1994

Kabat-Zinn, Jon, *Full Catastrophe Living*, New York, Dell Publishing, 1990

Kasl, Charlotte Davis, Ph.D., *Women, Sex, And Addiction,* New York, Harper and Row, 1989

Keen, Sam, and Valley-Fox, Anne, *Your Mythic Journey*, New York, Tarcher/Putnam, 1973

Keleman, Stanley, *Emotional Anatomy*, Center Press, Berkeley, Ca., 1985

Kepner, James I., *Body Process*, San Francisco, Jossey-Bass Inc., 1993

Kirsta, Alix, *The Book Of Stress Survival*, New York, Simon and Schuster, 1986

Kishline, *Moderate Drinking*, Tucson, See Sharp Press, 1994

Klein, Alan M., *Little Big Men*, Albany, State University of New York Press, 1993

Knaster, Mirka, *Discovering the Body's Wisdom*, New York, Bantam, 1996

Kornfield, Jack, *A Path With Heart*, New York, Bantam, 1993

Kramer, Joel, and Alstad, Diana, *The Guru Papers*, Frog, Ltd., Berkeley, Ca., 1993

Krogh, David, *Smoking: The Artificial Passion*, New York, W.H. Freeman and Co., 1991

Leonard, George, *Mastery*, New York, Plume, 1991

Levine, Peter A., *Waking the Tiger*, Berkeley, North Atlantic Books, 1997

Lewis, Dennis, *The Tao of Natural Breathing*, San Francisco, Mountain Wind Publishing, 1997

Liedloff, Jean, *The Continuum Concept*, New York, Addison-Wesley Publishing Co., 1977

Lowen, Alexander, M.D., *Pleasure*, New York, Penguin Books, 1970

Ludwig, Arnold M., M.D., *Understanding the Alcoholic's Mind,* Oxford, Oxford University Press, 1988

Martorano, Joseph, M.D., and Morgan, Maureen, C.S.W., R. N., with Fryer, William, *Unmasking PMS*, New York, The Berkeley Publishing Group, 1993

Masson, Jeffrey Moussaieff, *Dogs Never Lie About Love*, New York, Random House, 1997

Masson, Jeffrey Moussaieff and Susan McCarthy, *Why Elephants Weep*, New York, Dell Publishing, 1995

McGuire, Rev. Michael A., *Baltimore Catechism No.2,* New York, Benzinger Brothers, Inc., 1941

Morgan, Elaine, *The Descent of the Child,* New York, Oxford University Press, 1995

Muller, Wayne, *Legacy of the Heart*, New York, Fireside, 1992

Nathanielsz, Peter W., M.D., Ph.D., *Life in the Womb*, New York, Promethean Press, 1999

Norris, Ronald V., M.D. with Sullivan, Colleen, *PMS: Premenstrual Syndrome*, New York, Berkeley Publishing Group, 1983

Northrup, Christiane, M.D., *Women's Bodies, Women's Wisdom,* New York, Bantam, 1994

Novotny, Pamela Patrick, *Relief From PMS*, New York, Dell Publishing, 1992

Olson, Stuart Alve, *Cultivating the Ch'i*, St. Paul, Minnasota, Dragon Door Publications, Third Edition, 1993

Ornish, Dean, M.D., *Love and Survival*, New York, Harper Collins, 1998.

Ornish, Dean, M.D., *Dr. Dean Ornish's Program For Reversing Heart Disease*, New York, Ivy Books, 1996

Peele, Stanton, Ph. D., and Brodsky, Archie, *The Truth About Addiction and Recovery*, New York, Fireside, 1991

Peele, Stanton, *Diseasing of America*, New York, Lexinton Books, 1995

Pert, Candace B., Ph.D., *Molecules of Emotion*, New York, Scribner, 1997

Phelps, Janice Keller, M.D., and Nourse, Alan E., M.D., *The Hidden Addiction and How to Get Free*, Boston, Little, Brown and Company, 1986

Raabe, Tom, *Biblioholism*, Golden Colorado, Fulcrum Publishing, 1991

Rama, Swami, Ballentine, Rudolph, M.D., Hymes Alan, M.d., *The Science of Breath*, Honesdale, Pa., The Himalayan Institute Press, 1979, 1998

Robinson, Bryan, Ph.D., *Overdoing It*, Deerfield, Florida, Health Communications, Inc., 1992

Roth, Geneen, *When Food Is Love,* New York, Plume, 1991

Rothschild, Babette, *The Body Remembers,* New York, W.W. Norton, 2000

Rubel, Arthur J, O'Nell, Carl W., and Collado-Ardon, Rolando, *Susto, Folk Illness,* Berkeley, University of California Press, 1984

Ruchlis, Hy, *How Do You Know It's True,* Buffalo, New York, Prometheus Books, 1991

Sannella, Lee, M.D., *The Kundalini Experience*, Lower Lake, Ca., Integral Publishing, 1992

Schaef, Anne Wilson, and Fassel, Diane, *The Addictive Organization,* New York, Harper Collins, 1988

Schaef, Anne Wilson, *When Society Becomes An Addict*, New York, Harper Collins, 1987

Schaefer, Charles E., Ph.D. and Digeronimo, Theresa Foy, M. Ed., *How to Talk to Your Kids About Really Important Things*, San Francisco, Jossey-Bass Publishers, 1994

Shapiro, Debbie, *The Bodymind Workbook,* Rockport, MA., Element Books Inc., 1990

Sheppard, Kay, *Food Addiction: The Body Knows*, Deerfield Beach, Florida, Health Communications Inc., 1993

Shlain, Leonard, *The Alphabet Versus The Goddess*, New York, Viking Penguin, 1998

Small, Meredith F., *What's Love Got to Do with It?,* New York, Doubleday, 1995

Smith, Ann W., M. S., *Overcoming Perfectionism*, Deerfield Beach, Florida, Health Communications Inc., 1990

Smith, Margaret, *Ritual Abuse*, New York, Harper Collins, 1993

Snow, Candace, and Willard, David, R.N., *I'm Dying To Take Care Of You*, Redmond, WA., Professional Counselor Books, 1989

Somer, Elizabeth, M. A., R. D., *Food and Mood*, New York, Henry Holt and Company, Inc., 1995

Spock, Benjamin, M. D., and Parker, Steven J., *Dr. Spock's Baby And Child Care,* New York, Simon and Schuster, 1998

Sundermeyer, Colleen A., Ph.D., *Emotional Weight*, New York, Perigee Books, 1993

Tassi, Nina, Ph. D., *Urgency Addiction*, Dallas, Taylor Publishing Company, 1991

Thevenin, Tine, *The Family Bed*, Wayne, New Jersey, Avery Publishing Group, 1987

Trump, Donald J. and Schwartz, Tony, *Trump: The Art Of The Deal*, New York, Warner Books, Inc., 1987

Washton, Arnold, Ph.D. and Boundy, Donna, M.S.W., *Willpower's Not Enough*, New York, Harper and Row, 1989

Waterhouse, Debra, M.P.H., R.D., *Why Women Need Chocolate*, New York, Hyperion, 1995

Weil, Andrew, M.D., *Natural Health, Natural Medicine*, Boston, Houghton Mifflin Company, 1990

Weil, Andrew, M.D., and Rosen, Winifred, *From Chocolate To Morphine*, Boston, Houghton Mifflin Company, 1993

Wells, Patrick, and Rushkoff, Douglas, *Stoned Free*, Port Townsend, WA, Loompanics Unlimited, 1995

Wills, Christopher, *The Runaway Brain*, London, Harper Collins, 1993

Yogananda, Paramahansa, *Autobiography of a Yogi*, Self-Realization Fellowship, 1998

Zi, Nancy, *The Art Of Breathing*, New York, Bantam, 1986

For more information contact the author at

The Little Wellness Company
14 Monarch Bay Plaza #372
Monarch Beach, Ca. 92629

Email: ReturntoNature@JonBurras.com
JonBurras.com

About the Author

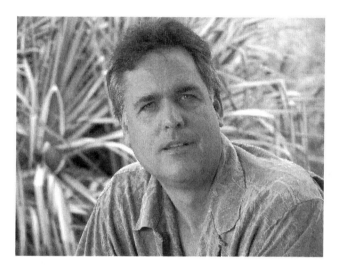

JON BURRAS
Author, yoga teacher, wellness consultant, bodyworker,
wilderness guide and international lecturer

Jon Burras is a true renaissance man. He is trained in many different disciplines and has great skill in blending those talents into many aspects. He believes that nature is our greatest teacher and attempts to understand and follow the natural rhythm of nature. He is a seeker of knowledge and teaches with compassion and insight. He believes that the true understanding of ourselves comes when we begin to honor the many relationships that unite everything together.

Made in the USA
San Bernardino, CA
13 July 2020

75388204R00250